Veterinary Laboratory Medicine: Small and Exotic Animals

CLINICS IN LABORATORY MEDICINE

www.labmed.theclinics.com

September 2015 • Volume 35 • Number 3

ELSEVIER

1600 John F. Kennedy Boulevard • Suite 1800 • Philadelphia, Pennsylvania, 19103-2899

http://www.theclinics.com

CLINICS IN LABORATORY MEDICINE Volume 35, Number 3
September 2015 ISSN 0272-2712, ISBN-13: 978-0-323-43027-2

Editor: Adrianne Brigido
Developmental Editor: Colleen Viola

Reprints. For copies of 100 or more, of articles in this publication, please contact the Commercial Reprints Department, Elsevier Inc., 360 Park Avenue South, New York, New York 10010-1710. Tel. 212-633-3874, Fax: 212-633-3820, E-mail: reprints@elsevier.com.

Clinics in Laboratory Medicine (ISSN 0272-2712) is published quarterly by Elsevier Inc., 360 Park Avenue South, New York, NY 10010-1710. Months of issue are March, June, September, and December. Business and Editorial offices: 1600 John F. Kennedy Blvd., Suite 1800, Philadelphia, PA 19103-2899. Periodicals postage paid at NewYork, NY and additional mailing offices. Subscription prices are $250.00 per year (US individuals), $419.00 per year (US institutions), $135.00 per year (US students), $305.00 per year (Canadian individuals), $510.00 per year (Canadian institutions), $185.00 per year (Canadian students), $390.00 per year (international individuals), $510.00 per year (international institutions), $185.00 (international students). Foreign air speed delivery is included in all Clinics subscription prices. All prices are subject to change without notice. POSTMASTER: Send address changes to *Clinics in Laboratory Medicine*, Elsevier Health Sciences Division, Subscription Customer Service, 3251 Riverport Lane, Maryland Heights, MO 63043. **Customer Service: 1-800-654-2452 (US). From outside of the US and Canada, call 1-314-447-8871. Fax: 1-314-447-8029. E-mail: journalscustomerservice-usa@elsevier.com (for print support) or journalsonlinesuppor-t-usa@elsevier.com (for online support).**

Clinics in Laboratory Medicine is covered in *EMBASE/Exerpta Medica, MEDLINE/PubMed (Index Medicus), Cinahl, Current Contents/Clinical Medicine, BIOSIS* and *ISI/BIOMED*.

Contributors

AUTHORS

KARIN ALLENSPACH, Dr med vet, FVH, PhD, FHEA
Diplomate, European College of Veterinary Internal Medicine (Companion Animals); Associate Professor and Reader in Internal Medicine, Department of Clinical Sciences and Services, Royal Veterinary College, University of London, North Mymms, United Kingdom

DOROTHEE BIENZLE, DVM, PhD
Diplomate, American College of Veterinary Pathologists (Clinical Pathology); Professor and Canada Research Chair in Veterinary Pathology, Department of Pathobiology, University of Guelph, Guelph, Ontario, Canada

ANDREA A. BOHN, DVM, PhD
Diplomate, American College of Veterinary Pathologists (Clinical Pathology); Associate Professor, Department of Microbiology, Immunology, and Pathology, College of Veterinary Medicine and Biomedical Sciences, Colorado State University, Fort Collins, Colorado

MARY JO BURKHARD, DVM, PhD
Diplomate, American College of Veterinary Pathologists (Clinical Pathology); Associate Professor, Department of Veterinary Biosciences, College of Veterinary Medicine, The Ohio State University, Columbus, Ohio

TERRY W. CAMPBELL, MS, DVM, PhD
Associate Professor, Department of Clinical Sciences, College of Veterinary Medicine and Biomedical Sciences, Colorado State University, Fort Collins, Colorado

SETH E. CHAPMAN, DVM, MS
Diplomate, American College of Veterinary Pathologists (Clinical Pathology); IDEXX Laboratories Inc, Worthington, Ohio

KRYSTAN R. GRANT, DVM
Department of Clinical Sciences, Colorado State University, Fort Collins, Colorado

ROGER A. HOSTUTLER, DVM, MS
Diplomate, American College of Veterinary Internal Medicine (Small Animal Internal Medicine); MedVet Medical and Cancer Centers for Pets, Worthington, Ohio

MICHAEL P. JONES, DVM
Diplomate, American Board of Veterinary Practitioners (Avian Practice); Associate Professor, Avian and Zoological Medicine, Department of Small Animal Clinical Sciences, University of Tennessee, College of Veterinary Medicine, Knoxville, Tennessee

ERIC KLAPHAKE, DVM
Diplomate, American College of Zoological Medicine; Diplomate, American Board of Veterinary Practitioners (Avian); Diplomate, American Board of Veterinary Practitioners (Reptile/Amphibian); Cheyenne Mountain Zoo, Colorado Springs, Colorado

NICOLE M. LINDSTROM, MS, DVM
Laboratory Animal Veterinary Program Specialist, Virginia Tech, Blacksburg, Virginia

CAROLINE MANSFIELD, BSc, BVMS, PhD, MANZCVS
Diplomate, European College of Veterinary Internal Medicine-Companion Animals; Hill's Associate Professor; Head of Small Animal Medicine, Faculty of Veterinary Science, The University of Melbourne, Werribee, Victoria, Australia

DAVID M. MOORE, MS, DVM
Diplomate, American College of Laboratory Animal Medicine; Associate Vice President for Research Compliance, Department of Biomedical Sciences and Pathobiology, Virginia Tech, Blacksburg, Virginia

MARK A. OYAMA, DVM
Diplomate, American College of Veterinary Internal Medicine; Professor and Chief, Section of Cardiology, Department of Clinical Studies-Philadelphia, School of Veterinary Medicine, University of Pennsylvania, Philadelphia, Pennsylvania

BARRAK M. PRESSLER, DVM, PhD
Diplomate, American College of Veterinary Internal Medicine; Assistant Professor of Small Animal Medicine, Department of Veterinary Clinical Sciences, College of Veterinary Medicine, The Ohio State University, Columbus, Ohio

LESLIE C. SHARKEY, DVM, PhD
Associate Professor, Veterinary Clinical Sciences Department, University of Minnesota College of Veterinary Medicine, St Paul, Minnesota

STEPHEN A. SMITH, MS, DVM, PhD
Professor of Aquatic, Wildlife and Pocket Pet Medicine, Department of Biomedical Sciences and Pathobiology, Virginia-Maryland Regional College of Veterinary Medicine, Virginia Tech, Blacksburg, Virginia

JOHN M. SYKES IV, DVM
Diplomate, American College of Zoological Medicine; Senior Veterinarian, Zoological Health Program, Wildlife Conservation Society, Bronx Zoo, Bronx, New York

MAXEY L. WELLMAN, DVM, MS, PhD
Diplomate, American College of Veterinary Pathologists (Clinical Pathology); Professor, Department of Veterinary Biosciences, College of Veterinary Medicine, The Ohio State University, Columbus, Ohio

KURT ZIMMERMAN, DVM, PhD
Diplomate, American College of Veterinary Pathologists; Associate Professor of Clinical and Anatomical Pathology, Department of Biomedical Sciences and Pathobiology, Virginia-Maryland Regional College of Veterinary Medicine, Virginia Tech, Blacksburg, Virginia

Contents

> Serum creatinine concentration is insensitive for detecting kidney injury and does not assist in differentiation between glomerular versus tubular damage. Advanced renal function tests, including glomerular filtration rate testing, determining fractional excretion of electrolytes, and assay of urine biomarkers, may allow earlier detection of reduced renal function mass, differentiation of renal from non-renal causes of azotemia, and assist with localization of damage. This article reviews the principles, indications, and limitations of these tests and describes their use in sample clinical scenarios.

> Routine biochemical tests generally include serum enzymes, proteins, and other markers useful for identifying hepatobiliary disease in dogs and cats. Obtaining results outside the reference intervals can occur with direct hepatocellular injury, enzyme induction by hepatocytes or biliary epithelium, or decreased hepatic function. However, detection of biochemical abnormalities does not necessarily indicate clinically significant disease. For a comprehensive approach to detection and treatment of hepatobiliary disease, the laboratory results must be correlated with the history and physical examination findings, diagnostic imaging results, and other assays.

> Laboratory tests are an important part of the workup of small intestinal diseases in dogs and cats. Especially in chronic cases, when extragastrointestinal causes need to be ruled out, it is important to adhere to a systematic workup. This article details the newest available data on tests to aid this diagnostic process. Once the diagnosis of a chronic enteropathy is made, there are many laboratory tests that can help in monitoring the disease and providing prognostic information. Several new tests being evaluated for clinical usefulness are discussed.

> The pancreas remains a difficult organ to evaluate using laboratory methods alone. No single laboratory test is diagnostic of pancreatitis (chronic or acute) without other diagnostic modalities concurring with the diagnosis or ruling out other diseases. The diagnosis of pancreatitis is particularly difficult in cats, and pancreatitis often occurs with other diseases. The use of pancreatic cytology may be useful in diagnosing both

inflammation and neoplasia. Exocrine pancreatic insufficiency (EPI) can be relatively easily diagnosed when clinically manifested by the measurement of trypsinlike immunoreactivity. Diagnosis is more difficult when EPI is subclinical.

Blood-based assays for various cardiac biomarkers can assist in the diagnosis of heart disease in dogs and cats. The two most common markers are cardiac troponin-I and N-terminal pro-B–type natriuretic peptide. Biomarker assays can assist in differentiating cardiac from noncardiac causes of respiratory signs and detection of preclinical cardiomyopathy. Increasingly, studies indicate that cardiac biomarker testing can help assess the risk of morbidity and mortality in animals with heart disease. Usage of cardiac biomarker testing in clinical practice relies on proper patient selection, correct interpretation of test results, and incorporation of biomarker testing into existing diagnostic methods.

Lactate is a product of anaerobic metabolism. Lactate concentration in blood is used clinically as an indicator of tissue hypoperfusion and hypoxia to determine disease severity, assess response to therapy, and predict outcome. This article reviews lactate physiology, sample collection and processing, and interpretation of lactate concentration in clinical practice.

Iron is an essential element and is used by every cell in the body. This article summarizes iron metabolism and disorders associated with iron metabolism in dogs and cats. The diagnostic tests currently in use for assessing iron status are discussed.

This article summarizes and compares the various assays available to aid in the diagnosis and characterization of lymphoma in small animal patients. These techniques include cytology, histopathology, immunocytochemistry and immunohistochemistry, immunophenotyping by flow cytometry, and polymerase chain reaction for clonal antigen receptor gene rearrangement.

Pet ferrets are presented to veterinary clinics for routine care and treatment of clinical diseases and female reproductive problems. In addition to obtaining clinical history, additional diagnostic testing may be required, including hematological assessments. This article describes common blood collection methods, including venipuncture sites, volume of blood that can be safely collected, and handling of the blood. Hematological parameters for normal ferrets are provided along with a description of the morphology of ferret leukocytes to assist in performing a differential count.

Pet rabbits are presented to veterinary clinics for routine care and treatment of clinical diseases. In addition to obtaining clinical history, additional diagnostic testing may be required, including hematological assessments. This article describes common blood collection methods, including venipuncture sites, volume of blood that can be safely collected, and handling of the blood. Hematological parameters for normal rabbits are provided for comparison with in-house or commercial test results. A description of the morphology of rabbit leukocytes is provided to assist in performing a differential count. Differential diagnoses are provided for abnormal values identified in the hemogram.

Hamsters, gerbils, rats, and mice are presented to veterinary clinics and hospitals for prophylactic care and treatment of clinical signs of disease. Physical examination, history, and husbandry practice information can be supplemented greatly by assessment of hematologic parameters. As a resource for veterinarians and their technicians, this article describes the methods for collection of blood, identification of blood cells, and interpretation of the hemogram in mice, rats, gerbils, and hamsters.

Pet guinea pigs are presented to veterinary clinics for routine care and treatment of clinical diseases. In addition to obtaining clinical history, diagnostic testing may be required, including hematological assessments. This article describes common blood collection methods, including venipuncture sites, the volume of blood that can be safely collected, and handling of the blood. Hematological parameters for normal guinea pigs are provided for comparison with in-house or commercial test results. A description of the morphology of guinea pig leukocytes is provided to assist in performing a differential count.

Avian veterinarians often rely heavily on the results of various diagnostic tests, including hematology results. As such, cellular identification and evaluation of the cellular response are invaluable tools that help veterinarians understand the health or condition of their patient, as well as to monitor severity and clinical progression of disease and response to treatment. Therefore, it is important to thoroughly understand how to identify and evaluate changes in the avian erythron and leukon, as well as to interpret normal and abnormal results.

Reptile Hematology

John M. Sykes IV and Eric Klaphake

The basic principles of hematology used in mammalian medicine can be applied to reptiles. The appearances of the blood cells are significantly different from those seen in most mammals, and vary with taxa and staining method used. Many causes for abnormalities of the reptilian hemogram are similar to those for mammals, although additional factors such as venipuncture site, season, hibernation status, captivity status, and environmental factors can also affect values, making interpretation of hematologic results challenging. Values in an individual should be compared with reference ranges specific to that species, gender, and environmental conditions when available.

Fish Hematology and Associated Disorders

Krystan R. Grant

Fish health is a growing concern as pets, education, and aquaculture evolves. For the veterinary staff, fish handling, diagnostics, medicine, and surgery may require specialized training and equipment in comparison with terrestrial and arboreal animals, simply because of their aquatic nature and diversity. Fish hematology is one diagnostic tool that may not require additional equipment, may be inexpensive, and provide useful information in guiding treatment options. Challenges involving hematology may include handling and restraint, venipuncture, evaluation, and interpretation. In this article, strategies for these challenges are discussed for teleost (bony fish) and elasmobranch (cartilaginous fish) fish types.

Evaluation of the Blood Film

Terry W. Campbell

Evaluation of hemic cell morphology in stained blood film may be the most important part of the hematologic evaluation of exotic animals. The blood film provides important information regarding red blood cell abnormalities, such as changes in cell shape and color, presence of inclusions, and, in the case of lower vertebrates, changes in the position of the cell nucleus. Stained blood film also provides information about changes in leukocyte numbers and morphology, and shows important hemic features of mammalian platelets and the thrombocytes of lower vertebrates. The blood film is needed in the detection and identification of blood parasites.

Erratum

In the September 2013 issue (Volume 33, number 3), for the article "Advanced techniques for detection and identification of microbial agents of gastroenteritis," the abstract states that traditional diagnostic methods can "be labor intensive and suffer from long turnaround times and, in some cases, poor and Yi-Wei Tang sensitivity." This statement should instead read, "…be labor intensive and suffer from long turnaround times and, in some cases, poor sensitivity."

Clin Lab Med 35 (2015) ix
http://dx.doi.org/10.1016/j.cll.2015.06.001
0272-2712/15/$ – see front matter © 2015 Elsevier Inc. All rights reserved.

labmed.theclinics.com

Clinical Approach to Advanced Renal Function Testing in Dogs and Cats

Barrak M. Pressler, DVM, PhD

KEYWORDS

- Biomarkers • Fractional excretion • Glomerular filtration rate
- γ-Glutamyl transpeptidase • Microalbuminuria • Urine

KEY POINTS

- Advanced renal function tests may allow earlier detection of reduced renal functional mass and localization of damage to a particular nephron segment, and are required for diagnosis or exclusion of some causes of kidney injury.
- Measurement of glomerular filtration rate (GFR) allows for precise quantitative assessment of remaining filtration and excretion ability by the kidneys.
- Spot samples of simultaneously collected urine and plasma provide clinically reasonable approximations of total daily urine electrolyte excretion.
- The majority of plasma albumin is size and charge excluded from the ultrafiltrate; glomerular damage results in increased filtration of albumin and excretion into the urine. Microalbuminuria may be detected prior to positive reactions on standard urine protein dipstick pads, and before the urine protein:creatinine (UPC) ratio increases above reference range.
- Urinary N-acetyl-β-D-glucosaminidase (NAG):creatinine ratio is increased in dogs with chronic kidney disease, pyelonephritis, uncontrolled diabetes mellitus, pyometra, or X-linked hereditary nephropathy but does not differ before versus after control of hyperadrenocorticism with trilostane or transphenoidal hypophysectomy.

Serum biochemical analysis and urinalysis are the mainstay diagnostic tests for initial detection and estimation of severity of kidney disease in dogs and cats. Increased serum creatinine concentration and impaired urine concentrating ability, however, are relatively insensitive for detecting early kidney injury and do not assist in differentiation between glomerular versus proximal or distal tubular damage. Advanced renal

This article originally appeared in Veterinary Clinics of North America: Small Animal Practice, Volume 43, Issue 6, November 2013.
Funding Sources: Morris Animal Foundation, International Renal Interest Society, and The Ohio State University College of Veterinary Medicine.
Conflict of Interest: Previous funding from FAST Diagnostics.
Department of Veterinary Clinical Sciences, College of Veterinary Medicine, The Ohio State University, 601 Vernon Tharp Street, Columbus, OH 43210, USA
E-mail address: pressler.21@osu.edu

function tests, including GFR testing, determining fractional excretion (FE) of electrolytes, and assay of urine biomarkers, may allow earlier detection of reduced renal functional mass and differentiation of various renal and nonrenal differential diagnoses and assist with localization of damage. This article reviews the principles, indications, and limitations of these tests and describes their use in sample clinical scenarios.

GLOMERULAR FILTRATION RATE

Serum creatinine concentration is insensitive for detecting kidney injury. Increases in serum creatinine concentration are mild and often remain within reference range, until approximately 60% to 75% of all nephrons are no longer functional. In contrast, measurement of GFR allows for precise quantitative assessment of remaining filtration and excretion ability by the kidneys. Example situations when GFR measurement may provide critical information regarding remaining kidney function beyond serum creatinine concentration alone include diagnostic evaluation of dogs and cats with unexplained polyuria and polydipsia, to avoid overdosing of medications that are excreted by the kidneys or that have potential nephrotoxic effects, and to predict risk of overt renal failure after nephrectomy in dogs or cats with unilateral kidney disease, such as tumors or pyonephrosis.

Several methods for determination of GFR have been validated in dogs and cats, all of which report the volume of plasma, which has been cleared over a given interval of time, per kilogram of patient body weight. After injecting a substance (the marker) that is eliminated solely via filtration through the glomeruli and which then passes into the urine without being reabsorbed or further secreted by the tubules, the rate at which the concentration of marker decreases in successive blood samples allows calculation of the plasma clearance and GFR.[1] Assays that measure the rate of marker appearance in urine are more accurate than those that assay marker disappearance in plasma (because few markers are solely excreted via glomerular filtration without any tubular reuptake or secretion); however, urine assays that allow calculation of renal clearance (vs plasma clearance) are more cumbersome to perform because they require collection of all urine produced in a 24-hour period. Fortunately, plasma clearance assays using blood sampling techniques are sufficiently close to renal clearance, such that in the clinical setting urine collection is not required.[1–4]

Several markers have been validated for measurement of GFR in dogs and cats, including creatinine, cystatin C (CysC), iohexol, and radiolabeled molecules. In people, GFR is most commonly estimated (rather than measured) using serum creatinine concentration, body weight, and correction factors based on a patient's gender and race. Unfortunately, formulae for estimating GFR from serum creatinine have not proved accurate in dogs and cats due to greater individual, gender, and breed variation than occurs in people.[5,6] Intravenous administration of a sterile creatinine bolus is safe and cost effective; however, comparison of various markers suggests that exogenous creatinine GFR assays underestimate true GFR, likely due to some excretion into the gastrointestinal tract and perhaps tubular reuptake.[2,7,8] CysC is an endogenous protein produced by all nucleated cells at a constant rate that undergoes glomerular filtration without tubular secretion; however, commercial assays are limited, and comparative studies in dogs have suggested lower specificity for detection of reduced kidney function than exogenous creatinine GFR.[9–11]

Iohexol GFR measurement uses a marker that can be easily obtained by veterinarians and has been well validated for use in dogs and cats, and a commercial assay is available at a reasonable cost to owners. After intravenous bolus injection of the same iodinated contrast agent used in diagnostic imaging studies, plasma samples are collected at predetermined times (usually 2, 3, and 4 hours after injection); the volume of injection is based on concentration of elemental iodine within the iohexol.[12] Iodinated compounds are stable for long periods, and plasma samples can be frozen for extended periods of time and assayed later if indicated.[13] Intravenous iohexol can induce acute kidney injury and renal failure in people, particularly in patients with pre-existing kidney damage; however, this idiosyncratic drug reaction is rare in dogs and cats.[14,15] Iohexol GFR assays have been safely used to study renal function in healthy dogs and cats,[16–21] in dogs with gentamicin-induced acute kidney injury,[22] in dogs and cats administered various nonsteroidal anti-inflammatory drugs (NSAIDs) after anesthesia,[20,23] and in cats with untreated or post-treated naturally occurring hyperthyroidism.[24–26] The most commonly used commercial assay for iohexol concentrations is offered by the Michigan State University Diagnostic Center for Population and Animal Health (http://www.animalhealth.msu.edu/); this diagnostic laboratory reports the calculated GFR after assaying serial plasma iohexol concentrations.

Radiolabeled markers validated for measurement of GFR currently used in clinical patients include chromium-51 ethylenediaminetetraacetic acid (EDTA) and technetium-99m diethylenetriamine pentaacetic acid (DTPA). These radionucleotides undergo glomerular filtration without tubular reabsorption or excretion and are stable in dog and cat blood samples but have short half-lives in vivo; this permits storage and shipping of samples to outside laboratories for assay of plasma clearance while patients are cleared of radioactivity and able to be released to owners within 24 to 48 hours.[27] Use of radiolabeled markers is limited, however, to specialty practices that are appropriately licensed to perform nuclear medicine–based testing. Radionucleotide GFR assays have been safely used to study renal function in anesthetized dogs,[28] in cats with solid tumors administered nephrotoxic chemotherapeutic agents,[29] and in dogs and cats with naturally occurring (cats with polycystic kidney disease[30] or azotemic chronic kidney disease[31]) or induced (cats with rejection of transplanted kidneys[32] or dogs that had previously undergone renal biopsy[33]) kidney disease (**Box 1**).

Although serial measurement of plasma iohexol or radionucleotides can be used to determine total, or global, GFR, these assays cannot determine the relative contributions of the right versus left kidney (ie, per-kidney GFR) to total renal excretion. Clinical use of per-kidney GFR is most commonly recommended in dogs or cats requiring unilateral nephrectomy (for example, due to presence of a renal tumor) but which have confirmed or suspected bilateral renal dysfunction. In these animals, determining both global and per-kidney GFR allows clinicians to predict the whether removal of the right or left kidney will result in renal failure and worsened quality of life.

Global and per-kidney GFR measurement can be determined using either iohexol or radionucleotide markers, when performed in tandem with advanced diagnostic imaging studies. CT of the abdomen in conjunction with iohexol allows per-kidney uptake of marker to be compared.[17] The ratio of uptake in the right versus left kidneys can then be used to calculate the per-kidney GFR. Gamma camera imaging of the abdomen after bolus administration of radionucleotide allows a similar comparison of marker uptake by each kidney over time and estimation of per-kidney GFR (**Box 2**).[8,34,35]

URINARY FRACTIONAL EXCRETION OF ELECTROLYTES

The kidneys are the primary organs responsible for excretion of electrolytes at times of excess and conservation at times of deficiency. Nonprotein-bound electrolytes are freely filtered through the glomeruli and then reabsorbed by electrolyte-specific exchange receptors throughout the proximal convoluted tubule, loop of Henle, and distal convoluted tubule. The rate of electrolyte reabsorption depends on multiple factors,

Box 1
Clinical scenarios: measurement of glomerular filtration rate

Case 1

An 8-year-old spayed female Shetland sheepdog was evaluated for polyuria and polydipsia of 3 months' duration. The owners reported that the dog had been urinating large volumes of clear urine every 2 to 3 hours and emptying the water bowl multiple times per day; however, the urine stream appeared normal without any associated straining, and the dog was otherwise acting normal with unchanged appetite and activity level. Physical examination of the dog was unremarkable, but the bladder was distended with a large volume of urine. All values on complete blood cell count and serum biochemistry panel were within reference range, although serum creatinine concentration were at the upper end of the reference range (1.2 mg/dL; reference range, 0.3–1.4 mg/dL). Urine specific gravity was 1.009 on 2 different occasions and the remainder of the urinalysis unremarkable. Abdominal radiography revealed that the kidneys were bilaterally smaller than expected and slightly misshapen.

Differential diagnoses for a dog with polyuria and polydipsia and unremarkable physical examination and minimum database may include atypical hypoadrenocorticism, central or primary nephrogenic diabetes insipidus, hyperadrenocorticism infections with lipopolysaccharide-producing bacteria, liver dysfunction, psychogenic polydipsia, and renal insufficiency. Loss of urine concentrating ability occurs in dogs with approximately 66% loss of total nephron function. Azotemia may not be noted, however, until 75% of nephrons are lost; during the intervening period (ie, damage to approximately 66%–75% of total nephrons) dogs may be polyuric and polydipsic due to kidney injury, but serum creatinine and blood urea nitrogen concentrations remain within reference ranges. This scenario, termed *renal insufficiency*, rather than *renal failure*, is of particular concern in this dog given the repeatable isosthenuria and appearance of the kidneys on abdominal radiographs.

Plasma iohexol clearance determination of GFR was performed in this dog using 1 mL/kg of iohexol containing 300 mg/mL elemental iodine/mL (Omnipaque 300 (iohexol) injection, GE Healthcare, Princeton, New Jersey); blood samples were collected 2, 3, and 4 hours after administration. Calculated GFR result was 0.9 mL/min/kg (reference range, 2.89–8.07 mL/min/kg), supporting a presumptive diagnosis of renal insufficiency. Ultrasonographic examination of the abdomen was recommended to better characterize the dog's kidney disease; bilateral dilatation of the renal pelves was noted with echogenic debris. Aerobic bacterial culture of urine resulted in greater than 100,000 colony-forming units/mL of *Staphylococcus aureus* and a 6-week course of amoxicillin-clavulanic acid was prescribed for a presumptive diagnosis of bilateral pyelonephritis. The owners reported that after 2-weeks of therapy, the dog's polyuria and polydipsia had resolved, and 2 weeks after the end of antibiotic therapy, repeat aerobic culture of urine did not result in any growth, and repeat GFR measurement revealed plasma iohexol clearance had increased to 3.27 mL/min/kg.

Case 2

An 11-year-old castrated male Labrador retriever was evaluated for a gradual decrease in activity level over the previous year and left hind limb lameness after playing with the other dogs in the household. Orthopedic examination and radiographs of both hind limbs were consistent with moderate osteoarthritis of both stifles and hocks. Two years before the current evaluation, this dog had been diagnosed with leptospirosis-induced acute renal failure (serum creatinine concentration 5.7 mg/dL); aggressive treatment with intravenous fluids and antibiotics were successful in resolving the azotemia (current serum creatinine concentration is 1.3 mg/dL).

NSAIDs are the mainstay treatment of osteoarthritis in dogs but may induce or exacerbate kidney injury. Unfortunately, these owners declined treatment with alternative analgesics due to cost concerns. Although serum creatinine concentration is within the laboratory reference range, there is a concern that sufficient residual chronic kidney injury may be present from the previous leptospirosis infection, such that there is an increased likelihood of drug nephrotoxicity but not enough to currently result in azotemia. Samples were submitted for determination of plasma iohexol clearance, and calculated GFR was 1.4 mL/min/kg, or approximately 50% of the lower end of the laboratory reference range (2.89–8.07 mL/min/kg). The prescribed NSAID was, therefore, reduced by 50% of the recommended milligram/kilogram dosage; 2 years later, the owners reported that the dog's lameness and activity level were much improved, and serum creatinine concentration remained within reference range.

Box 2
Clinical scenario: measurement of global and per-kidney glomerular filtration rate

An 11-year-old, spayed female domestic shorthaired cat was evaluated for gross hematuria of 2 weeks' duration. On physical examination, a midabdominal mass was palpated in the region of the left kidney, and the right kidney was slightly smaller than expected. Ultrasonographic examination of the abdomen revealed a large mass completely effacing the normal left kidney parenchyma, and several hyperechoic, wedge-shaped lesions in the right kidney extending from the renal medulla up to the cortical surface, consistent with chronic infarction. Serum creatinine concentration was 1.9 mg/dL (reference range, 0.2–1.6 mg/dL).

Based on the serum creatinine concentration and ultrasonographic abnormalities, this cat likely had International Renal Interest Society stage 2 chronic kidney disease. Unilateral nephrectomy was recommended after further diagnostic evaluation failed to reveal any metastases; however, there was concern that further reduction in functional nephrons after nephrectomy would result in worsening of azotemia, uremia, and unacceptable quality of life. Global and per-kidney GFR were, therefore, measured via technetium-99m DTPA and gamma camera imaging to determine both the current total renal function and the percent contribution of the mass-containing kidney.

Global GFR in this cat was 0.6 mL/min/kg (reference range, 1.15–2.73 mL/min/kg). The ratio of nucleotide uptake in the left, mass-containing kidney versus the right kidney was 1:9 (ie, 10% of total GFR vs 90% of total GFR). Based on the low contribution of the left kidney to total renal function, nephrectomy was performed. One month after surgery, the cat's serum creatinine was 2.7 mg/dL, and the owners report no abnormal clinical signs.

---

including dietary concentrations, renal function, various hormones (including parathyroid hormone and aldosterone), rate of ultrafiltrate flow through the nephron, and need to conserve or excrete water based on intravascular volume status.[36] Calculating the percent excretion of an electrolyte in relation to that electrolyte's serum concentration and correcting for filtration rate based excretion of creatinine is FE.

Although urine collection over a 24-hour period is most accurate for determining FE of electrolytes, spot samples of simultaneously collected urine and plasma provide clinically reasonable approximations of total daily excretion despite some variability.[37] The formula for calculating FE of a given electrolyte, E, is

$$\%FE = \frac{(\text{Urine concentration of E}) \times (\text{Plasma concentration of creatinine})}{(\text{Urine concentration of creatinine}) \times (\text{Plasma concentration of E})} \times 100$$

Because of the many factors that may influence FE, there are no definable reference ranges for dogs or cats with plasma electrolyte concentrations within reference range; however, as a general rule, FE of sodium should be low (<1%) whereas FE of potassium is high (up to 25%).[38,39]

Clinical use of electrolyte FE is limited due to the variety of influencing endogenous and exogenous factors. In select cases of increased or decreased serum electrolyte concentrations, however, FE may allow clinicians to prioritize differential diagnoses. Most laboratories that perform serum biochemical analyses are able to assay urine concentrations of creatinine and electrolytes. Dogs and cats in which FE of 1 or more electrolytes is considered should be fed a consistent diet before testing (the author suggests at least 1 week before submission of samples) to minimize food-associated fluctuations in urine electrolyte excretion. Dehydration should also be corrected and normal hydration should persist for several days, because healthy kidneys reabsorb excess sodium in an effort to restore water balance (under the influence of aldosterone). Interpretation of results requires forehand consideration of (1) serum electrolyte concentrations: animals with a given electrolyte concentration greater than reference range should have greater-than-expected FE of that electrolyte and vice versa; (2) possible endocrine diseases: several endocrine diseases alter renal excretion and reabsorption of electrolytes—for example, excess parathyroid hormone (ie, in animals with primary hyperparathyroidism) promotes calcium reabsorption from the urine and phosphorus excretion, whereas insufficient aldosterone (ie, in animals with hypoadrenocorticism) results in decreased sodium reabsorption and excessive potassium reuptake in the distal convoluted tubule; and (3) renal function: in most dogs and cats with either acute or chronic kidney failure, serum electrolyte concentrations remain within reference range despite widespread nephron injury; this likely occurs because remaining nephrons and undamaged segments of diseased nephrons are able to compensate for the increased per-nephron excretion or reabsorption requirements—a potassium-wasting nephropathy, however, has been historically reported in cats (although the prevalence of this disease is now low for unknown reasons), renal secondary hyperparathyroidism unpredictably alters FE of calcium and phosphorus, and animals with severe polyuria may be unable to appropriately reabsorb electrolytes due to high rate of ultrafiltrate flow through the nephron. Because of these many interrelated factors and the difficulty predicting total expected effect on electrolyte excretion in a given patient, the clinical use of FE is limited; nevertheless, on occasion these tests may be cost-effective when prioritizing a limited number of differential diagnoses (**Box 3**).

URINARY BIOMARKERS OF KIDNEY INJURY

Biomarkers are physiologic molecules (usually proteins) that increase or decrease in association with normal or pathologic processes.[40] As discussed previously, serum creatinine concentration is relatively insensitive for early detection of renal injury; therefore, serum and urinary biomarkers that increase with early kidney damage have been the focus of many studies in people with naturally occurring disease and laboratory animal models of nephrotoxicity. Serum and plasma biomarkers seem less sensitive and have poorer correlation with presence or severity of kidney injury than urinary biomarkers. Clinical use of these biomarker proteins requires normalization to urine creatinine (ie, urine biomarker:creatinine ratio) to correct for changes rate and volume of urine production: with changes in urine volume, biomarker and creatinine concentrations are expected to proportionally increase or decrease.[41] A few urinary biomarker assays are offered by diagnostic laboratories, although clinical validation in dogs and cats is still limited.

Commercially Available Urinary Biomarkers of Renal Injury

Urine albumin/microalbuminuria
The majority of plasma albumin is size excluded and charge excluded from the ultrafiltrate; glomerular damage results in increased passage of albumin into the urine.[42] Although conventional urine dipsticks are the standard initial screening test for detection of proteinuria, urine albumin concentration must be approximately 30 mg/dL or greater to be detected by this method. Normal urine albumin concentration in dogs and cats, however, is significantly lower than this limit of detection: although there are slight differences between these species, the upper end of the reference range is approximately 1 mg/dL.[43] The range between these numbers (1–30 mg/dL) is referred to as mALB, whereas proteinuria greater than 30 mg/dL is termed *overt proteinuria*. Detection of mALB may allow earlier diagnosis of pathologically increased urine protein excretion, which can occur with primary glomerular diseases or extrarenal inflammatory diseases that secondarily damage the kidneys. Just as with overt

---

Box 3
Clinical scenario: fractional excretion of electrolytes

A 12-year-old spayed female Persian cat was evaluated for routine dental cleaning. The owner reported that the cat was healthy and active and the appetite normal and on physical examination the body condition was appropriate, despite the owner reporting that for the previous 6 months she had been feeding a home-prepared organic, vegetarian mixture of rice, tofu, and blenderized carrots and green beans. She had been previously instructed to supplement the diet with an adult human-strength multivitamin once per day but admits that she has difficulty administering medications by mouth to the cat and has not followed this recommendation for at least 2 months. Complete blood cell count, serum biochemical analysis, and urinalysis were performed before anesthesia for the dental cleaning; the only abnormality noted was moderate hypokalemia (2.1 mEq/L, reference range, 3.2–5.3 mEq/L). Serum concentration of creatinine was within the reported reference range (0.9 mg/dL; reference range, 0.2–1.6 mg/dL), and indirect systolic blood pressure was 175 mm Hg.

Differential diagnoses for hypokalemia in cats included hyperaldosteronism (due to an aldosterone-secreting adrenal tumor), potassium wasting renal disease, diet-related causes (ie, insufficient dietary concentration), and gastric or proximal duodenal obstruction with protracted vomiting and secondary metabolic alkalosis. In a patient with diet-related hypokalemia (as was suspected in this cat) or protracted vomiting (which was unlikely given the reported history), the kidneys would be expected to maximize potassium reabsorption, resulting in a very low to negligible FE of this electrolyte. In contrast, cats with hyperaldosteronism or potassium wasting renal disease would be expected to have an inappropriate FE of potassium. Ultrasonographic examination of the abdomen was recommended to determine whether or not an adrenal mass was present, because hyperaldosteronism in cats often results in hypertension (which was noted during the initial examination). The owner was reluctant to consent to this diagnostic test, however, due to expense.

Given the primary differentials for this cat's hypokalemia (insufficient dietary concentration of potassium or primary hyperaldosteronism), FE of potassium was determined. Urine concentration of creatinine was 250 mg/dL, and urine potassium of creatinine was 15.2 mEq/L. Substituting these values into the FE formula,

$$\%FE = \frac{(\text{Urine concentration of } K^+) \times (\text{Plasma concentration of creatinine})}{(\text{Urine concentration of creatinine}) \times (\text{Plasma concentration of } K^+)} \times 100$$

$$\%FE = \frac{(15.2 \text{ mEq/L}) \times (0.9 \text{ mg/dL})}{(250 \text{ mg/dL}) \times (2.1 \text{ mEq/L})} \times 100 = 2.6\%$$

The low FE of potassium was more consistent with increased reabsorption of electrolytes by the kidneys in response to hypokalemia, and therefore, a presumptive diagnosis of insufficient dietary potassium, resulting in hypokalemia was made. Conversely, hyperaldosteronism would have been expected to result in an inappropriately high potassium FE, because this hormone induces potassium excretion in the distal convoluted tubule. The owner was advised to supplement the cat with a potassium gluconate paste (she declined to feed a more balanced diet). Reevaluation of serum potassium concentration after 3 weeks of paste administration confirmed that all electrolytes were now within the laboratory reference range.

---

proteinuria, however, mALB may be due to preglomerular, glomerular, or postglomerular causes.[43]

There are strong associations between presence and magnitude of mALB and poor outcome in people. mALB is a strong prognostic indicator for later development of renal failure in diabetic patients; presence of mALB is also correlated with cardiovascular disease and death in patients with type 1 or type 2 diabetes mellitus.[44–46] Successful therapy with angiotensin-converting ednzyme inhibitors and better glycemic control slow the progression of mALB to overt proteinuria and decreases the likelihood of eventual azotemia and end-stage renal disease.[45] Other inflammatory diseases associated with mALB in people include some neoplasms, inflammatory bowel disease, and acute inflammatory conditions, such as pancreatitis and myocardial infarction; in many of these diseases, the magnitude of mALB correlates with severity.[46] This correlation is particularly evident in people with lung or breast cancer or lymphoma, where presence and magnitude of mALB are associated with histologic subtype, tumor burden, presence or absence of metastatic disease, and median survival time.

The E.R.D.-HealthScreen (Heska, Loveland, Colorado) is a point-of-care test for detection of mALB. These assays are species specific, and separate kits must be purchased for detection of mALB in dogs versus cats. Urine samples are diluted to a standard concentration, thus correcting for urine specific gravity. Unfortunately, the E.R.D.-HealthScreen is only semiquantitative rather than providing a precise measurement of mALB: results are reported as negative, low positive, medium positive, or high positive. Additionally, these tests were developed for use in all dogs and cats, but mALB reference ranges for mALB may vary based on breed and age.[47]

mALB occurs in approximately one-third of dogs and cats presenting to veterinary teaching hospitals for a variety of conditions, and greater than 50% of critically ill dogs have urine protein in the mALB range but do not have increased urine protein:creatinine ratios.[48–50] mALB has been demonstrated to occur before overt proteinuria in dogs with hereditary X-linked nephritis[51] and in soft-coated wheaten terriers with protein-losing nephropathy.[52] Dogs with lymphoma or osteosarcoma have normal urine protein:creatinine ratios but often have mALB; whether urine protein correlates with tumor burden or remission status is unknown.[53] Dogs with heartworm disease develop mALB before overt proteinuria, and histologic evidence of glomerular disease is evident at the time of mALB development.[54] Other inflammatory conditions found in dogs with mALB include renal failure, pancreatitis, and cardiovascular disease, although it is unknown whether presence of mALB correlates with prognosis or glomerular injury.[48,55] Unlike in people, strenuous exercise does not cause transient mALB in dogs.[56] mALB is more common in cats with chronic kidney disease, hypertension, or hyperthyroidism, and presence and greater magnitude of mALB are associated with decreased survival time.[49,50,57–60]

It is still unclear when or how much further diagnostic investigation or therapeutic intervention is indicated in mALB-positive animals. Dogs and cats in which mALB has been detected should first have urine protein:creatinine ratios determined to quantitate the severity of proteinuria. Breeds known to develop hereditary glomerular diseases should likely be monitored regularly, and if magnitude of mALB increases, then further steps should be considered. In dogs or cats with unexpected, persistently positive E.R.D.-HealthScreen results, it may be advised to screen for glomerular diseases and/or extrarenal inflammatory diseases. No doubt, long-term longitudinal studies evaluating the benefit of these recommendations are still needed. It is unknown whether antiproteinuria therapies in animals with mALB are of any benefit.

Urine γ-glutamyl transpeptidase:creatinine ratio

Serum concentrations of the transmembrane amino acid transporter γ-glutamyl transpeptidase (GGT) are commonly used in the diagnostic evaluation of dogs and cats with hepatic or biliary tract disease. GGT is expressed in several other tissues, however, including the apical surface of proximal convoluted tubular epithelial cells, which release small amounts of GGT into the urine. Several studies in dogs with naturally occurring or experimentally induced kidney disease have demonstrated that the urine GGT:creatinine ratio is a sensitive early marker of tubular injury, oftentimes increasing before rises in serum creatinine concentration, decreases in GFR or urine specific gravity, or appearance of casts in urine sediment. Dogs with gentamicin-induced renal failure have increased urine GGT activity 24 hours after initial dosing, whereas serum creatinine concentration did not increase above reference range until 7 days of drug administration[61–63]; 50% of intact female dogs with pyometra have moderate to high increases in urine GGT:creatinine ratios before ovariohysterectomy, which then gradually decrease over the 10 days after surgery.[64]

Urine GGT is labile, and samples should be assayed within 24 hours or frozen. Reference range in normal dogs for urine GGT:creatinine ratio is wide (1.93–28.57 IU/g), likely due to interindividual variation rather than circadian changes in excretion.[65,66] Anecdotally, and in the personal experience of the author, baseline assay of urine GGT:creatinine in patients of interest followed by serial measurement is of greater clinical utility than comparison to the suggested reference range (**Box 4**).

Selected Investigational Urinary Biomarkers of Renal Injury

Cystatin C

CysC is an inhibitor of endogenous extracellular proteinases that is produced by all nucleated cells, freely filtered across the glomerulus, and reabsorbed by renal tubular cells. Serum concentrations of CysC increase as GFR decreases, and urine concentrations increase after tubular injury. Utility of absolute urine CysC concentrations and CysC:creatinine ratio in the prediction of presence, severity, and outcome of acute kidney injury in people is unclear, because prospective studies have yielded conflicting results. A single study in dogs with either acute kidney injury or chronic kidney disease evaluated urine CysC:creatinine ratio and confirmed greater excretion than in healthy dogs.[67] Several CysC assays are available for research studies using canine plasma or urine but not clinical patients.

Interleukin 18

Interleukin 18 (IL-18) is a proinflammatory cytokine that polarizes helper T cells toward a T_H1 phenotype, induces interferon-γ production and release, and enhances

---

Box 4
Clinical scenario: urine GGT:creatinine ratio

A 6-year-old castrated male Rottweiler was evaluated for tachypnea associated with aspiration pneumonia due to idiopathic megaesophagus. The dog had been appropriately treated for multiple episodes of bacterial pneumonia over the preceding 2 years, with antibiotic therapy guided by sensitivity testing of aerobic bacterial cultures of transtracheal washings. The most recent culture indicated infection with Escherichia coli, resistant to all tested antibiotics other than aminoglycosides and carbapenems. Because of cost concerns, the owners elected home subcutaneous administration of amikacin for treatment; they also voiced monetary concerns when told that repeat thoracic radiographs would be required to guide duration of antibiotic therapy.

Before the first dose of amikacin, urine GGT:creatinine ratio was 3.72 IU/g, urine specific gravity was 1.042 without any casts noted, and serum creatinine concentration was 0.9 mg/dL. Two days after the first injection, the owners reported by tachypnea had resolved; urine GGT:creatinine ratio was 4.55 IU/g with a specific gravity of 1.045 and no casts were noted. Five days after beginning treatment, urine GGT:creatinine ratio had increased further to 7.21 IU/g, urine specific gravity was 1.035, and urine sediment remained benign. Eight days after initiating antibiotic therapy, urine specific gravity was 1.039, but GGT:creatinine ratio had tripled from baseline to 10.48, so amikacin administration was discontinued. Two weeks after discontinuing treatment, a lateral thoracic radiograph revealed resolution of previously noted interstitial and alveolar radio-opacities.

production of complement-activating IgG subclasses. Serum and urinary IL-18 concentrations increase in people with acute kidney injury, chronic kidney disease, and glomerular disease.[68–72] Increased IL-18 mRNA or serum concentrations have been reported in dogs with various inflammatory diseases, including autoimmune thyroiditis,[73] immune-mediated hemolytic anemia,[74] and sinonasal aspergillosis[75]; increased serum concentrations of this cytokine are associated with greater likelihood of death in dogs with immune-mediated hemolytic anemia.[74] Although IL-18 expression has been demonstrated in Madin-Darby canine kidney cells (a commonly used laboratory cell line),[76] in vivo investigations have not been performed in dogs with experimentally induced or naturally occurring kidney disease as yet.

Kidney injury molecule-1
Kidney injury molecule-1 (KIM-1) is a transmembrane protein normally found in healthy proximal convoluted tubular cells and shed into the urine at low concentrations. KIM-1 expression is rapidly up-regulated, however, by tubular epithelium after kidney injury, and KIM-1:creatinine concentration increases. Urinary KIM-1 increases in people with ischemic, nephrotoxic, or septic renal damage, polycystic kidney disease, and renal neoplasia.[77–79] Although in vitro expression of KIM-1 has been confirmed in Madin-Darby canine kidney cells, there are as yet no published in vivo studies of KIM-1 in dogs or cats.[79] A KIM-1 assay is available for canine urine (MILLIPLEX MAP Canine Kidney Toxicity Magnet Bead Panel 1, EMD Millipore Corporation, Billerica, Massachusetts) in conjunction with CysC and clusterin (a proposed biomarker not discussed in this article) but is only marketed for research purposes.

N-acetyl-β-D-glucosaminidase
N-acetyl-β-D-glucosaminidase (NAG) is an intracellular protein that participates in glycosaminoglycan catabolism; glycoproteins reabsorbed by proximal convoluted tubular cells are degraded by NAG and other lysosomal enzymes.[80] Increased urine excretion occurs in people with proximal tubular epithelial cell damage, particularly with acute kidney injury. Urinary NAG:creatinine ratio is increased in dogs with chronic kidney disease,[81,82] pyelonephritis,[81] uncontrolled diabetes mellitus,[81] pyometra,[81] or X-linked hereditary nephropathy[83] but does not differ before versus after control of hyperadrenocorticism with trilostane or transphenoidal hypophysectomy.[84] In cats, urinary NAG:creatinine ratio increases with chronic kidney disease.[85,86] Assays for urine retinol binding protein (RBP) are marketed for research use only.

Neutrophil gelatinase–associated lipocalin
Neutrophil gelatinase–associated lipocalin (NGAL) is an intracellular protein of hepatocytes, neutrophil granules, and epithelial cells, including the tubular epithelium of the thick ascending loop of Henle and collecting ducts.[87] Expression of NGAL is low in healthy tissues but in response to inflammation is up-regulated and plays a role in stabilizing and potentiating matrix metalloproteinases and sequestering iron, thereby inhibiting bacterial growth. Urinary NGAL:creatinine ratio is more sensitive than serum creatinine concentration for detection of acute kidney injury in people, and increases with progression of chronic kidney disease.[88,89] A few studies in dogs have investigated the utility of NGAL as a biomarker of renal damage; increases before serum creatinine concentration have been reported in laboratory dogs with gentamicin nephrotoxicity[90] or X-linked hereditary nephropathy[83] and in privately owned dogs with naturally occurring acute kidney injury or chronic kidney disease.[91] A canine-specific urine NGAL assay is available for research use only (BioPorto Diagnostics, Gentofte, Denmark).

Retinol binding protein

RBPs complex with and transport retinol (vitamin A). The plasma isoenzyme–retinol complex binds to transthyretin, which prevents passage of the low-molecular-weight (21-kDa) RBP protein across the glomerular filtration barrier.[92] In the absence of retinol, RBP undergoes a conformational change that prevents binding to transthyretin, passes into the glomerular ultrafiltrate, and is reabsorbed by proximal convoluted tubule cells. Tubular epithelial injury of any cause in people impairs RBP reabsorption and increases the urine RBP:creatinine ratio. Similarly, increased urinary excretion of RBP has been demonstrated in dogs with chronic kidney disease,[82] untreated hyperadrenocorticism,[84] and X-linked hereditary nephropathy[83] and in cats with untreated hyperthyroidism.[26,93] Assays for RBP can be purchased for laboratory use but are not offered by commercial laboratories for clinical patients.

REFERENCES

1. Von Hendy-Willson VE, Pressler BM. An overview of glomerular filtration rate testing in dogs and cats. Vet J 2011;188:156–65.
2. Watson AD, Lefebvre HP, Concordet D, et al. Plasma exogenous creatinine clearance test in dogs: comparison with other methods and proposed limited sampling strategy. J Vet Intern Med 2002;16:22–33.
3. La Garreres AL, Laroute V, De La Farge F, et al. Disposition of plasma creatinine in non-azotemic and moderately azotemic cats. J Feline Med Surg 2007;9:89–96.
4. van Hoek I, Vandermeulen E, Duchateau L, et al. Comparison and reproducibility of plasma clearance of exogenous creatinine, exo-iohexol, and endo-iohexol and ^{51}Cr-EDTA in young adult and aged healthy cats. J Vet Intern Med 2007;21:950–8.
5. Lefebvre HP, Craig AJ, Braun JP. GFR in the dog: breed effect [abstract]. In: Proceedings of the 16th ECVIM-CA Congress. Munich, Germany: European College of Veterinary Internal Medicine–Companion Animals; 2006. p. 261.
6. Robinson T, Harbison M, Bovee KC. Influence of reduced renal mass on tubular secretion of creatinine in dog. Am J Vet Res 1974;35:487–91.
7. Ross LA, Finco DR. Relationship of selected clinical renal function tests to glomerular filtration rate and renal blood flow in cats. Am J Vet Res 1981;42:1704–10.
8. Uribe D, Krawiec DR, Twardock AR, et al. Quantitative renal scintigraphic determination of the glomerular filtration rate in cats with normal and abnormal kidney function, using 99mTc-diethylenetriaminepentaacetic acid. Am J Vet Res 1992;53:1101–7.
9. Antognoni MT, Siepi D, Porciello F, et al. Serum cystatin-C evaluation in dogs affected by different diseases associated or not with renal insufficiency. Vet Res Commun 2007;31:269–71.
10. Wehner A, Hartmann K, Hirschberger J. Utility of serum cystatin C as a clinical measure of renal function in dogs. J Am Anim Hosp Assoc 2008;44:131–8.
11. Miyagawa Y, Takemura N, Hirose H. Evaluation of the measurement of serum cystatin C by an enzyme-linked immunosorbent assay for humans as a marker of the glomerular filtration rate in dogs. J Vet Med Sci 2009;71:1169–76.
12. Sanderson SL. Measuring glomerular filtration rate: practical use of clearance tests. In: Bonagura JD, Twedt DC, editors. Kirk's veterinary therapy XIV. St Louis (MO): Saunders Elsevier; 2009. p. 868–71.
13. Mutzel W, Speck U. Pharmacokinetics and biotransformation of iohexol in the rat and the dog. Acta Radiol Suppl 1980;362:87–92.

14. Nossen JO, Jakobsen JA, Kjaersgaard P, et al. Elimination of the non-ionic X-ray contrast media iodixanol and iohexol in patients with severely impaired renal function. Scand J Clin Lab Invest 1995;55:341–50.
15. Rudnick MR, Goldfarb S, Wexler L, et al. Nephrotoxicity of ionic and nonionic contrast media in 1196 patients: a randomized trial. The iohexol cooperative study. Kidney Int 1995;47:254–61.
16. Goy-Thollot I, Chafotte C, Besse S, et al. Iohexol plasma clearance in healthy dogs and cats. Vet Radiol Ultrasound 2006;47:168–73.
17. O'Dell-Anderson KJ, Twardock R, Grimm JB, et al. Determination of glomerular filtration rate in dogs using contrast-enhanced computed tomography. Vet Radiol Ultrasound 2006;47:127–35.
18. Bexfield NH, Heiene R, Gerritsen RJ, et al. Glomerular filtration rate estimated by 3-sample plasma clearance of iohexol in 118 healthy dogs. J Vet Intern Med 2008;22:66–73.
19. Miyamoto K. Use of plasma clearance of iohexol for estimating glomerular filtration rate in cats. Am J Vet Res 2001;62:572–5.
20. Goodman LA, Brown SA, Torres BT, et al. Effects of meloxicam on plasma iohexol clearance as a marker of glomerular filtration rate in conscious healthy cats. Am J Vet Res 2009;70:826–30.
21. Heiene R, Reynolds BS, Bexfield NH, et al. Estimation of glomerular filtration rate via 2- and 4-sample plasma clearance of iohexol and creatinine in clinically normal cats. Am J Vet Res 2009;70:176–85.
22. Von-Hendy-Willson VE, Pressler BM, Sandoval RM, et al. Rapid determination of GFR in dogs with acute kidney injury using a portable fluorescence ratiometric analyzer [abstract N/U 5]. J Vet Intern Med 2011;25:717–8.
23. Kongara K, Chambers P, Johnson CB. Glomerular filtration rate after tramadol, parecoxib and pindolol following anaesthesia and analgesia in comparison with morphine in dogs. Vet Anaesth Analg 2009;36:86–94.
24. Becker TJ, Graves TK, Kruger JM, et al. Effects of methimazole on renal function in cats with hyperthyroidism. J Am Anim Hosp Assoc 2000;36:215–23.
25. Boag AK, Neiger R, Slater L, et al. Changes in the glomerular filtration rate of 27 cats with hyperthyroidism after treatment with radioactive iodine. Vet Rec 2007;161:711–5.
26. van Hoek I, Lefebvre HP, Peremans K, et al. Short- and long-term follow-up of glomerular and tubular renal markers of kidney function in hyperthyroid cats after treatment with radioiodine. Domest Anim Endocrinol 2009;36:45–56.
27. Krawiec DR, Twardock AR, Badertscher RR 2nd, et al. Use of 99mTc diethylenetriaminepentaacetic acid for assessment of renal function in dogs with suspected renal disease. J Am Vet Med Assoc 1988;192:1077–80.
28. Fusellier M, Desfontis J, Madec S, et al. Influence of three anesthetic protocols on glomerular filtration rate in dogs. Am J Vet Res 2007;68:807–11.
29. Bailey DB, Rassnick KM, Erb HN, et al. Effect of glomerular filtration rate on clearance and myelotoxicity of carboplatin in cats with tumors. Am J Vet Res 2004;65:1502–7.
30. Reichle JK, DiBartola SP, Leveille R. Renal ultrasonographic and computed tomographic appearance, volume, and function of cats with autosomal dominant polycystic kidney disease. Vet Radiol Ultrasound 2002;43:368–73.
31. Deguchi E, Akuzawa M. Renal clearance of endogenous creatinine, urea, sodium, and potassium in normal cats and cats with chronic renal failure. J Vet Med Sci 1997;59:509–12.

32. Halling KB, Graham JP, Newell SP, et al. Sonographic and scintigraphic evaluation of acute renal allograft rejection in cats. Vet Radiol Ultrasound 2003;44: 707–13.

33. Groman RP, Bahr A, Berridge BR. Effects of serial ultrasound-guided renal biopsies on kidneys of healthy adolescent dogs. Vet Radiol Ultrasound 2004;45: 62–9.

34. Barthez PY, Hornof WJ, Cowgill LD, et al. Comparison between the scintigraphic uptake and plasma clearance of Tc-99mdiethylenetriaminepentacetic acid (DTPA) for the evaluation of the glomerular filtration rate in dogs. Vet Radiol Ultrasound 1998;39:470–4.

35. Kampa N, Lord P, Maripuu E. Effect of observer variability on glomerular filtration rate measurement by renal scintigraphy in dogs. Vet Radiol Ultrasound 2006;47: 212–21.

36. Lefebvre HP, Dossin D, Trumel C, et al. Fractional excretion tests: a critical review of methods and applications in domestic animals. Vet Clin Pathol 2008; 37:4–20.

37. Finco DR, Brown SS, Barsanti JA, et al. Reliability of using random urine samples for "spot" determination of fractional excretion of electrolytes in cats. Am J Vet Res 1997;58:1184–7.

38. Adams LG, Polzin DJ, Osborne CA, et al. Comparison of fractional excretion and 24-hour urinary excretion of sodium and potassium in clinically normal cats and cats with induced chronic renal failure. Am J Vet Res 1991;52:718–22.

39. Corea M, Seeliger E, Boemke W, et al. Diurnal pattern of sodium secretion in dogs with and without chronically reduced renal perfusion pressure. Kidney Blood Press Res 1996;19:16–23.

40. Biomarkers Definitions Working Group. Biomarkers and surrogate endpoints: preferred definitions and conceptual framework. Clin Pharmacol Ther 2001;69: 89–95.

41. Waikar SS, Sabbisetti VS, Bonventre JV. Normalization of urinary biomarkers to creatinine during changes in glomerular filtration rate. Kidney Int 2010;78: 486–94.

42. Russo LM, Sandoval RM, McKee M, et al. The normal kidney filters nephrotic levels of albumin retrieved by proximal tubule cells: retrieval is disrupted in nephrotic states. Kidney Int 2007;71:504–13.

43. Grauer GF. Proteinuria: measurement and interpretation. Top Companion Anim Med 2011;26:121–7.

44. Mogensen CE, Chachati A, Christensen CK, et al. Microalbuminuria: an early marker of renal involvement in diabetes. Uremia Invest 1985–1986;9:85–95.

45. Viberti GC, Hill RD, Jarrett RJ. Microalbuminuria as a predictor of clinical nephropathy in insulin-dependent diabetes melilitus. Lancet 1982;1:1430–2.

46. Gosling P. Microalbuminuria: a marker of systemic disease. Br J Hosp Med 1995;54:285–90.

47. Radecki S, Donnelly RE, Jensen WA, et al. Effect of age and breed on the prevalence of microalbuminuria in dogs [abstract 110]. J Vet Intern Med 2003;17:406.

48. Whittemore JC, Gill VL, Jensen WA, et al. Evaluation of the association between microalbuminuria and the urine albumin-creatinine ratio and systemic disease in dogs. J Am Vet Med Assoc 2006;229:958–63.

49. Whittemore JC, Miyoshi Z, Jensen WA, et al. Association of microalbuminuria and the urine albumin-to-creatinine ratio with systemic disease in cats. J Am Vet Med Assoc 2007;230:1165–9.

50. Vaden SL, Turman CA, Harris TL, et al. The prevalence of albuminuria in dogs and cats in an ICU or recovering from anesthesia. J Vet Emerg Crit Care (San Antonio) 2010;20:479–87.

51. Hsieh OF, Lees GE, Clark SE, et al. Development of albuminuria and overt proteinuria in heterozygous (carrier) female dogs with X-linked hereditary nephropathy (XLHN) [abstract 118]. J Vet Intern Med 2005;19:432.

52. Vaden SL, Jensen WA, Longhofer S, et al. Longitudinal study of microalbuminuria in soft-coated wheaten terriers [abstract 115]. J Vet Intern Med 2001;15:300.

53. Pressler BM, Proulx DR, Williams LE, et al. Urine albumin concentration is increased in dogs with lymphoma or osteosarcoma [abstract 101]. J Vet Intern Med 2003;17:404.

54. Grauer GF, Oberhauser EB, Basaraba RJ, et al. Development of microalbuminuria in dogs with heartworm disease [abstract 103]. J Vet Intern Med 2002;16:352.

55. Pressler BM, Vaden SL, Jensen WA, et al. Detection of canine microalbuminuria using semiquantitative test strips designed for use with human urine. Vet Clin Pathol 2002;31:56–60.

56. Gary AT, Cohn LA, Kerl ME, et al. The effects of exercise on urinary albumin excretion in dogs. J Vet Intern Med 2004;18:52–5.

57. Jepson RE, Brodbelt D, Vallance C, et al. Evaluation of predictors of the development of azotemia in cats. J Vet Intern Med 2009;23:806–13.

58. Chakrabarti S, Syme H, Elliott J. Clinicopathological variables predicting progression of azotemia in cats with chronic kidney disease. J Vet Intern Med 2012;26:275–81.

59. Jepson RE, Elliott J, Brodbelt D, et al. Effect of control of systolic blood pressure on survival in cats with systemic hypertension. J Vet Intern Med 2007;21:402–9.

60. Syme HM, Markwell PJ, Pfeiffer D, et al. Survival of cats with naturally occurring chronic renal failure is related to severity of proteinuria. J Vet Intern Med 2006;20:528–35.

61. Cronin RE, Bulger RE, Southern P, et al. Natural history of aminoglycoside nephrotoxicity in the dog. J Lab Clin Med 1980;95:463–74.

62. Frazier DL, Aucoin DP, Riviere JE. Gentamicin pharmacokinetics and nephrotoxicity in naturally acquired and experimentally induced disease in dogs. J Am Vet Med Assoc 1988;192:57–63.

63. Rivers BJ, Walter PA, O'Brien TD, et al. Evaluation of urine gamma-glutamyl transpeptidase-to-creatinine ratio as a diagnostic tool in an experimental model of aminoglycoside-induced acute renal failure in the dog. J Am Anim Hosp Assoc 1996;32:323–36.

64. Heiene R, Moe L, Mølmen G. Calculation of urinary enzyme excretion, with renal structure and function in dogs with pyometra. Res Vet Sci 2001;70:129–37.

65. Brunker JD, Ponzio NM, Payton ME. Indices of urine N-acetyl-β-D-glucosaminidase and γ-glutamyl transpeptidase activities in clinically normal adult dogs. Am J Vet Res 2009;70:297–301.

66. Uechi M, Uechi H, Nakayama T. The circadian variation of urinary N-acetyl-β-D-glucosaminidase and γ-glutamyl transpeptidase in clinically healthy cats. J Vet Med Sci 1998;60:1033–4.

67. Monti P, Benchekroun G, Berlato D, et al. Initial evaluation of canine urinary cystatin C as a marker of renal tubular function. J Small Anim Pract 2012;53:254–9.

68. Lonnemann G, Novic D, Rubinstein M, et al. Interleukin-18, interleukin-18 binding protein and impaired production of interferon-γ I in chronic kidney failure. Clin Nephrol 2003;60:327–34.

69. Parikh CR, Jani A, Melnikov VY, et al. Urinary interleukin-18 is a marker of human acute tubular necrosis. Am J Kidney Dis 2004;43:405–14.
70. Parikh CR, Abraham E, Ancukiewicz M, et al. Urine IL-18 is an early diagnostic marker for acute kidney injury and predicts mortality in the intensive care unit. J Am Soc Nephrol 2005;16:3046–52.
71. Hewins P, Morgan MD, Holden N, et al. IL-18 is upregulated in the kidney and primes neutrophil responsiveness in ANCA-associated vasculitis. Kidney Int 2006;69:605–15.
72. Pressler BM, Falk RJ, Preston CA. Interleukin-18, neutrophils, and ANCA. Kidney Int 2006;69:424–5.
73. Choi EW, Shin LS, Bhang DH, et al. Hormonal change and cytokine mRNA expression in peripheral blood mononuclear cells during the development of canine autoimmune thyroiditis. Clin Exp Immunol 2006;146:101–8.
74. Kjelgaard-Hansen M, Goggs R, Wiinberg B, et al. Use of serum concentrations of interleukin-18 and monocyte chemoattractant protein-1 as prognostic indicators in primary immune-mediated hemolytic anemia in dogs. J Vet Intern Med 2011;25:76–82.
75. Peeters D, Peters IR, Clercx C, et al. Quantification of mRNA encoding cytokines and chemokines in nasal biopsies from dogs with sino-nasal aspergillosis. Vet Microbiol 2006;114:318–26.
76. Jalilian I, Spildrejorde M, Seavers A, et al. Functional expression of the damage-associated molecular pattern receptor P2X7 on canine kidney epithelial cells. Vet Immunol Immunopathol 2012;150:228–33.
77. Huang Y, Don-Wauchope AC. The clinical utility of kidney injury molecule 1 in the prediction, diagnosis, and prognosis of acute kidney injury: a systematic review. Inflamm Allergy Drug Targets 2011;10:260–71.
78. Lim AI, Tang SC, Lai KN, et al. Kidney injury molecule-1: more than just an injury marker of tubular epithelial cells? J Cell Physiol 2012;228:917–24.
79. Kotsis F, Nitschke R, Boehlke C, et al. Ciliary calcium signaling is modulated by kidney injury molecule-1 (Kim1). Pflugers Arch 2007;453:819–29.
80. Reeko S, Soeta S, Syuto B, et al. Urinary excretion of N-acetyl-β-D-glucosaminidase and its isoenzymes in cats with urinary disease. J Vet Med Sci 2002;64: 367–71.
81. Reeko S, Soeta S, Miyazaki M, et al. Clinical availability of urinary of N-acetyl-β-D-glucosaminidase index in dogs with urinary diseases. J Vet Med Sci 2002;64: 361–5.
82. Smets PM, Meyer E, Maddens BE, et al. Urinary markers in healthy young and aged dogs and dogs with chronic kidney disease. J Vet Intern Med 2010;24: 65–72.
83. Nabity MG, Lees GE, Cianciolo R, et al. Urinary biomarkers of renal disease in dogs with X-linked hereditary nephropathy. J Vet Intern Med 2012;26: 282–93.
84. Smets PM, Lefebvre HP, Meij BP, et al. Long-term follow-up of renal function in dogs after treatment for ACTH-dependent hyperadrenocorticism. J Vet Intern Med 2012;26:565–73.
85. Jepson RE, Vallance C, Syme HM, et al. Assessment of urinary N-acetyl-β-D-glucosaminidase activity in geriatric cats with variable plasma creatinine concentrations with or without azotemia. Am J Vet Res 2010;71:241–7.
86. Lapointe C, Bélanger MC, Dunn M, et al. N-acetyl-β-D-glucosaminidase index as an early biomarker for chronic kidney disease in cats with hyperthyroidism. J Vet Intern Med 2008;22:1103–10.

87. Paragas N, Qiu A, Zhang Q, et al. The Ngal reporter mouse detects the response of the kidney to injury in real time. Nat Med 2011;17:216–22.

88. Giasson J, Li GH, Chen Y. Neutrophil gelatinase-associated lipocalin (NGAL) as a new biomarker for non-acute kidney injury (AKI) diseases. Inflamm Allergy Drug Targets 2011;10:272–82.

89. Nickolas TL, Forster CS, Sise ME, et al. NGAL (Lcn2) monomer is associated with tubulointerstitial damage in chronic kidney disease. Kidney Int 2012;82: 718–22.

90. Kai K, Yamaguchi T, Yoshimatsu Y, et al. Neutrophil gelatinase-associated lipocalin, a sensitive urinary biomarker of acute kidney injury in dogs receiving gentamicin. J Toxicol Sci 2013;38:269–77.

91. Lee YJ, Hu YY, Lin YS, et al. Urine neutrophil gelatinase-associated lipocalin (NGAL) as a biomarker for acute canine kidney injury. BMC Vet Res 2012;8:248.

92. Raila J, Mathews U, Schweigert FJ. Plasma transport and tissue distribution of β-carotene vitamin A and retinol-binding protein in domestic cats. Comp Biochem Physiol A Mol Integr Physiol 2001;130:849–56.

93. van Hoek I, Meyer E, Duchateau L, et al. Retinol-binding protein in serum and urine of hyperthyroid cats before and after treatment with radioiodine. J Vet Intern Med 2009;23:1031–7.

A Laboratory Diagnostic Approach to Hepatobiliary Disease in Small Animals

Seth E. Chapman, DVM, MS[a],*, Roger A. Hostutler, DVM, MS[b]

KEYWORDS

- Hepatic disease • Enzymes • Bile acids • Bilirubin • Proteins

KEY POINTS

- Liver enzymes can be classified as leakage or induction enzymes; although they are sensitive indicators for detection of disease and/or cholestasis, they often are not specific for a primary cause.
- Increased serum enzyme activities can occur in clinically normal animals, and in animals with hepatic and nonhepatic disease.
- Serum bile acids and ammonia can be measured to evaluate hepatic function.
- Detection of other biochemical abnormalities, such as hypoproteinemia, hypoglycemia, or hypocholesterolemia, may be useful. However, these analytes are often not sensitive indicators of liver disease.

TESTING AND REFERENCE INTERVALS

Understanding the limitations of laboratory diagnostic tests for hepatobiliary disease is important in avoiding misinterpretation of results. Most of these tests are quantitative assays performed on serum or plasma samples and measured on a continuous scale. Clinical interpretation of tests results is guided by reference intervals (RI), but there is inherent overlap in results between clinically healthy and diseased animals. Animals with clinically significant disease can have "normal" test results, and clinically healthy animals can have "abnormal" results.

Determination of RI varies based on the number of test subjects (minimum of 40 based on The American Society for Veterinary Clinical Pathology guidelines) and distribution of data (Gaussian vs nonparametric).[1] Intervals are often established based

This article originally appeared in Veterinary Clinics of North America: Small Animal Practice, Volume 43, Issue 6, November 2013.

Disclosures: The authors have nothing to disclose.

[a] IDEXX Laboratories Inc, 300 East Wilson Bridge Road, Suite 200, Worthington, OH 43085, USA; [b] MedVet Medical and Cancer Centers for Pets, 300 East Wilson Bridge Road, Worthington, OH 43085, USA

* Corresponding author.

E-mail address: seth-chapman@idexx.com

on results from the central 95% of the reference group. Therefore, values from 5% of the test population of clinically healthy animals will fall outside the established interval. In effect, 2.5% of the reference population will have values above or below the RI. RI for a given analyte may vary between laboratories, and comparison of results obtained from different instruments or using different methodology must be done with caution. Adherence to quality-control guidelines and instrument maintenance with proper sample collection and handling are paramount for consistently obtaining accurate results and minimizing variation attributable to instrument or operator error.

OVERVIEW OF HEPATIC ENZYMES

- Enzymes are categorized into leakage enzymes (alanine aminotransferase [ALT], aspartate aminotransferase [AST]) indicating hepatocellular injury, and induction enzymes (alkaline phosphatase [ALP], γ-glutamyltransferase [GGT]) associated with increased synthesis.
- The severity of serum-activity elevation for leakage enzymes depends on the cellular concentration and the subcellular location. Elevation of serum activity from enzymes found within the cytosol and mitochondria suggests a greater degree of cell injury than elevation of activity from enzymes found within the cytosol alone.
- Induction enzymes are typically associated with the cell membrane, and severity of the serum-activity elevation depends on the capacity for enzyme production.
- The severity of increase of serum enzyme activity may be interpreted as a fold elevation above the upper limit of the RI. A 2-fold to 3-fold elevation is often considered of mild severity. A 4-fold to 5-fold elevation and greater than 10-fold elevation may be considered of moderate and marked severity, respectively.[2]
- The finding of elevated liver enzyme activity is commonly encountered during routine biochemical testing. Detection of a single elevated liver enzyme, particularly of mild severity, may be nonspecific and insufficient for the diagnosis of hepatobiliary disease. In a study of biochemical abnormalities detected in a large population of healthy and diseased canines of various ages, elevations of serum activity for both leakage enzymes (ALT, AST) and induction enzymes (ALP, GGT) was observed in approximately 17%, 11%, 39%, and 19% of the cases, respectively.[3]
- The diagnostic utility of serum enzyme measurement for detection of hepatobiliary disease is enhanced by evaluation of both leakage and induction enzymes, as well as correlation with additional diagnostics such as hepatic function tests or histopathology.
- The duration of increase for leakage and induction enzymes depends on the rate of clearance or half-life, and on the nature and severity of the inciting cause.

Alanine Aminotransferase

ALT is found in high concentrations in the cytoplasm of canine and feline hepatocytes, and is a useful marker of hepatocellular injury in dogs and cats. This enzyme is a catalyst in a reaction resulting in deamination of alanine with production of pyruvate for entry into the Krebs cycle or gluconeogenesis pathway.[4] The enzyme is also found in cardiac and skeletal muscle cells, renal epithelial cells, and red blood cells (RBCs). The primary clinical utility of this enzyme is detection of hepatocellular injury, although enzyme distribution in other tissues can present a diagnostic challenge. Examples include differentiating elevation of serum enzyme activity due to hepatic disease from artifactual elevation (ie, in vitro hemolysis, lipemia) or extrahepatic origin (severe muscle trauma). Enzyme activity in skeletal and cardiac muscle is substantially less (approximately 5% and 25%) than in hepatocytes, but the capacity for elevated serum activity is considerable when factoring total body muscle mass as a potential source of ALT.[5] Correlation with serum creatine kinase (CK) activity is often useful in differentiating a muscle origin from a hepatic origin for ALT. CK activity increases quickly after muscle injury, with peak levels occurring at approximately 6 to 12 hours, although activity decreases within 24 to 48 hours owing to a short half-life.[6]

Increased serum activity of this enzyme is typically associated with alterations of permeability of the hepatocellular membrane, with potential causes including toxic insult, inflammatory disease, hypoxia, tissue trauma, and neoplasia (**Box 1**). Elevations of ALT associated with corticosteroids or phenobarbital therapy may be multifactorial because of increased enzyme synthesis and cell injury.[7] Increased ALT activity is not specific for a particular disease process, and can occur with reversible or irreversible hepatocellular injury. Although the degree of serum elevation may be roughly proportional to severity of disease and hepatic mass affected, underlying abnormality may be present in the absence of elevated enzyme activity resulting from a quantitative decrease in hepatocytes (eg, advanced cirrhosis, portosystemic shunting with atrophy). Inflammatory or necrotizing disorders are often associated with the most severe serum enzyme elevations, while moderate elevations can occur with hepatic neoplasia, biliary tract disease (obstructive or nonobstructive), and cirrhosis.[8] Mild serum enzyme elevation is nonspecific and can occur with a wide spectrum of metabolic, neoplastic, vascular, and (chronic) inflammatory disorders. There are also multiple disorders or drugs that can result in elevated serum ALT activity without the presence of significant primary hepatocellular disease (**Box 2**).

Box 1
Potential causes for elevated serum activity of ALT and AST

Hepatocellular Injury or Necrosis:

Cirrhosis

Corticosteroid hepatopathy (endogenous or exogenous)

Drug toxicity/idiosyncratic reaction

> Acetaminophen, anesthetic agents, arsenical compounds, carprofen, diazepam/oxazepam, griseofulvin, itraconazole, ketoconazole, lomustine, phenobarbital, phenytoin, primidone, mebendazole, methimazole, oxibendazole-diethylcarbamazine, tetracycline, trimethoprim-sulfadiazine

Diabetes mellitus

Hepatic lipidosis

Hypoxia (cardiac insufficiency, hepatic congestion, anemia)

Hyperthyroidism (feline)

Inflammatory disease (hepatitis, cholangiohepatitis)

> Infectious: ascending enteric bacterial infection, feline infectious peritonitis virus, liver fluke, histoplasmosis, leptospirosis

> Noninfectious: copper-associated hepatopathy (Bedlington terrier, Dalmatian, Doberman Pinscher, Labrador retriever), idiopathic chronic hepatitis

Portosystemic shunt

Toxin ingestion (aflatoxin, amanita mushroom, blue-green algae, copper, herbicides or insecticides, iron, sago palm, zinc, xylitol)

Neoplasia (primary hepatobiliary or metastatic)

Trauma

Myocyte Injury or Necrosis:

Canine musculodystrophy

Ischemia

Myositis

Trauma

Data from Refs.[4,9,10]

Box 2
Nonhepatic causes for elevated serum activity of hepatic leakage enzymes (ALT and AST)

Inflammation

Pancreatitis

Enteritis

Myositis

Infection

Urinary tract infections

Endocarditis

Pneumonia

Septic peritonitis

Pyothorax

Pyometra

Endocrine Disease

Hyperthyroidism/hypothyroidism

Hyperadrenocorticism

Diabetes mellitus

Drugs

Corticosteroids (dogs)

Antiepileptic drugs

Other

Hemolysis (AST)

Following hepatocellular injury, serum ALT levels increase within 12 hours and reach peak concentration in approximately 24 to 48 hours.[4,11] Resolution of the elevated serum enzyme activity depends on the nature of disease, such as an acute toxic insult versus an ongoing inflammatory or infectious process. ALT has a half-life of approximately 40 to 61 hours in dogs, and approximately 3.5 hours in cats.[7]

Aspartate Aminotransferase

AST is an enzyme that is present in marked quantities in the mitochondria of hepatocytes. Therefore, its elevation may indicate significant hepatocellular damage, given the mitochondria are not as readily injured as the cell membrane in many disease processes. This aspect is important because AST determined in serial samples will often normalize before ALT with resolution of hepatocellular abnormality.

However, AST is not specific to the liver, and is present in significant quantities in myocytes and RBCs. Should an elevated AST be noted, a CK, ALT, and hematocrit may be useful in determining true hepatic origin. Hemolysis can be associated with significant increases in serum AST activity.[4] The causes of an elevated AST are similar to those of ALT (see **Box 1**). There are no significant causes of a decreased AST. It is important to bear in mind that other disease processes or drugs may cause elevated AST without the presence of significant primary hepatocellular disease (see **Box 2**). AST has a half-life of approximately 12 hours in dogs and 1.5 hours in cats.[7,11]

Alkaline Phosphatase

ALP is an enzyme found in the membranes of hepatocytes that line bile canaliculi and sinusoids. An increased ALP can indicate primary hepatic disease such as cholestatic liver disease, canalicular cell necrosis, and increased hepatic synthesis. An elevated ALP in cats always warrants further investigation into underlying primary hepatic disease, because cats have less hepatocellular ALP than dogs and ALP is readily excreted by the kidneys. However, in dogs ALP is not liver specific. The elevation may be due to extrahepatic sources (kidney, pancreas, brain, bone marrow, spleen, testes, lymph node, placenta, cardiac and skeletal muscle). However, it should be noted that the magnitude of elevation resulting from extrahepatic sources is likely to be minimal, or may be secondary to endogenous or exogenous glucocorticoids and other drugs such as phenobarbital. The most common drugs that cause an elevation in ALP are shown in **Box 3**. Liver-specific ALP has a serum half-life of approximately 70 hours in the dog and 6 hours in the cat.[7]

Other than drug induction, causes for an elevated ALP can be grouped into 4 primary categories: (1) primary biliary tract disease; (2) hepatic parenchymal disease; (3) systemic disease; and (4) normal for growing dogs younger than 8 months. In these individuals, the ALP typically is increased 2 to 3 times the upper end of the RI. Common causes of ALP increases associated with categories (1) to (3) for dogs and cats are shown in **Box 4**.

Given the vast array of diseases that may be associated with an elevated ALP, systemic disease should be ruled out before more invasive diagnostics such as a liver biopsy. This aspect is important because many concurrent diseases can imitate primary liver disease in presenting clinical signs or client complaints.

γ-Glutamyltransferase

GGT is a membrane-associated enzyme found in biliary epithelial cells and hepatocytes, as well as in pancreatic, renal tubular, and mammary gland epithelial cells. The enzyme acts as a catalyst for transfer of glutamyl groups to amino acids or peptides, and is involved in glutathione synthesis and degradation.[4] Elevations of serum levels are generally attributed to cholestasis or biliary hyperplasia resulting in enzyme induction. GGT may be a more sensitive indicator than ALP of hepatobiliary disease in cats, owing to the short half-life of ALP in cats. A notable exception is hepatic lipidosis, as moderate to marked elevation of ALP may be present with minimal, if any, elevation of GGT. In dogs, GGT is often considered more specific but less sensitive than ALP for

---

Box 3
Common drugs causing elevated ALP

Azathioprine

Barbiturates[a]

Cephalosporins

Cyclophosphamide

Doxycycline

Estrogens

Glucocorticoids[a]

Griseofulvin

Halothane

Ibuprofen

Methimazole (cats)

Methotrexate

Nitrofurantoin

Oxacillin

Phenobarbital[a]

Primidone[a]

Progesterone

Salicylates

Testosterone

Tetracycline

Thiabendazole

Trimethoprim-sulfamethoxazole–based drugs

[a] Drugs that most consistently increase ALP.

---

the detection of hepatobiliary disease. Corticosteroid administration or elevated endogenous corticosteroid levels may result in increased serum GGT activity in dogs, likely due to enzyme induction. Mild to modest increases of serum GGT can also occur with anticonvulsant therapy (phenobarbital, phenytoin, primidone). GGT has a half-life of approximately 72 hours in dogs.[7]

Lactate Dehydrogenase

Lactate dehydrogenase (LDH) is an enzyme that catalyzes the conversion of lactate to pyruvate. It is non–tissue specific and can be found in liver, heart, and skeletal muscle. Therefore, there are 5 isoenzymes identified with LDH. LDH1 is found in cardiac muscle and erythrocytes in small animals, LDH2, LDH3, and LDH4 are found in all tissues, and LDH5 is found in the liver and skeletal muscle of small animals. LDH may be reported on routine serum biochemical profiles for dogs and cats. However, its diagnostic value is of limited significance because it may be found in multiple body tissues as outlined here. Artifactual elevations can be seen with excessive exercise and hemolysis. Therefore, if an elevated LDH is noted, other liver indices should be

Box 4
Common diseases associated with an increased ALP

Primary Biliary Tract Disease (Dog and Cat)

Cholangitis

Pancreatitis

Cholelithiasis

Biliary neoplasia

Ruptured biliary tract

Cholecystitis

Parenchymal Disease (Dog)

Cholangiohepatitis (septic and immune mediated)

Chronic active hepatitis

Cirrhotic liver disease

Neoplasia

    Lymphoma

    Hepatoma

    Hepatocellular carcinoma

    Hemangiosarcoma

    Histiocytic sarcoma

    Metastatic carcinoma (secondary to localized cholestasis)

Toxins

Parenchymal Disease (Cat)

Neoplasia: lymphoma (most common), mast-cell tumor

Biliary sludging (especially in anorexic cats)

Cholangiohepatitis (septic and immune mediated)

Hepatic lipidosis (hallmark of diagnosis is an elevated ALP with a normal GGT)

Feline infectious peritonitis

Toxins

Systemic Disease (Dog)

Hyperadrenocorticism

Diabetes mellitus

Cholestasis associated with sepsis

Tick-borne disease such as ehrlichiosis

Osteomyelitis

Osteosarcoma

Hepatic entrapment as seen with diaphragmatic hernia

Right-sided heart failure

Primary and secondary hyperparathyroidism

Healing fracture

Systemic Disease (Cat)

Hyperthyroidism

Diabetes mellitus

evaluated before an extensive diagnostic workup, because inexplicable elevations of great magnitude are not uncommon. It should be noted that the isoenzymes are not routinely available, and its measurement does not provide any additional information to that provided from evaluation of CK, AST, and ALT.

Bilirubin

Bilirubin is predominantly formed during removal of senescent RBCs through the mononuclear phagocyte system, primarily through the action of intracellular microsomal heme oxygenase. This enzyme catalyzes degradation of hemoglobin to iron, carbon monoxide, globin, and biliverdin, with biliverdin further reduced to bilirubin and released from the cell for protein-bound transport (albumin) to the liver.[7] Following transfer of bilirubin into hepatocytes, mediated by the transport proteins ligandin or fatty-acid binding protein, bilirubin is conjugated with glucuronide via the enzyme uridine diphosphate glucuronyl transferase.[4,7] The conjugated water-soluble form of bilirubin is actively transported from hepatocytes across the bile canalicular membrane and, following entry into the intestine as a component of bile, is subsequently degraded by colonic bacteria into urobilogen.[4] Hyperbilirubinemia can be caused by prehepatic (hemolytic) disease, primary hepatic disease, and post-hepatic disease.

Prehepatic hyperbilirubinemia is secondary to hemolysis of RBCs. This process is easily distinguishable from other causes because marked concurrent anemia is also present. RBC morphology should be evaluated in all anemic hyperbilirubinemic patients for spherocytosis, autoagglutination, Heinz bodies, and hemotropic parasites. Common causes of hemolysis include immune-mediated disease processes, hemotropic parasites, drugs and toxins (**Box 5**), disseminated intravascular coagulation, vasculitis, and microangiopathic disease. Concurrent elevation in ALT is often noted because of hypoxic injury to hepatocytes.

Primary hepatic hyperbilirubinemia is often secondary to concurrent decreased hepatocyte function and intrahepatic cholestasis. This condition leads to decreased bilirubin uptake, conjugation, and excretion. However, significant hepatic disease must be present to result in hyperbilirubinemia. There are numerous diseases associated with hyperbilirubinemia in dogs and cats, and the most common disease processes are listed in **Box 6**.

Post-hepatic hyperbilirubinemia is secondary to obstruction of the extrahepatic bile duct. The most common causes include pancreatitis, cholelithiasis, biliary neoplasia,

---

Box 5
Common drugs and toxins that may cause hemolysis

Acetaminophen

β-Lactam antibiotics (penicillins and cephalosporins)

Lead

Macrodantin

Onions

Sulfonamides

Vitamin K (cats)

Zinc

Box 6
Common hepatic diseases causing hyperbilirubinemia

Dogs:

Chronic hepatitis with interface hepatitis with or without fibrosis (chronic active hepatitis)

Cirrhosis

Infectious disease (leptospirosis)

Hepatic necrosis (toxins)

Septicemia

Round-cell neoplasia such as lymphoma, histiocytic sarcoma, and mast-cell disease

Cholangiohepatitis

Cats:

Hepatic lipidosis

Cholangitis

Cholangiohepatitis

Feline infectious peritonitis

Round-cell neoplasia (lymphoma, mast-cell tumor)

---

and pancreatic neoplasia. With extrahepatic biliary duct obstruction there often are disproportionate increases in cholestatic enzymes (ALP and GGT) in comparison with hepatocellular enzymes (ALT and AST). In addition, serum cholesterol levels are often elevated with biliary obstruction. Imaging of the liver with ultrasonography is often helpful in confirming the diagnosis and further directing therapy.

Serum Bile Acids

Bile acids are amphipathic steroids primarily synthesized in the liver from cholesterol via the enzyme 7α-hydroxylase, with cholic acid as the predominant type in the dog and cat.[7] Through micelle formation, bile acids enhance solubilization of lipids within the intestine, facilitating digestion and absorption of fats. Serum bile acids often are used to assess hepatic function. Serum bile acids are indicated for further evaluation of persistently elevated serum liver enzyme activity, suspected portosystemic shunts or cirrhosis, and monitoring the therapy of inpatients with hepatic diseases (**Box 7**). To obtain maximum sensitivity, both a 12-hour fasting preprandial sample and a 2-hour postprandial sample should be obtained. Patients should be fed a diet that has a moderate fat density to stimulate gallbladder contraction after obtaining the preprandial sample.

Multiple factors may affect the results of bile acids testing. Hemolysis and lipemia may falsely decrease or increase serum bile acid concentrations measured by spectrophotometric methods. Therefore, one should not feed an extremely fat-dense food or use a radioimmunoassay. In addition, patients that have had a cholecystectomy or have ileal disease may have unreliable results because the ileum is the primary source of bile-acid absorption. Therefore, results may be unreliable in animals that have had ileal resection or are suspected to have significant ileal or lower gastrointestinal tract disease. Spontaneous gallbladder contraction may occur during the fasting period, and can result in a fasting value exceeding the postprandial sample. However, both values should be within the RI unless hepatic abnormality is present.

Box 7
Causes of decreased and increased serum bile acids

Decreased Bile Acids

Decreased gastric motility

Hypermotile gastrointestinal tract

Gastrointestinal malabsorption

Ileal resection

Ileal disease

Increased Bile Acids

Hepatocellular disease

- Hepatic lipidosis
- Toxic insult
- Necrosis (toxic, ischemic, heat, and so forth)
- Inflammatory (cirrhosis, immune mediated, infectious)
- Infectious, primary hepatic
- Cholangiohepatitis (septic and nonseptic)
- Infectious, nonhepatic origin
- Neoplastic

Cholestatic disease (bile acids need not be performed in patients with hyperbilirubinemia)

Portosystemic shunting

Microvascular disease

Although bile acids are an excellent indicator of hepatic function, the magnitude of the increase is not specific to an underlying particular diagnosis or prognosis. Bile acids typically are not often elevated with nonhepatic disease, antiepileptic therapy, or glucocorticoid administration.

Urine bile acids have a diagnostic utility similar to that of serum bile acids in dogs and cats. Advantages of performing urine bile acids testing include: sensitivity and specificity comparable with those of serum bile acids for detecting liver dysfunction in both dogs and cats; a nonfasted sample is acceptable; a sample may be collected at home; sampling avoids shortcomings of serum bile acids such as delayed gastric emptying, spontaneous gallbladder contraction, and delayed intestinal transit time. Urine bile acids may be beneficial for routine monitoring of patients on potentially hepatotoxic drugs such as phenobarbital.

Ammonia

Ammonia is derived mostly from colonic bacteria through digestion of dietary protein, gastrointestinal mucosa, and gastrointestinal hemorrhage. The ammonia is then transported to the liver via the portal vein. With normal liver function, the liver metabolizes most of the ammonia to urea. As with serum bile acids, ammonia levels can be a sensitive and specific indicator of liver function, and should be performed on a fasted sample. Samples must be kept in an ice bath and analyzed within 30 minutes for reliable results. Decreased ammonia levels can be seen with administration of aminoglycosides such as neomycin, lactulose, probiotics, and enemas. A decreased ammonia level in patients not on concurrent therapy is of no clinical significance.

Common causes of increased ammonia levels are shown in **Box 8**.

Indirect Markers of Hepatobiliary Disease

Hepatobiliary disease can result in decreased protein synthesis as well as altered glucose and lipid metabolism. However, a reduction of approximately 70% to 80% of hepatic function must be present before these biochemical abnormalities are detected. As such, these are typically not considered sensitive indicators for detection of disease, and fluctuations can occur with some analytes depending on the specific disease process.

Coagulation Factors
- Enzymatic and nonenzymatic coagulation factors are synthesized in the liver, and hepatic insufficiency can result in hemostatic defects caused by decreased production.
- Enzymatic factors include II (prothrombin), VII, IX, X, XI, XII, and XIII.
- Nonenzymatic factors include I (fibrinogen), V, and VIII.
- Prolongation of activated clotting time, prothrombin time, and activated partial thromboplastin time can occur with severe hepatic insufficiency; thromboelastography may reveal tracings consistent with a hypocoagulable state.
- Cholestasis rarely results in hemostatic defects, attributed to maldigestion with decreased absorption of fat-soluble vitamins, and diminished vitamin K–dependent carboxylation of factors II, VII, IX, and X.
- Investigation for a coagulopathy should always be performed before fine-needle aspiration or biopsy of the liver, given the potential complication of hemorrhage.

Albumin and Globulins:
- Hypoalbuminemia can occur as a result of decreased protein synthesis.
- Hyperalbuminemia has rarely been reported with hepatocellular carcinoma.[12]
- α- and β-globulin hepatic synthesis may be decreased; γ-globulin production is primarily dependent on B lymphocytes and plasma cells.
- Hyperglobulinemia can potentially occur as a result of diminished filtration and clearance of toxins and microbial agents from the portal circulation. This process can occur with vascular anomalies (eg, shunts) or with decreased hepatic mass resulting in fewer Kupffer cells.

Blood Urea Nitrogen (BUN) and Ammonia:
- Altered circulation or hepatic insufficiency can result in decreased delivery of ammonia from the portal circulation for entry into the urea cycle, resulting in hyperammonemia and decreased serum BUN.

Box 8
Causes of increased ammonia levels

High-protein meals

Excessive exercise

Improper sample handling or delayed submission

Hepatic insufficiency

Inherited disorders of the urea cycle

Drugs: narcotics, diuretics leading to alkalosis

Glucose:
- Hypoglycemia can occur as a result of reduction of hepatic glycogen stores, delayed insulin clearance, or decreased gluconeogenesis.
- Hyperglycemia can potentially occur as a result of decreased absorption from the portal circulation or hyperglucagonemia associated with hepatocutaneous syndrome.

Cholesterol:
- Hypercholesterolemia can occur as a result of cholestasis.
- Hypocholesterolemia can occur from diminished synthesis associated with decreased hepatic function or portosystemic shunts.

HEMATOLOGY

There are relatively few abnormalities specific for hepatobiliary disease that can be detected on a complete blood count with a blood smear review.

- Microcytosis can occur with portosystemic shunts or potentially with severe hepatic insufficiency, likely due to altered iron transport or metabolism.
- Acanthocytes can occur with lipid disorders and disruption of normal vasculature (eg, hemangiosarcoma).
- Ovalocytes (elliptocytes) can occur in cats with hepatic lipidosis.

URINALYSIS ABNORMALITIES SECONDARY TO HEPATIC DISEASE

One of the most common, and earliest, clinical signs of liver disease is polyuria and polydipsia. Therefore, the specific gravity of urine in patients with liver disease is often markedly decreased. Bilirubinuria and urate urolithiasis or crystalluria are also indicators that hepatic disease may be present.

For bilirubin to be excreted in the urine, it must be conjugated. Bilirubinuria greater than 2+ in a urine dipstick in a dog, and any bilirubinuria in cats, should raise the index of suspicion for underlying hepatic disease. Bilirubinuria may be seen in dogs without hepatic or hemolytic disease, owing to loss of unconjugated bilirubin (in patients with proteinuric renal disease) or conjugation and production of bilirubin in renal tubular cells (primarily in males). Cats have a much higher renal threshold for bilirubin than dogs, and any degree of bilirubinuria warrants investigation into hepatic or hemolytic disease.

Urate urolithiasis or crystalluria is seen in approximately 40% to 70% of patients with portosystemic shunts (both intrahepatic and extrahepatic); this may also be breed related in Dalmatians, English bulldogs, miniature schnauzers, Shih Tzus, and Yorkshire terriers, in which no underlying portosystemic shunt is present. Acidic urine may lead to urate urolithiasis in both dogs and cats.

CYTOLOGY

Fine-needle aspiration cytology can be useful in the diagnosis of several hepatic diseases, but there are other disorders or lesions that typically require histopathology for diagnosis. The greatest utility is typically for metabolic or neoplastic disorders with multifocal or diffuse distribution throughout the liver. Multiple studies have been performed comparing the accuracy of fine-needle aspiration cytology of the liver with histopathology.

In a study by Roth[13] comparing liver cytology and biopsy diagnoses, 56 cases (25 canine, 31 feline) were reviewed, with complete agreement noted in approximately 60% of the cases, partial agreement in approximately 20% of the cases, and disagreement in the remaining 20%. Agreement was most common with lipidosis, lymphoma, and epithelial neoplasia. Disagreement was most common for cases of hepatitis, although disagreement was also observed in cases of fibrosis, amyloidosis, lymphoma, and hemangiosarcoma.

Another study by Wang and colleagues[14] compared accuracy of ultrasound-guided fine-needle aspiration cytology with histopathology in 97 cases (56 canine, 41 feline). Overall agreement was observed in approximately 30% of the canine cases and 51% of the feline cases. A cytologic diagnosis of vacuolar change was confirmed by histopathology as a predominant disease process in approximately 64% and 83% of the canine and feline cases, respectively. Vacuolar change was also reported as the disorder most often misdiagnosed cytologically. Such misdiagnosis was partially attributed to cases of vacuolar change occurring as a secondary process, and the limitation of cytology in detecting the primary underlying disorder (such as metabolic or nutritional disease, hypoxia, inflammation). Inflammatory disease was accurately identified cytologically in approximately 25% and 27% of canine and feline cases.

A large study by Bahr and colleagues[15] was conducted on the accuracy of ultrasound-guided fine-needle aspiration cytology of focal liver lesions in dogs. In comparison with histology, cytology had the highest sensitivity for detection of vacuolar change (58%) and neoplasia (52%). Cytology had lower sensitivity for detection of inflammation (31%), necrosis (20%), and hyperplasia (14%). Within the category of neoplasia, cytology had the highest sensitivity for detection of round-cell tumors (60%), and lowest sensitivity for detection of sarcomas (17%). The sensitivity for detection of carcinomas varied based on tumor type, with higher sensitivity for identification of nonhepatocellular carcinoma (55%) than for hepatocellular carcinoma (35%). Cytology carried the highest positive predictive value (87%) for neoplasia, and although limited in detection of disease (depending on tumor type), a cytologic diagnosis of neoplasia could be interpreted with a high degree of confidence. Regarding inflammatory disease, cytology had limited sensitivity for detection of nonsuppurative inflammation (31%), with poor sensitivity for identification of suppurative (14%) or mixed-cell inflammation (8%).

Neoplasia

Diagnosis of round-cell neoplasia is often possible, including lymphoma, histiocytic sarcoma, plasma cell neoplasia, and mast-cell disease. In some cases, distinction between the various tumor types can be difficult if the cells are poorly differentiated. Regarding lymphoma, cytology is often useful when there is a predominance of large lymphocytes or large granular lymphocytes (**Figs. 1** and **2**). Small-cell or intermediate-cell predominant forms of lymphoma can be cytologically indistinguishable from hyperplastic or inflammatory populations, requiring collection of samples for histopathology or polymerase chain reaction for clonality.

For epithelial neoplasia, aspiration of solitary nodules for the purpose of differentiating nodular hyperplasia from neoplasia may be of limited value. There can be considerable overlap in the cytologic appearance of hepatocellular hyperplasia and neoplasia (hepatoma, well-differentiated hepatocellular carcinoma). A diagnosis of carcinoma can be made cytologically, particularly in cases when there is moderate to marked cellular anaplasia (**Fig. 3**). However, correlation with other clinical findings and imaging results is often necessary to help differentiate a primary hepatobiliary tumor from a metastatic lesion. Similarly, a cytologic diagnosis of neuroendocrine neoplasia is possible in some cases, but specific tumors in this category can be cytologically indistinguishable, thus limiting the differentiation of a primary tumor (hepatic or biliary neuroendocrine carcinoma) from a metastatic process (eg, insulinoma,

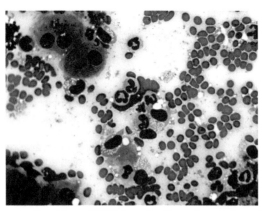

Fig. 1. Fine-needle aspiration biopsy (FNA) from the liver of a cat shows lymphoma of large granular lymphocytes (Diff-Quik, original magnification ×100).

gastrinoma, pheochromocytoma). Mesenchymal neoplasms often do not exfoliate well, and cytology may be poorly sensitive for detection of these lesions. For hemangiosarcoma in particular, fine-needle aspiration may be of limited utility because definitive cytologic diagnosis is often not achieved, and there may be considerable risk of complication with sample collection (eg, rupture of cavitated mass, hemorrhage due to thrombocytopenia).

Lipid and Nonlipid Vacuolar Change

Cytology is useful in identifying vacuolar change such as occurs with feline hepatic lipidosis (**Fig. 4**), although a cause is often not identified. Canine nonlipid vacuolar hepatopathy (**Fig. 5**) is a common finding, but this is a nonspecific process that can occur with a variety of metabolic disorders, hypoxia, toxin ingestion, inflammation, nodular hyperplasia, and neoplasia.

Infectious and Inflammatory Disease

Lesions such as a bacterial abscess or fungal infection (eg, histoplasmosis) are often amenable to cytologic diagnosis. Diagnosis of viral disease (eg, feline infectious

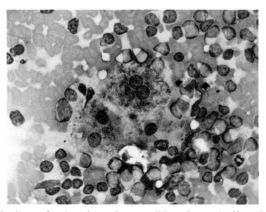

Fig. 2. FNA from the liver of a dog shows large-cell lymphoma (Diff-Quik, original magnification ×100).

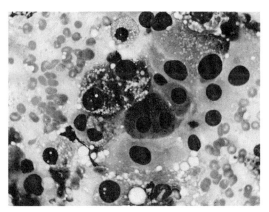

Fig. 3. FNA from the liver of a dog shows hepatocellular carcinoma (Diff-Quik, original magnification ×100).

peritonitis, infectious canine hepatitis), protozoal disease (eg, toxoplasmosis, neosporosis), leptospirosis, mycobacteriosis, and parasitic disease often requires additional diagnostics such as serology, polymerase chain reaction, and/or histopathology with special stains.

HISTOPATHOLOGY

Histopathology is necessary in many cases for the differentiation of benign from malignant lesions, identification of vascular anomalies (eg, microvascular dysplasia, portosystemic shunts) or cirrhosis, diagnosis of inflammatory conditions, and detection of storage disorders (eg, glycogen storage disease, copper hepatopathy). Additional stains may necessary for diagnosis (eg, rhodanine for copper, immunohistochemistry for tumor identification). Collection of a wedge biopsy via exploratory laparotomy or laparoscopic biopsy is preferred over ultrasound-guided Tru-Cut biopsy. Tru-Cut biopsy may be useful in cases with diffuse disease (eg, lymphoma, lipidosis), but microscopic evaluation may be limited by small sample size or because of

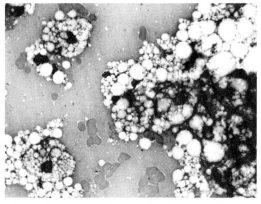

Fig. 4. FNA from the liver of a cat shows hepatic lipidosis (Wright stain, original magnification ×100).

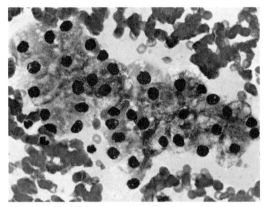

Fig. 5. FNA from the liver of a dog shows nonlipid vacuolar change (Diff-Quik, original magnification ×100).

fragmentation. Collection of samples containing a minimum of 15 portal triads has been recommended to help ensure the tissue is representative of acinar units.[10]

In a study by Cole and colleagues,[16] morphologic diagnosis from liver samples obtained by needle biopsy from dogs and cats were compared with those obtained by wedge biopsy, with the diagnosis obtained from the wedge biopsy considered the definitive diagnosis. The morphologic diagnosis from the needle-biopsy specimen was in agreement with the diagnosis from the wedge biopsy in 40% of animals with hepatic disease, and in 48% of all animals in the study (including 33 animals without hepatic disease). The results of this study suggest that caution must be exercised when interpreting histopathologic findings from needle-biopsy specimens.

REFERENCES

1. Friedrichs KR, Harr KE, Freeman KP, et al. ASVCP reference interval guidelines: determination of de novo reference intervals in veterinary species and other related topics. Vet Clin Pathol 2012;41(4):441–53.
2. Bunch SE. Diagnostic tests for the hepatobiliary system. In: Nelson RW, Couto CG, editors. Small animal internal medicine. 3rd edition. St. Louis, Missouri: Mosby; 2003. p. 483–505.
3. Comazzi S, Pieralisi C, Bertazzolo W. Haematological and biochemical abnormalities in canine blood: frequency and associations in 1022 samples. J Small Anim Pract 2004;45(7):343–9.
4. Stockham SL, Scott MA. Fundamentals of veterinary clinical pathology. Ames, Iowa: Iowa State Press; 2002. p. 435–86.
5. Lassen ED. Laboratory evaluation of the liver. In: Thrall MA, editor. Veterinary hematology and clinical chemistry. Baltimore, Maryland: Lippincott Williams & Wilkins; 2004. p. 355–75.
6. Steinberg J. Creatine Kinase. In: Vaden SL, Knoll JS, Smith FW, et al, editors. Blackwell's five minute veterinary consult: laboratory tests and diagnostic procedures: canine and feline. Ames, Iowa: Wiley-Blackwell; 2009. p. 196–7.
7. Meyer DJ, Harvey JW. Veterinary laboratory medicine. 2nd edition. Philadelphia, Pennsylvania: W. B. Saunders and Co.; 1998. p. 157–86.
8. Washbau RJ, Day MJ. Canine and feline gastroenterology. St. Louis, Missouri: Elsevier Saunders; 2013. p. 849–957.

9. Bain PJ. Alanine aminotransferase. In: Vaden SL, Knoll JS, Smith FW, et al, editors. Blackwell's five minute veterinary consult: laboratory tests and diagnostic procedures: canine and feline. Ames, Iowa: Wiley-Blackwell; 2009. p. 32–3.

10. Center SA. Hepatic disease in small animals. In: The Merck veterinary manual. Available at: http://www.merckmanuals.com/vet/digestive_system/hepatic_disease_in_small_animals/overview_of_hepatic_disease_in_small_animals.html. Accessed June 1, 2013.

11. Bain PJ. Liver. In: Latimer KS, editor. Duncan and Prasse's veterinary laboratory medicine clinical pathology. 5th edition. Ames, Iowa: Wiley-Blackwell; 2011. p. 211–30.

12. Cooper ES, Wellman ML, Carsillo ME. Hyperalbuminemia associated with hepatocellular carcinoma in a dog. Vet Clin Pathol 2009;38(4):516–20.

13. Roth L. Comparison of liver cytology and biopsy diagnoses in dogs and cats: 56 cases. Vet Clin Pathol 2001;30(1):35–8.

14. Wang KY, Panciera DL, Al-Rukibat RK, et al. Accuracy of ultrasound-guided fine-needle aspiration of the liver and cytologic findings in dogs and cats: 97 cases (1990-2000). J Am Vet Med Assoc 2004;224(1):75–8.

15. Bahr KL, Sharkey LC, Murakami T, et al. Accuracy of US-guided FNA of focal liver lesions in dogs: 140 cases (2005-2008). J Am Anim Hosp Assoc 2013;49(3): 190–6.

16. Cole TL, Center SA, Flood SN, et al. Diagnostic comparison of needle and wedge biopsy specimens of the liver in dogs and cats. J Am Vet Med Assoc 2002; 220(10):1483–90.

Diagnosis of Small Intestinal Disorders in Dogs and Cats

Karin Allenspach, Dr med vet, FVH, PhD, FHEA

KEYWORDS

• Diagnostic workup • Chronic diarrhea • Small intestine • Laboratory tests

KEY POINTS

• A serum albumin concentration of less than 2 g/L is an indicator of poor prognosis in dogs with inflammatory bowel disease (IBD).
• Cobalamin should be supplemented in all cases with decreased serum cobalamin concentrations.
• Increased canine pancreatic lipase in dogs with IBD is associated with a worse outcome.
• In cases of suspected intestinal lymphoma, polymerase chain reaction for antigen receptor rearrangements and immunophenotyping by flow cytometry or immunohistochemistry should be used in conjunction with clinical signs to help establish a diagnosis.
• Evaluation of intestinal biopsies for expression of CD11c using immunofluorescence may be a helpful diagnostic test for IBD in dogs.
• Genetic testing for mutations in innate immunity receptors is available for German Shepherd dogs, and could become a useful test for other breeds of dogs in the future.

INTRODUCTION: DIAGNOSTIC WORKUP OF SMALL INTESTINAL DISORDERS

The last decade has brought numerous advances in our knowledge about the pathogenesis of chronic intestinal disorders in people, particularly regarding inflammatory bowel disease (IBD), which comprises Crohn disease and ulcerative colitis. Specifically, the interplay of innate immunity receptors with commensals of the intestinal microbiome plays an important role in the disease pathogenesis. Molecular studies have identified specific disbalances in the microbiome of people with IBD. In addition, genetic polymorphisms that are associated with an increased risk of development of IBD have been identified. These data promise to be helpful in the development of new diagnostic options and targeted molecular treatment strategies for IBD. New findings

This article originally appeared in Veterinary Clinics of North America: Small Animal Practice, Volume 43, Issue 6, November 2013.
Current Funding Sources: Morris Animal Foundation, British Biotechnology and Bioscience Research Fund, Probiotics Ltd UK, Laboklin GmbH Germany.
Conflict of Interests: None.
Department of Clinical Sciences and Services, Royal Veterinary College, University of London, Hawkshead Lane, North Mymms, Hatfield AL9 7PT, UK
E-mail address: kallenspach@rvc.ac.uk

in chronic enteropathies in dogs and cats suggest a pathogenesis similar to that in people with IBD. Recent studies have detected disbalances in expression of innate immunity receptors (so-called toll-like receptors [TLRs]) in the intestines of dogs with IBD[1,2] that are similar to those seen in people with IBD. The expression of some of these receptors also has been correlated with severity of clinical disease in dogs with IBD, which makes it likely that they are causally implicated in the pathogenesis.[3] In addition, disbalances in the microbiome (so-called dysbiosis) have been identified using molecular methods in dogs and cats with IBD.[4–6] These findings point toward a pathogenesis of IBD in dogs and cats similar to that in people, even if the clinical manifestations of these diseases are different. There is hope that similar advances regarding diagnostic options and new therapeutic modalities will be made for canine and feline IBD as has been done for IBD in humans.

A thorough history is important in the evaluation of small animal patients exhibiting signs of intestinal disorder. The first differentiation should be to establish whether the disease is acute or chronic. Diarrhea, vomiting, dehydration, weight loss, lethargy, and melena all can be signs of small intestinal disease. The disease is acute if clinical signs have been present for only a few days. However, if clinical signs persist for more than 3 weeks or are intermittently present for more than 3 weeks, the disease is defined as chronic.

If the animal has diarrhea, the next step is to determine whether it has small intestinal, large intestinal, or a combination of small and large intestinal diarrhea (**Table 1**).

Differential Diagnoses for Acute Small Intestinal Diseases

Systemically well

- Dietary indiscretion
- Intestinal parasites (*Ancylostoma caninum*, *Toxocara*, *Giardia*, *Tritrichomonas fetus*)

Systemically unwell, abnormal abdominal palpation, severe diarrhea with hematochezia, melena, and frequent vomiting

- Dietary indiscretion
- Toxicity
- Viral infection (parvovirus, coronavirus, distemper, feline leukemia virus [FeLV]/feline immunodeficiency virus [FIV])
- Bacterial infection (*Salmonella*, *Campylobacter*, *Clostridium*)
- Intestinal parasites (*Giardia*, *Tritrichomonas*)

Table 1 Differentiation of small-bowel and large-bowel diarrhea		
	Small	Large
Volume	+++	+
Mucus	−	+++
Frequency	+	+++
Tenesmus	−	+++
Dyschezia	−	+
Weight loss	++	+
Vomiting	+	+
General condition	+	−

- Acute pancreatitis
- Intestinal obstruction
- Hypoadrenocorticism (Addison disease)

DIAGNOSTIC WORKUP OF CHRONIC SMALL INTESTINAL DIARRHEA

Once clinical signs persist for more than 3 weeks, additional workup is required to establish the diagnosis. In chronic cases it is more common for systemic, nongastrointestinal problems to cause the signs, and therefore the first diagnostic steps must be directed at excluding these extragastrointestinal causes.

Causes of Chronic Small Intestinal Disease

Extragastrointestinal (Metabolic) Causes
- Hepatic disease (portosystemic shunt)
- Hyperthyroidism (cats)
- Hypoadrenocorticism (Addison disease) (dogs)
- Renal insufficiency
- Pancreatitis (acute or chronic)
- Exocrine pancreatic insufficiency (EPI)

Gastrointestinal Causes
- Intestinal parasites (*Giardia* infection, *Tritrichomonas* infection) (cats)
- Chronic partial obstruction of the small intestine
- Lymphangiectasia
- Neoplasia: lymphosarcoma
- Food intolerance/food allergy
- Chronic enteropathies/IBD
  - Eosinophilic enteritis
  - Lymphoplasmacytic enteritis

The diagnosis of chronic gastrointestinal causes is one of exclusion, and a full diagnostic workup needs to be done first to rule out all known causes of extragastrointestinal inflammation. This workup commonly involves a complete blood cell count, serum biochemical analysis, urinalysis, and fecal analysis for helminth and protozoal parasites (*Giardia* and *Tritrichomonas* in cats). Further tests are indicated if none of these tests are abnormal: trypsin-like immunoreactivity to exclude EPI, canine pancreatic lipase immunoreactivity (cPLI) to assess the possibility of pancreatitis or pancreatic tumors, corticotropin stimulation test or basal cortisol concentration to exclude hypoadrenocorticism, and cobalamin concentrations to assess the absorptive function of the distal small intestine. Total thyroxine (T4) and FeLV/FIV infection also should be assessed in cats. Abdominal ultrasonography will be more helpful than endoscopy in determining whether the small and/or large intestine is affected and whether there are mass lesions that need surgical intervention. If the results of these tests do not determine the cause for the clinical signs and the patient is stable (ie, has a normal appetite, is not lethargic, there is no or minimal weight loss, the serum protein concentration is normal, and there is no intestinal thickening on diagnostic imaging), a well-conducted therapeutic trial with an elimination diet or hydrolyzed diet for at least 2 weeks can be performed. If there is no response to a well-conducted dietary trial within 2 weeks after starting the diet, it is unlikely that the patient is suffering from food-responsive disease (FRD) (food allergy or food intolerance).[7] If the dietary trial is unsuccessful, antimicrobials (metronidazole, 10–15 mg/kg by mouth twice a day or tylosin, 10 mg/kg by mouth once to twice a day) for 2 to 3 weeks can be administered. Intestinal biopsies for histopathology are collected from those patients that either fail to respond to empiric therapy or have worsening of their clinical signs. Most patients with chronic enteropathies can be diagnosed by obtaining endoscopic biopsies, as long as at least 12 to 15 biopsies from the small intestine are taken (**Fig. 1**). In rare cases, a diagnosis of lymphoma can be missed if no full-thickness biopsies are obtained, especially in cats, and if the ileum has not been sampled.

INTERPRETATION OF LABORATORY TESTS TO AID THE DIAGNOSIS OF CHRONIC SMALL INTESTINAL DIARRHEA
Serum Albumin Concentrations

Dogs
Decreased serum albumin concentration has been described as a negative prognostic indicator in retrospective and prospective studies of IBD in dogs. Protein-losing enteropathy (PLE) accounts for the loss of albumin through the gut mucosa in severely affected dogs with IBD. PLE in dogs can be associated with severe lymphoplasmacytic IBD, intestinal lymphoma, or, rarely, primary lymphangiectasia. In one study of dogs with IBD, 12 of 80 (16%) dogs had hypoalbuminemia and 4 of 80 (5%) had panhypoproteinemia.[8] Seven of 12 dogs with hypoalbuminemia had to be euthanized for intractable IBD, identifying decreased serum albumin concentration as a major risk factor associated with a worse outcome. In another recent prospective study of dogs with IBD, 12 of 58 (21%) dogs initially presented with hypoalbuminemia.[7] Of these 12 dogs, 7 were panhypoproteinemic with severe hypoalbuminemia (mean albumin level 11 g/L), and 3 of these dogs eventually had to be euthanized. However, it must be noted that relatively mild reductions in serum albumin (<2 g/L) previously

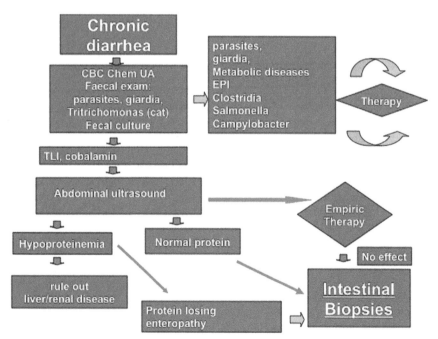

Fig. 1. Diagnostic workup for dogs and cats presenting with signs of chronic small intestinal disease. CBC, complete blood cell count; Chem, serum biochemical profile; EPI, exocrine pancreatic insufficiency; UA, urinalysis.

had been associated with an increased risk of refractoriness to treatment. At this level, most patients will not yet show any clinical signs of hypoalbuminemia, such as ascites, peripheral edema, or pleural effusion.

Furthermore, another study found that severely hypoalbuminemic dogs that failed to improve on immunosuppressive doses of steroids were successfully treated with cyclosporine.[9] This finding suggests that early aggressive treatment in hypoalbuminemic dogs may potentially decrease mortality rates in severely ill animals. Serum albumin concentration also can be used to monitor patients, as improvement of serum albumin concentrations higher than 2 g/L usually indicates treatment success, even if clinical improvement can be seen earlier in some cases. It is therefore recommended to evaluate serum albumin concentrations every 2 to 3 weeks to assess when treatment can be tapered off or discontinued.

Cats

There is not much published information regarding serum albumin concentrations in cats with chronic intestinal disease. PLE as a clinical syndrome does not exist in cats, as clinical signs such as ascites and peripheral edema do not usually occur in cats with hypoalbuminemia caused by intestinal disease. In addition, the hypoalbuminemia seen in such cases is usually mild. In cats with IBD, the prevalence of hypoalbuminemia ranged from 5% to 24%.[10–12] However, there is evidence that cats with chronic intestinal disease and decreased serum albumin concentrations may have concurrent pancreatic disease.

In one recent retrospective study, cats with IBD and serum feline pancreatic lipase (fPLI) concentrations of 2.0 µg/L or higher had a lower median serum albumin concentration than cats with IBD and a normal fPLI.[13] However, hypoalbuminemia was not a negative predictor of survival in this study. Another study found that cats with moderate to severe pancreatitis were significantly more likely to be hypoalbuminemic than were healthy cats and cats with mild pancreatitis.[14]

Therefore, hypoalbuminemia in cats with chronic intestinal disease should prompt the clinician to measure fPLI concentrations and/or to perform abdominal ultrasonographic examination to determine if there is concurrent pancreatitis. Depending on the severity of the hypoalbuminemia, the clinician's approach to treatment might be altered.

Serum Cobalamin Concentrations in Dogs and Cats

Serum cobalamin concentrations should be measured in any small animal patient with chronic small intestinal disease. Cobalamin absorption is receptor-mediated in the ileum, and decreased serum cobalamin concentrations are most commonly seen when this part of the small intestine is affected. However, absorption of cobalamin also involves intrinsic factor, which in dogs and cats is produced primarily in the pancreas. For this reason most small animals with EPI have low serum cobalamin concentrations (**Fig. 2**). The author's group[7] has shown recently that serum cobalamin also is very important for prognosis in dogs with chronic enteropathies. If cobalamin serum concentration is below the reference interval, the risk for later euthanasia increases by a factor of 10. It is therefore important to supplement dogs with hypocobalaminemia while they undergo treatment of IBD, as this "risk of euthanasia" can be reversed by cobalamin supplementation.

Cats

Serum cobalamin concentration has long been known to be an important negative prognostic factor in cats with chronic enteropathies.[15] The prevalence of decreased serum cobalamin concentrations in cats with chronic gastrointestinal signs has

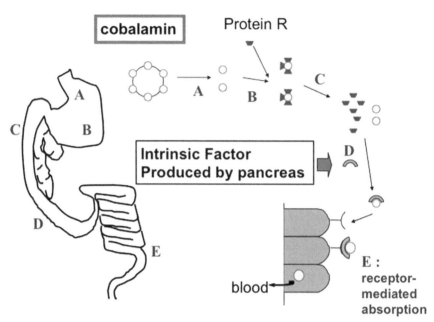

Fig. 2. Absorption of cobalamin is a complex process involving several steps. Cobalamin is released from food protein in the stomach (A) and immediately bound to R-binder proteins (B). In the proximal small intestine, the cobalamin-R-binder complex is cleaved after digestion of the R-binder by pancreatic proteases (C). Free cobalamin can now bind to intrinsic factor (IF) (D), the majority of which is secreted by the pancreas in cats and dogs. This cobalamin-IF complex is subsequently absorbed by specialized receptors in the ileum (E).

been reported to be up to 16.5%.[16] In cats, it has also been reported that cobalamin supplementation can improve clinical signs regardless of the underlying diagnosis, and even if given as the sole treatment for their disease.[15] It is therefore recommended that cats with chronic intestinal disease are supplemented with cobalamin regardless of whether a specific cause for the disease can be identified.

Supplementation recommendations for dogs and cats
Supplementation of cobalamin should be given parenterally (subcutaneously) as a weekly injection for at least 6 weeks. Exact dosages are not reported, as it is a water-soluble vitamin and cannot be overdosed. For tested recommendations, please visit the Web site of the Texas GI Laboratory (http://vetmed.tamu.edu/gilab).

Canine Pancreatic Lipase

cPLI has recently become available as a commercial test and is useful in the assessment of pancreatitis in dogs.[17] However, cPLI also can be elevated in dogs with chronic enteropathy. In a retrospective study of 50 dogs with IBD, the author's group[18] evaluated clinical signs, age, serum lipase and amylase activities, albumin and cobalamin concentrations, abdominal ultrasonography results, histopathologic review of intestinal biopsies, management of IBD, and follow-up in dogs with IBD, either with or without concurrent chronic pancreatitis. Sixteen dogs with increased cPLI and 32 dogs with normal cPLI values were compared. No significant differences were found for clinical activity score, serum amylase activity, serum lipase activity, serum cobalamin concentration, serum albumin concentration, abdominal ultrasonography scores, and histopathology scores for IBD. There was no difference in the frequency of steroid treatment between the groups. Dogs with IBD and concurrent elevated cPLI were significantly older than dogs without elevated cPLI. Moreover, dogs with elevated cPLI had a higher risk of a poor follow-up score and were significantly more likely to be euthanized at follow-up. These data show that elevated cPLI in canine IBD may indicate that a subset of these patients could also have chronic subclinical pancreatitis. In patients that have been diagnosed with IBD and also have elevated cPLI without overt imaging evidence of acute pancreatitis, it is recommended to discuss treatment options for IBD that also will treat possible autoimmune pancreatitis. The author has had anecdotal success with cyclosporine at 5 mg/kg daily for 8 weeks in such cases.

C-Reactive Protein

C-reactive protein (CRP) is a serum acute-phase protein that can be elevated in many different diseases. In people with IBD, several calculated indices of clinical activity of disease incorporate measurements of CRP.[19] In dogs, a similar correlation between the canine IBD activity index (CIBDAI) and serum CRP concentration has been found in one large study of 58 dogs.[20] CRP was elevated in the 28 dogs with CIBDAI scores greater than 5 (which comprises mild to moderate disease activity) in comparison with normal dogs, and CRP decreased significantly after treatment.[20]

In the author's experience, CRP is not very helpful when assessing dogs with chronic enteropathies. CRP was measured in 21 dogs with IBD before treatment and in 18 dogs after treatment.[7] CRP was elevated in only 6 of 21 dogs before treatment, and did not correlate with CIBDAI or histologic scoring.

A large percentage of dogs with IBD do not show any elevations in CRP. Interpretation of elevated levels also may be hampered by increases related to diseases other than IBD.

Fecal α_1-Proteinase Inhibitor

Fecal α_1-proteinase inhibitor (α_1-PI) can be used as a test for dogs in which the clinician suspects PLE although the clinical signs are not yet overtly visible. α_1-PI is a plasma protein similar in size to albumin. If the intestinal mucosal barrier is compromised and loss of protein into the intestinal lumen occurs, α_1-PI is lost at approximately the same rate as albumin. Unlike albumin, however, its proteinase inhibitor properties protect α_1-PI from degradation by intestinal proteases, and can be measured in feces. The test recently has been validated for dogs.[21]

Prompt diagnosis of PLE in a patient with IBD is important because hypoalbuminemia is a risk factor for negative outcome,[7] and the cause should be treated aggressively to improve survival. The α_1-PI assay is especially valuable in patients with intestinal disease that have concurrent renal or hepatic disease. In these patients, measurement of fecal α_1-PI can help assess which portion, if any, of the protein loss can be attributed to the intestine. This test is available only at the Texas GI Laboratory. Ideally, 3 consecutive fresh fecal samples should be submitted to improve test accuracy, which means that fecal α_1-PI is not a useful test for practitioners outside North America.

Histology and World Small Animal Veterinary Association (WSAVA) Scoring of Intestinal Biopsies

Sampling of intestinal biopsies is an essential step in the evaluation of small intestinal disorders, to exclude neoplastic causes and confirm the presence of intestinal inflammation. However, interpretation of intestinal biopsies is difficult and subject to controversy. In several recent studies looking at conventional histologic interpretation of intestinal biopsies, there was no correlation between clinical activity and histologic grading either before or after therapy.[7,20,22] In addition, total lymphocyte counts as well as the number of infiltrating CD3 cells in the lamina propria cannot be used as markers for clinical activity of disease, as there is no difference in cell counts before and after treatment.[23] These findings suggest that the type and degree of histologic infiltrates in canine IBD may not be as helpful as in human medicine, in which clinical scores correlate very well with histologic grading. Therefore, a new grading scheme for the histologic interpretation of endoscopically obtained biopsies from dogs and cats with IBD has recently been published by the WSAVA Working Group.[24] The findings in this study suggest that microarchitectural changes seem to be much more important than cellular infiltrates when assessing histologic severity. However, there is limited information on how well this new grading system correlates with clinical disease. In one retrospective study, the interpathologist variability was still very high even when using the picture guide from the original publication.[25] In addition, it is of concern that the only parameter that correlated with clinical disease was the presence of lymphangiectasia and hypoalbuminemia. Further prospective studies are warranted before the WSAVA scoring can be adopted as a useful tool for clinicians.

PARR in Intestinal Biopsies

The polymerase chain reaction for antigen receptor rearrangements (PARR) amplifies the highly variable T- or B-cell antigen receptor genes, and is used to detect the presence of a clonally expanded population of lymphocytes. This test has been advocated as useful when applied on endoscopically sampled biopsies if a diagnosis of intestinal lymphoma is suspected but not confirmed by conventional histopathology. In a study at the Royal Veterinary College, the author prospectively evaluated the accuracy of PARR for the diagnosis of intestinal lymphoma in biopsies obtained endoscopically from dogs in a comparison with the gold standard of histopathology and clinical outcome determined by follow-up information of at least 2 years. Samples from 39 dogs were included. PARR results indicated a clonal expansion in 7 of 36 dogs. However, these dogs were clinically healthy after dietary treatment 2 years after the endoscopy, so they clearly did not have lymphoma. The data from this study indicate a false-positive rate of almost 20% for PARR when performed on endoscopic biopsies. Another recent study has confirmed these findings, showing that in dogs with IBD, PARR results showed at least one oligoclonal pattern in 38% of dogs, and an immunoglobulin (7 of 47; 14.9%) or T-cell receptor (1 of 47: 2.1%) monoclonal pattern in 17% of dogs.[26] The conclusion that a positive PARR test on an endoscopic biopsy means a diagnosis of lymphoma must therefore be made cautiously in a clinical situation, and clinical signs, response to treatment, and immunohistochemistry must also be taken into account.

Perinuclear Antineutrophilic Cytoplasmic Antibodies

Perinuclear antineutrophilic cytoplasmic antibodies (pANCA) have been useful in the diagnosis of human IBD for decades.[27] These antibodies are serum autoantibodies similar to antinuclear antibodies (ANA), but seem to be more specific for intestinal disease than for ANA. pANCA are detected by immunofluorescence by visualizing a typical pattern of perinuclear staining.

In the first study to assess the clinical usefulness of pANCA in dogs with IBD, sensitivity for pANCA was 0.51 and specificity ranged between 0.56 and 0.95. pANCA proved to be a highly specific marker for IBD in dogs when the group of dogs with chronic diarrhea of other causes were tested against dogs with IBD (specificity 0.95).[28] This finding is in agreement with reports from human medicine that show a specificity of up to 94% for pANCA when distinguishing between IBD and healthy controls, as well as patients with non–IBD-related diarrhea from other causes.[29] When pANCA were tested in a group of dogs with FRD and compared with pANCA in dogs with steroid-responsive disease, a positive pANCA titer was significantly associated with FRD.[30]

The pANCA assay might be helpful in differentiating dogs with chronic diarrhea caused by FRD or IBD: If the result is positive, a food-responsive chronic enteropathy is highly likely, however, if the result is negative, IBD cannot be excluded.

pANCA also may be associated with the syndrome of familial PLE in soft-coated wheaten terriers (SCWT).[31] pANCA were detectable in the serum of dogs an average 1 to 2 years before the onset of clinical disease, and were highly correlated with hypo-albuminemia. This test could be a useful screening test for this specific disease in SCWT.

Care must be taken in interpreting a positive pANCA test result if other inflammatory or immune-mediated diseases are present. A recent study showed that many dogs with various vector-borne diseases or immune-mediated hemolytic anemia were positive for pANCA.[32]

Calprotectin and S100A12

Calprotectin and S100A12 are calcium-binding proteins that are abundant in the granules of neutrophils and macrophages. In people with IBD, serum and fecal concentrations of these proteins are increased in comparison with healthy people. In addition, fecal concentrations of calprotectin correlate very well with clinical disease activity in children with IBD.[33]

An immunoassay for measurement of canine calprotectin in serum and fecal samples is available.[34] A serum calprotectin concentration of 296.0 μg/L or higher has sensitivity of 82.4% and specificity of 68.4% for distinguishing dogs with idiopathic IBD from healthy dogs. However, calprotectin concentrations were not significantly correlated with clinical severity, serum CRP concentration, or severity of histopathologic changes. The clinical usefulness of this test needs further evaluation.

Immunohistochemistry for P-Glycoprotein on Intestinal Biopsies

P-glycoprotein (P-gp) is a transmembrane protein that functions as a drug-efflux pump in the intestinal epithelium. Human patients with IBD who fail to respond to treatment with glucocorticosteroids express high levels of P-gp in lamina propria lymphocytes.[35] Two research groups have evaluated P-gp expression in biopsies of dogs with IBD. In one study,[36] duodenal biopsies from 48 dogs were evaluated by immunohistochemistry. Biopsies were evaluated after treatment with prednisolone in 15 dogs and after dietary therapy alone in 16 dogs. Dogs treated with prednisolone showed significantly higher P-gp expression in lamina propria lymphocytes after treatment compared with expression before treatment. By contrast, the group treated solely with an elimination diet showed no difference in P-gp scores before and after treatment. Moreover, a statistically significant association between refractoriness to steroid treatment and high P-gp expression was found in the glucocorticosteroid-treated group.[36] In another recent study, P-gp expression was higher in duodenal epithelial cells of dogs with IBD compared with healthy control dogs.[37] However, there was no difference in P-gp expression in colonic epithelial cells between IBD and control groups. These results indicate that epithelial and lamina propria lymphocyte expression of P-gp is upregulated in dogs with IBD, and they are even higher after prednisolone treatment. In addition, high P-gp expression could indicate possible multidrug resistance and should be taken into account when managing dogs that have failed steroid treatment previously.

Immunohistochemistry for CD11c in Intestinal Biopsies

CD11c is a marker of human and murine dendritic cells (DCs), and cells expressing this marker have been shown to have similar morphologic and functional characteristics in dogs. DCs are important in determining the outcome of an immune reaction in the gut, that is, whether a pathogen will elicit a massive immune response or whether a commensal will induce tolerance.[38] Specific subsets of inducible DCs are decreased in the diseased tissues of people with IBD.[39] It is plausible that the number of DCs in the intestine could be used as a surrogate marker of inflammation in dogs with IBD. In one recent study, endoscopic biopsies from the duodenum, ileum, and colon were obtained from dogs with IBD and healthy dogs.[40] CD11c expression was assessed by immunofluorescence using a canine monoclonal antibody (**Fig. 3**). The number of CD11c-positive cells in the duodenum, ileum, and colon of dogs with IBD was significantly reduced in comparison with controls. There was a significant negative correlation between the number of CD11c-positive cells in the colon of dogs with IBD and clinical severity. This marker therefore holds promise as a useful test to assess histologic samples. However, additional prospective studies are needed to evaluate the clinical utility of this test.

Genetic Testing

Over the last decade, numerous genes have been associated with an increased risk of development of IBD in humans, many of them implicated in the innate immune response in the intestine.[41] Dogs with IBD may have a similar genetic component, especially because there are breeds predisposed to certain forms of IBD. Boxers are predisposed to histiocytic ulcerative colitis, and German shepherd dogs (GSD) are predisposed to lymphoplasmacytic IBD.[42] The author's group[43] recently performed a mutational analysis of the canine genes for TLR2, TLR4, TLR5, and NOD2 in GSD with IBD, and then further evaluated these in a case-control study with more than 50 cases and healthy GSD controls. Several mutations in TLR4 and TLR5 were found to be significantly associated with an increased risk of development of IBD. Moreover, these results were replicated in 38 other non-GSD breeds for the TLR5 mutation.[44] A follow-up study showed that peripheral blood cells of dogs carrying

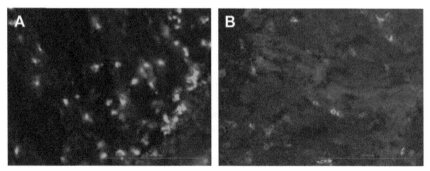

Fig. 3. Immunofluorescence for CD11c on intestinal biopsies from (A) a healthy dog and (B) a dog with IBD. CD11c expression in the intestinal mucosa is more abundant in healthy dogs than in dogs with IBD (original magnification ×100).

the mutation are hyperresponsive to flagellin, which is the natural ligand for TLR5.[45] This finding proves for the first time that a genetic mutation implicated in the pathogenesis of dogs with IBD has functional consequences at the protein level. Taken together, these findings make it very likely that TLR5 mutations are causally associated with canine IBD. Genetic testing for these polymorphisms currently is available only at the Royal Veterinary College. Such tests could become important for breeders and practitioners in the future. However, it is likely that in a multifactorial disease such as IBD in dogs, other genetic mutations and environmental factors also play a role in the pathogenesis. With the advent of genome-wide association studies, it is possible that more causative mutations will be identified.

SUMMARY

Many laboratory tests are available to aid the diagnostic workup of cats and dogs with chronic small intestinal disorders. Some of these have been available for many years, such as serum albumin and cobalamin concentrations, as well as canine pancreatic lipase, and new data now show that these tests also may be prognostic indicators in animals with chronic enteropathy. Other tests have only relatively recently become available to practitioners, such as serum CRP, fecal α_1-PI, WSAVA standardization of histopathology readings, and PARR. The value of these tests needs to be evaluated in every clinical situation. New tests that are not yet widely available, such as pANCA, calprotectin, CD11c immunofluorescence, and genetic testing, may become very useful tests in the future.

REFERENCES

1. Burgener IA, Konig A, Allenspach K, et al. Upregulation of toll-like receptors in chronic enteropathies in dogs. J Vet Intern Med 2008;22:553–60.
2. Allenspach K, House A, Smith K, et al. Evaluation of mucosal bacteria and histopathology, clinical disease activity and expression of Toll-like receptors in German shepherd dogs with chronic enteropathies. Vet Microbiol 2010;146: 326–35.
3. McMahon LA, House AK, Catchpole B, et al. Expression of Toll-like receptor 2 in duodenal biopsies from dogs with inflammatory bowel disease is associated with severity of disease. Vet Immunol Immunopathol 2010;135:158–63.
4. Janeczko S, Atwater D, Bogel E, et al. The relationship of mucosal bacteria to duodenal histopathology, cytokine mRNA, and clinical disease activity in cats with inflammatory bowel disease. Vet Microbiol 2008;128:178–93.
5. Xenoulis PG, Palculict B, Allenspach K, et al. Molecular-phylogenetic characterization of microbial communities imbalances in the small intestine of dogs with inflammatory bowel disease. FEMS Microbiol Ecol 2008;66:579–89.
6. Suchodolski JS, Camacho J, Steiner JM. Analysis of bacterial diversity in the canine duodenum, jejunum, ileum, and colon by comparative 16S rRNA gene analysis. FEMS Microbiol Ecol 2008;66(3):567–78.
7. Allenspach K, Wieland B, Grone A, et al. Chronic enteropathies in dogs: evaluation of risk factors for negative outcome. J Vet Intern Med 2007;21:700–8.
8. Craven M, Simpson JW, Ridyard AE, et al. Canine inflammatory bowel disease: retrospective analysis of diagnosis and outcome in 80 cases (1995-2002). J Small Anim Pract 2004;45:336–42.
9. Allenspach K, Rufenacht S, Sauter S, et al. Pharmacokinetics and clinical efficacy of cyclosporine treatment of dogs with steroid-refractory inflammatory bowel disease. J Vet Intern Med 2006;20:239–44.

10. Jergens AE. Feline idiopathic inflammatory bowel disease: What we know and what remians to be unraveled. J Fel Med Surg 2012;14(7):445–58.
11. Dennis JS, Kruger JM, Mullaney TP. Lymphocytic/plasmacytic colitis in cats: 14 cases (1985-1990). J Am Vet Med Assoc 1993;202:313–8.
12. Baez JL, Hendrick MJ, Walker LM, et al. Radiographic, ultrasonographic, and endoscopic findings in cats with inflammatory bowel disease of the stomach and small intestine: 33 cases (1990-1997). J Am Vet Med Assoc 1999;215: 349–54.
13. Bailey S, Benigni L, Eastwood J, et al. Comparisons between cats with normal and increased fPLI concentrations in cats diagnosed with inflammatory bowel disease. J Small Anim Pract 2010;51:484–9.
14. Forman MA, Marks SL, De Cock HE, et al. Evaluation of serum feline pancreatic lipase immunoreactivity and helical computed tomography versus conventional testing for the diagnosis of feline pancreatitis. J Vet Intern Med 2004;18: 807–15.
15. Ruaux CG, Steiner JM, Williams DA. Early biochemical and clinical responses to cobalamin supplementation in cats with signs of gastrointestinal disease and severe hypocobalaminemia. J Vet Intern Med 2005;19:155–60.
16. Reed N, Gunn-Moore D, Simpson K. Cobalamin, folate and inorganic phosphate abnormalities in ill cats. J Feline Med Surg 2007;9:278–88.
17. Mansfield C. Acute panceatitis in dogs: Advances in understanding, diagnostics and treatment. Top Compan Anim Med 2012;27(3):123–32.
18. Kathrani A, Steiner JM, Suchodolski J, et al. Elevated canine pancreatic lipase immunoreactivity concentration in dogs with inflammatory bowel disease is associated with a negative outcome. J Small Anim Pract 2009;50:126–32.
19. Nielsen OH, Vainer B, Madsen SM, et al. Established and emerging biological activity markers of inflammatory bowel disease. Am J Gastroenterol 2000;95: 359–67.
20. Jergens AE, Schreiner CA, Frank DE, et al. A scoring index for disease activity in canine inflammatory bowel disease. J Vet Intern Med 2003;17:291–7.
21. Heilmann RM, Paddock CG, Ruhnke I, et al. Development and analytical validation of a radioimmunoassay for the measurement of alpha1-proteinase inhibitor concentrations in feces from healthy puppies and adult dogs. J Vet Diagn Invest 2011;23:476–85.
22. Garcia-Sancho M, Rodriguez-Franco F, Sainz A, et al. Evaluation of clinical, macroscopic, and histopathologic response to treatment in nonhypoproteinemic dogs with lymphocytic-plasmacytic enteritis. J Vet Intern Med 2007;21:11–7.
23. Schreiner NM, Gaschen F, Grone A, et al. Clinical signs, histology, and CD3-positive cells before and after treatment of dogs with chronic enteropathies. J Vet Intern Med 2008;22:1079–83.
24. Day MJ, Bilzer T, Mansell J, et al. Histopathological standards for the diagnosis of gastrointestinal inflammation in endoscopic biopsy samples from the dog and cat: a report from the World Small Animal Veterinary Association Gastrointestinal Standardization Group. J Comp Pathol 2008;138(Suppl 1):S1–43.
25. Willard M, Mansell J. Correlating clinical activity and histopathologic assessment of gastrointestinal lesion severity: current challenges. Vet Clin North Am Small Anim Pract 2011;41:457–63.
26. Olivero D, Turba ME, Gentilini F. Reduced diversity of immunoglobulin and T-cell receptor gene rearrangements in chronic inflammatory gastrointestinal diseases in dogs. Vet Immunol Immunopathol 2011;144:337–45.

27. Vermeire S, Peeters M, Rutgeerts P. Diagnostic approach to IBD. Hepatogastroenterology 2000;47:44–8.
28. Allenspach K, Luckschander N, Styner M, et al. Evaluation of assays for perinuclear antineutrophilic cytoplasmic antibodies and antibodies to *Saccharomyces cerevisiae* in dogs with inflammatory bowel disease. Am J Vet Res 2004;65: 1279–83.
29. Dubinsky MC, Ofman JJ, Urman M, et al. Clinical utility of serodiagnostic testing in suspected pediatric inflammatory bowel disease. Am J Gastroenterol 2001;96: 758–65.
30. Luckschander N, Allenspach K, Hall J, et al. Perinuclear antineutrophilic cytoplasmic antibody and response to treatment in diarrheic dogs with food responsive disease or inflammatory bowel disease. J Vet Intern Med 2006;20:221–7.
31. Allenspach K, Lomas B, Wieland B, et al. Evaluation of perinuclear antineutrophilic cytoplasmic autoantibodies as an early marker of protein-losing enteropathy and protein-losing nephropathy in soft coated wheaten terriers. Am J Vet Res 2008;69:1301–4.
32. Karagianni AE, Solano-Gallego L, Breitschwerdt EB, et al. Perinuclear antineutrophil cytoplasmic autoantibodies in dogs infected with various vector-borne pathogens and in dogs with immune-mediated hemolytic anemia. Am J Vet Res 2012; 73:1403–9.
33. Aadland E, Fagerhol MK. Faecal calprotectin: a marker of inflammation throughout the intestinal tract. Eur J Gastroenterol Hepatol 2002;14:823–5.
34. Heilmann RM, Jergens AE, Ackermann MR, et al. Serum calprotectin concentrations in dogs with idiopathic inflammatory bowel disease. Am J Vet Res 2012;73: 1900–7.
35. Farrell RJ, Menconi MJ, Keates AC, et al. P-glycoprotein-170 inhibition significantly reduces cortisol and cyclosporin efflux from human intestinal epithelial cells and T lymphocytes. Aliment Pharmacol Ther 2002;16:1021–31.
36. Allenspach K, Bergman PJ, Sauter S, et al. P-glycoprotein expression in lamina propria lymphocytes of duodenal biopsy samples in dogs with chronic idiopathic enteropathies. J Comp Pathol 2006;134:1–7.
37. Van der Heyden S, Vercauteren G, Daminet S, et al. Expression of P-glycoprotein in the intestinal epithelium of dogs with lymphoplasmacytic enteritis. J Comp Pathol 2011;145:199–206.
38. Ng SC, Benjamin JL, McCarthy NE, et al. Relationship between human intestinal dendritic cells, gut microbiota, and disease activity in Crohn's disease. Inflamm Bowel Dis 2011;17:2027–37.
39. Ng SC, Kamm MA, Stagg AJ, et al. Intestinal dendritic cells: their role in bacterial recognition, lymphocyte homing, and intestinal inflammation. Inflamm Bowel Dis 2010;16:1787–807.
40. Kathrani A, Schmitz S, Priestnall SL, et al. CD11c+ cells are significantly decreased in the duodenum, ileum and colon of dogs with inflammatory bowel disease. J Comp Pathol 2011;145:359–66.
41. Lees CW, Barrett JC, Parkes M, et al. New IBD genetics: common pathways with other diseases. Gut 2011;60:1739–53.
42. Kathrani A, Werling D, Allenspach K. Canine breeds at high risk of developing inflammatory bowel disease in the south-eastern UK. Vet Rec 2011;169:635.
43. Kathrani A, House A, Catchpole B, et al. Polymorphisms in the TLR4 and TLR5 gene are significantly associated with inflammatory bowel disease in German shepherd dogs. PLoS One 2010;5:e15740.

44. Kathrani A, House A, Catchpole B, et al. Breed-independent toll-like receptor 5 polymorphisms show association with canine inflammatory bowel disease. Tissue Antigens 2011;78:94–101.
45. Kathrani A, Holder A, Catchpole B, et al. TLR5 Risk-associated haplotype for canine inflammatory bowel disease confers hyper-responsiveness to flagellin. PLoS One 2012;7:e30117.

Practical Interpretation and Application of Exocrine Pancreatic Testing in Small Animals

Caroline Mansfield, BSc, BVMS, PhD, MANZCVS

KEYWORDS

- Specific canine pancreatic lipase (spec-cPL) • SNAP®-cPL™
- Trypsinlike immunoreactivity (TLI) • Pancreatic elastase (PE-1)

KEY POINTS

- A positive specific canine pancreatic lipase (spec-cPL) or SNAP-cPL in dogs should be considered in conjunction with other clinical signs and diagnostic imaging to ensure acute pancreatitis is the main cause of the clinical presentation.
- A negative spec-cPL or SNAP-cPL result means acute pancreatitis is unlikely to be the cause of the dog's presenting signs.
- Serum canine pancreatic elastase-1 (cPE-1) has a high specificity (92%) for the diagnosis of pancreatitis; increases in serum cPE-1 are more likely to be seen in severe acute pancreatitis.
- Feline acute pancreatitis is best diagnosed by a combination of clinical signs, feline pancreatic lipase immunoreactivity, and abdominal ultrasound.
- Close evaluation of cats with pancreatitis for concurrent disease is essential.
- Chronic pancreatitis is difficult to diagnose with laboratory testing.
- Pancreatic cytology may be of benefit in diagnosing pancreatic neoplasia.

INTRODUCTION

The assessment of the pancreas can be difficult in clinical situations because the pancreas is located adjacent to many other abdominal organs (**Fig. 1**). As a result, disease located within the abdomen can cause bystander pancreatic inflammation. The clinical signs of primary acute pancreatitis are indistinguishable from other acute abdominal crises, such as septic peritonitis or intestinal obstruction. The diagnosis of acute

This article originally appeared in Veterinary Clinics of North America: Small Animal Practice, Volume 43, Issue 6, November 2013.

Disclosures: The author received no incentive or payment from a commercial company in the preparation of this article.

Faculty of Veterinary Science, The University of Melbourne, 250 Princes Highway, Werribee, Victoria 3030, Australia

E-mail address: cmans@unimelb.edu.au

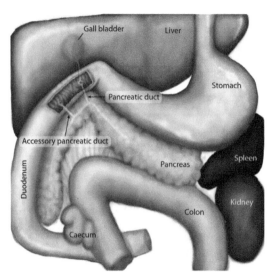

Fig. 1. The regional anatomy of the cranial abdomen in the dog. (*From* Mansfield C. Acute pancreatitis in dogs: advances in understanding, diagnostics and treatment. Top Companion Anim Med 2012;27:125; with permission.)

pancreatitis generally relies on a combination of investigations rather than one single test. Chronic inflammation of the pancreas is even more difficult to diagnose because there is often an association with other abdominal disease and biochemical testing is less useful. A strong index of suspicion, ideally pancreatic histology, and evaluation for intestinal or hepatic disease is generally required for a diagnosis of chronic pancreatitis.

The clinical assessment of exocrine pancreatic insufficiency is more straightforward, with most clinical cases capable of being diagnosed readily. There is a subset of animals whereby there are equivocal results of pancreatic function testing that can pose a diagnostic challenge.

ACUTE PANCREATITIS IN THE DOG

Dogs with acute pancreatitis generally present with a sudden onset of anorexia, abdominal pain, and vomiting, as detailed in **Table 1**.[1–3] The onset of pancreatic inflammation and/or necrosis can set up a wide array of inflammatory pathways, which may progress to cause hypovolemia, systemic inflammatory response syndrome (SIRS), or multiple organ dysfunction.[4] Even in very severe cases, the clinical signs of acute pancreatitis in dogs are not pathognomonic. It is essential, therefore, to ensure that differential diagnoses for acute pancreatitis, such as intestinal obstruction, closed pyometron, or septic peritonitis, that all are life threatening and require surgical intervention, are eliminated as a priority (**Box 1**). The next essential step is to eliminate diabetes ketoacidosis, liver disease, uremia and other metabolic causes of vomiting that require specific intervention. A typical diagnostic algorithm for acute pancreatitis is shown in **Fig. 2**.

Routine Clinical Pathology

Because of the need to rule out metabolic disease and to establish the baseline clinical status before treatment, routine clinical pathology (complete blood count, serum biochemical profile, urinalysis) should be obtained. Most laboratory abnormalities in dogs with pancreatitis result from hypovolemia or inflammation and are, therefore,

Table 1
Summary of clinical findings of 60 dogs with fatal acute pancreatitis

Historical Finding	Number of Cases	Percentage (%)
Anorexia	64	91
Vomiting	63	90
Weakness	55	79
Diarrhea	23	33
Polyuria/polydipsia	35	50
Neurologic abnormalities	14	20
Melena	11	16
Weight loss	8	11
Hematemesis	7	10
Hematochezia	3	4

Data from Hess RS, Saunders HM, Van Winkle TJ, et al. Clinical, clinicopathologic, radiographic, and ultrasonographic abnormalities in dogs with fatal acute pancreatitis: 70 cases (1986–1995). J Am Vet Med Assoc 1998;213:665–70.

not specific for pancreatitis.[5,6] Many of the differential diagnoses for pancreatitis, such as uremia or gastrointestinal inflammation, will also result in similar laboratory changes. In brief, these changes include leucocytosis, azotemia, and increased liver enzymes (eg, alanine transferase, alkaline phosphatase). Decreased calcium has also been documented in dogs with acute pancreatitis and has been suggested to carry a poorer prognosis.[7,8] Many dogs with acute pancreatitis have gross lipemia, whether as a cause or consequence of the disease (**Fig. 3**). However, the exact percentage of dogs with acute pancreatitis that have lipemia is not known.

Fluid Cytology

Because one of the major differential diagnoses for acute pancreatitis in dogs is septic peritonitis, the evaluation of free fluid should be performed early in the investigation. Fluid can be obtained by abdominocentesis using a 22- to 25-G needle or by using ultrasound guidance. In cases of small-volume free fluid, the areas between the bladder and the abdominal wall and between liver lobes seem to be frequent sites of initial fluid accumulation. Once fluid has been obtained, it should be stained and assessed for the presence of bacteria as well as having routine fluid analysis

Box 1
Suggested criteria for diagnosis of acute pancreatitis in dogs

- Absence of surgical disease on abdominal radiographs or analysis of abdominal fluid **AND**
- Abdominal ultrasound with evidence of primary pancreatitis **AND**
- One or more of the following:
  - Spec-cPL greater than 400 µg/L
  - Positive SNAP-cPL
  - Gross lipemia
  - Serum PE-1 greater than 17.24 ng/mL
  - Total lipase greater than 3 times the upper reference interval

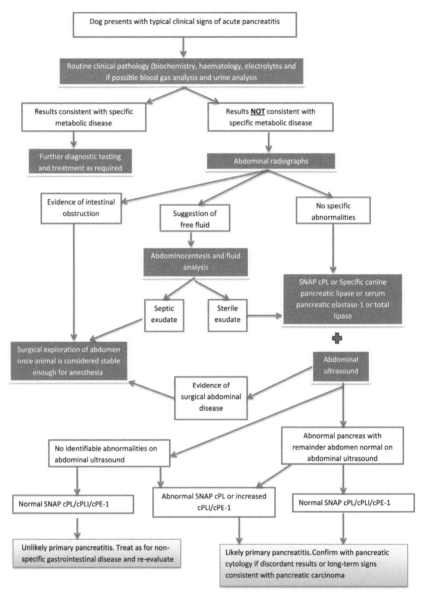

Fig. 2. A diagnostic algorithm for the diagnosis of acute pancreatitis in the dog. cPE-1, canine pancreatic elastase; cPL, canine pancreatic lipase; cPLI, canine pancreatic-lipase immunoreactivity.

(**Fig. 4**). Fluid from dogs with acute pancreatitis will also be a neutrophilic exudate (see **Fig. 4**), but bacteria are not present cytologically or on culture.

Serum Lipase and Amylase

Serum lipase and amylase concentrations have been shown to increase in experimental and naturally occurring canine pancreatitis.[5,8,9] However, neither enzyme is specific to the pancreas because they also originate from gastrointestinal mucosa

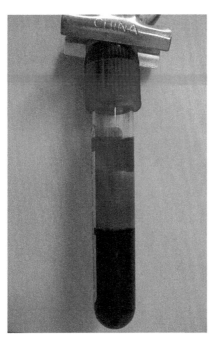

Fig. 3. A blood sample obtained from a dog with acute pancreatitis following centrifugation. The serum sits on top of a lipid layer, indicating gross lipemia.

and are excreted by the kidneys. It has been shown that serum lipase activity is markedly increased in dogs with acute enteritis, gastroenteritis, liver disease, and in renal failure.[10–12] Lipase concentration can also be elevated up to 5 times by the administration of dexamethasone in dogs with no pancreatic inflammation.[13] Serum lipase and amylase concentrations can also be normal in dogs that do have pancreatitis. In one retrospective review by Hess and colleagues,[1] (1998) less than 50% of dogs with acute fatal pancreatitis had increased lipase concentrations, whereas only 30.8% had increased amylase concentrations. Other estimates place the value more conservatively at 15% to 20% of dogs with acute pancreatitis having normal serum lipase and amylase concentrations.[10,14]

Trypsinogen Activation Peptide

Trypsinogen activation peptide (TAP) is the cleavage peptide produced when trypsinogen is cleaved to trypsin (**Fig. 5**). Theoretically, in pancreatitis, TAP will be released into the abdominal cavity and then the circulation in high concentrations and subsequently be cleared through the kidneys.[15] Several studies in people showed a high correlation between the severity of pancreatitis and urinary TAP concentration and a high degree of specificity and sensitivity for diagnosis.[16,17] A reference interval for the measurement of TAP in healthy dogs was established, and its utility as a diagnostic test for canine pancreatitis was assessed.[10] Unfortunately, TAP measurement was specific but not highly sensitive for the diagnosis of pancreatitis in dogs; because it is not readily available for routine clinical use, it cannot be recommended.

Trypsin-like Immunoreactivity

Serum trypsin-like immunoreactivity (TLI) is an accurate and specific indicator of pancreatic function and is thought to be entirely pancreatic in origin.[18] Serum TLI

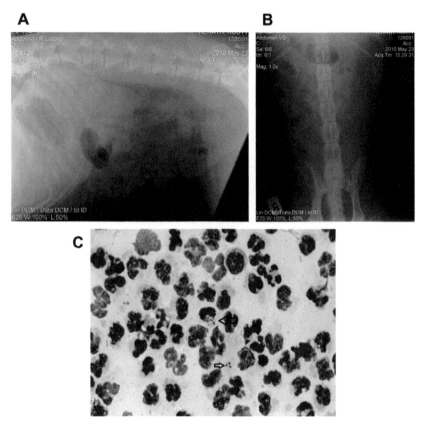

Fig. 4. Abdominal radiographs obtained from a dog ([A] lateral, [B] ventrodorsal) with abdominal pain. There is decreased contrast, suggesting effusion within the abdomen. Abdominocentesis should be performed. Septic peritoneal fluid (C) would have large numbers of activated neutrophils, with both free (*small solid arrow*) and intracellular (*large open arrow*) bacteria (Wright's stain, ×100 magnification).

has been shown in experimental canine models of acute pancreatitis to increase early in the course of the disease, followed by a rapid decrease.[19] In acute pancreatitis, the TLI concentration is often decreased by the time of sampling, so it is seldom useful clinically.[10,20] This reason, along with an often-lengthy delay in receiving results, makes the usefulness of TLI for the diagnosis of pancreatitis questionable.

Canine Pancreatic Lipase

Canine pancreatic lipase (cPL) is one of the most recently established laboratory tests in veterinary medicine, and its use is now widespread. The premise of this test is that it measures lipase that originates solely in the pancreas, and so it will only be increased in pancreatic inflammation.[21] Immunolocalization studies showed pancreatic lipase was present only within pancreatic tissue of dogs, and serum concentrations in dogs with absent exocrine pancreatic function were decreased.[22,23] The pancreatic lipase assay itself (first a radioimmunoassay and then an enzyme immunoassay) has been well validated.[24,25]

The canine pancreatic-lipase immunoreactivity (cPLI) assay was further developed into a commercially available specific canine pancreatic lipase (spec-cPL) sandwich

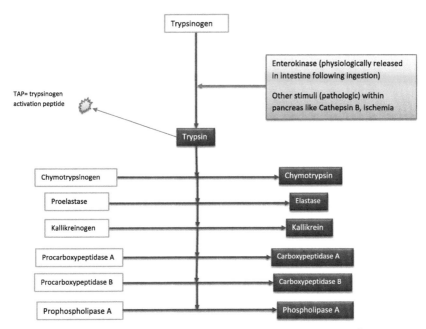

Fig. 5. Trypsin activating the pancreatic cascade and then perpetuating the activation of inert pancreatic zymogens (*blue boxes*) to active digestive pancreatic enzymes (*blue boxes*). TAP is one of the small peptides cleaved during the normal activation of trypsinogen, which normally should only occur within the intestine mediated by enterokinase; however, in pancreatitis, it occurs within the acinar cells themselves.

enzyme-linked immunosorbent assay (ELISA), using a recombinant peptide as the antigen and monoclonal antibody for measurement. This new commercially available assay shows a good correlation to the original assay as well as high reproducibility.[26] The newer assay has caused a change in the reference intervals for the diagnosis of pancreatitis, with results less than 200 μg/L expected in healthy dogs, and results more than 400 μg/L considered consistent with a diagnosis of pancreatitis.[27] A new in-clinic rapid semiquantitative assay (SNAP-cPL; Iddex Laboratories, Westbrook, ME) has also been developed and shows good alignment and reproducibility with the laboratory-based fully quantitative assay.[28] The current manufacturer recommendations are to follow up an in-house SNAP-cPL with a quantitative spec-cPL in order to be able to monitor the response to treatment. However, there are no studies to show that following pancreatic enzymes alters clinical management.

There have been several studies of cPLI and cPL, with most relying on histologic evidence of pancreatic inflammation as their gold standard. The results of these studies are summarized in **Table 2**. The sensitivity of cPLI/cPL for diagnosing pancreatic inflammation in dogs ranges from 21% to 88%.[29–33] The sensitivity of pancreatic lipase is greatly increased when more severely affected dogs are assessed.

The specificity of pancreatic lipase has been reported to range from to 80.0% to 97.5%, which is greater than for total lipase in some studies but comparable in others.[30,32–34] Again, studies assessing the specificity of pancreatic lipase have largely been based on histologic evaluation. Most of these samples were obtained at post mortem, but the primary cause of death was seldom reported. Therefore, it is important to bear in mind that the high specificities relate to histologic evidence of pancreatitis and not a primary clinical diagnosis of acute pancreatitis.

Table 2
Summary of sensitivity and specificity for various laboratory testing in dogs from various studies

Study	Number of Dogs	Method of Diagnosis	Analyte Assessed	Sensitivity (%)	Specificity (%)
McCord et al,[32] 2012	n = 84 AP = 57 Non-AP = 27	Combination of clinical and imaging results	Spec-cPL >400 µg/L Lipase Amylase	71.7–77.8 43.4–53.6 52.4–56.0	80.5–88.0 89.3–92.5 76.7–80.6
Trivedi et al,[33] 2011	n = 70 Mild AP = 56 Moderate-severe AP = 7 Normal pancreas = 7	Histology	Spec-cPL >400 µg/L cTLI Lipase Amylase	21 (mild) 71 (moderate-severe) 30 (mild) 29 (moderate-severe) 54 (mild) 71 (moderate-severe) 7 (mild) 14 (moderate-severe)	100 100 43 100
Mansfield et al	n = 32 Minimal/no inflammation = 20	Histology	Spec-cPL >400 µg/L	NA	90
Mansfield et al	n = 61 AP = 41 CP = 3 Pancreatic carcinoma = 5 Nonpancreatitis = 12	Histology	cPE-1 >17.24 ng/mL	61.4 (all) 66 (AP) 78 (severe AP)	91.7

Steiner et al	n = 11 (Severe AP)	Clinical findings and histology	Spec-cPL >400 µg/L	88	NA
Steiner et al	n = 22	Gross evidence at post mortem	Spec-cPL >400 µg/L Lipase Amylase	63.6 31.8 40.9	NA NA NA
Neilson-Carley et al,[34] 2011	n = 64 AP = 20 Other disease = 17 Healthy = 27	Histology	Spec-cPL >400 µg/L	NA	95
Haworth et al,[36]	n = 38 AP = 11 Non-AP = 26	Clinical evaluation of dogs presenting with acute abdominal disease	SNAP-cPL Spec-cPL >400 µg/L	82 70	59 77
Mansfield & Jones,[10] 2000	n = 42 AP = 15 Non-AP = 27	Clinical findings and histology	Lipase >3 × RI Amylase >3 × RI TLI >100 µ/L	63.6 22.7 37.5	54.6 78.1 89.3

Abbreviations: AP, acute pancreatitis; CP, chronic pancreatitis; cPE-1, serum canine pancreatic-elastase-1; cPL, canine pancreatic lipase (or canine pancreatic lipase immunoreactivity in earlier studies); NA, not assessed; RI, reference interval.

Data from Refs.[10,29–34,36,45]

In many of the initial studies of pancreatic lipase, dogs with renal failure were not expressly evaluated. However, one study that assessed dogs with experimentally induced chronic renal failure showed no increase in pancreatic lipase.[35] Further evaluation in animals with an acute decline in glomerular filtration rate is required.

One recent study showed a poor correlation between a positive SNAP-cPL test and a primary presentation of AP in dogs presenting with acute abdomen ($\kappa = 0.33$).[36] This study assessed dogs presenting to an emergency center with signs of acute abdominal disease and found a sensitivity of 82% but a specificity of 59% for SNAP-cPL. Another way of interpreting this is that approximately 40% of dogs with a positive SNAP-cPL had disease other than pancreatitis as their primary presenting problem. The conditions most commonly associated with this false-positive finding were small intestinal foreign-body obstruction, septic peritonitis, and hepatic disease (**Box 2**, **Fig. 6**). As previously discussed, it is possible that those dogs indeed did have histologic pancreatic inflammation that occurred secondary to the primary problem. However, failure to correctly identify the primary cause of the presentation would lead to inadequate treatment and management. Indeed, when assessing the specificity of pancreatic laboratory testing using histology as the gold standard, the presence of pancreatic bystander inflammation obscures the clinical relevance of such results. This idea is borne out in one study of dogs undergoing postmortem examination at a referral center that determined that 92% had pancreatic inflammation of some sort,[37] which is likely a gross overestimation of pancreatitis as the clinical cause of death.

A negative result for SNAP-cPL, on the other hand, seems to have a good correlation to dogs having disease other than acute pancreatitis.[36] This correlation is also demonstrated in a multicenter study that used Bayesian statistics to overcome the need for pancreatic histology as a gold standard, which also determined that dogs with Spec-cPL of 200 µg/L or less and/or a negative SNAP-cPL were unlikely to have clinical acute pancreatitis.[32]

Serum Pancreatic Elastase

Pancreatic elastase (PE-1) is released immediately after trypsin activation and also plays a role in perpetuating inflammation (see **Fig. 5**).[38] In a study in people, a sensitivity

---

Box 2
Case study

Tiny, a 5-year-old male neutered Australian cattle dog, was referred with a history of vomiting and abdominal pain. He had shown similar clinical signs 2 weeks before the referral and was diagnosed with pancreatitis based on a positive SNAP-cPL test. Routine clinical pathology was also consistent with pancreatitis. Nonspecific treatment (fluid, antibiotics, and analgesia) resulted in improvement, but he had deteriorated clinically in the last 2 days.

Physical examination findings: Tiny was moribund, had poor systolic blood pressure, was tachycardic, and had prolonged capillary refill time (>3 seconds). There was abdominal pain and free abdominal fluid.

Further testing: An abdominal ultrasound was performed that showed distended loops of bowel, large volume of abdominal effusion, and a foreign body within the small intestine.

Diagnosis: Septic peritonitis secondary to perforated small intestine was the diagnosis.

Outcome: After stabilization, Tiny underwent exploratory surgery, whereby a tennis ball was removed from his small intestine. Extensive parts of the small intestine required resection, and recovery was prolonged.

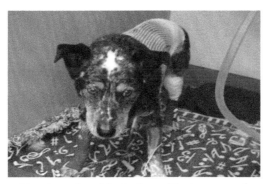

Fig. 6. Tiny, a 5-year-old male neutered Australian cattle dog, was referred with a history of vomiting and abdominal pain.

of 100% and specificity of 96% for the measurement of serum PE-1 to diagnose acute pancreatitis was reported.[39] These results were similar to a larger study that found that people with acute pancreatitis had significantly increased concentrations.[40]

Early medical studies used a radioimmunoassay that detected polyclonal elastase (bound to 1-α-antitrypsin complex) with a half-life of 2.2 days. The ELISA that has been more recently developed detects free or unbound elastase and has a half-life of 0.4 days.[41] The use of the ELISA narrows the window of opportunity for the detection of increased serum PE-1; there is a reasonable variation in the reference interval in healthy people.[42]

The canine PE-1 (cPE-1) assay used in these studies is an ELISA (ScheBo Elastase 1-Canine, ScheBo Biotech AG, Netanyastrasse 3, D-35394, Giessen, Germany), but it is less readily available than the fecal test. One study of dogs reported a serum cPE-1 interval of 32.1 to 659.3 ng/mL (median 55.8 ng/mL) in 16 healthy dogs; 24 to 1720 ng/mL (median 160 ng/mL) in 14 dogs with pancreatitis; and 5 to 182 ng/mL (median 43.3 ng/mL) in 6 dogs with renal disease.[43] A further study from the same investigators assessed the measurement of serum cPE-1, along with amylase, lipase, and TLI in 7 healthy beagles after endoscopic retrograde pancreatography, a procedure that is commonly associated with the development of pancreatic inflammation.[44] There was no difference between the baseline and any subsequent measurement of cPE-1 in any dog, although there was in the other 3 enzymes. Additionally, the range at baseline for the 7 healthy dogs was quite wide (0.1–411.6 ng/mL) with a median of 5.5 ng/mL. It is possible that the wide variation in normal dogs was caused by hemolysis, or the storage of blood samples in temperatures greater than 8°C for more than 72 hours caused a false increase in some samples, as advised by the assay manufacturer.

A later study that assessed 61 dogs that all had pancreatic histology determined overall a sensitivity of 61.4% and specificity of 91.7% when using a cutoff value for cPE-1 of 17.24 ng/mL.[45] The sensitivity of this test increased to 78.26% when only dogs with severe acute pancreatitis were assessed. Therefore, this assay seems to have a high positive likelihood ratio and low negative likelihood ratio.

There is a strong suggestion that serum PE-1 is not affected by renal clearance, as compared with many other pancreatic enzymes.[46] The proposed reason for this is that elastase circulates in the serum bound to inhibitor proteins, such as α-macroglobulin, and is too large to pass through the glomeruli, relying on extrarenal metabolic pathways for clearance. Again, in the larger cPE-1 study, there were 3 dogs with severe renal failure (urea 70.4 mmol/L, reference <12; creatinine 804 μmol/L, reference <120), and none had increased cPE-1.

Determining Severity

Early detection of severe pancreatitis is considered particularly important in people because this enables rapid transfer to intensive care units and improves outcome.[47] A similar conclusion could be made for canine acute pancreatitis. However, extrapolating from the studies that have been performed extensively in people, and to some extent in dogs, there is unlikely to be a single laboratory test that can differentiate severe from mild disease. Indeed, in the largest human study (more than 18,000 people in more than 200 centers), it was determined that SIRS, age greater than 60 years, and the presence of pleural effusion were most associated with prognosis.[48] This concept is similar to a severity score developed in dogs using clinical and laboratory data that could easily be obtained in general practice within 24 hours of admission.[3] The poor prognostic indicators identified in that study are outlined in **Table 3**. It is likely that other critical care parameters may be added to this scheme once further validation of the criteria is undertaken in larger cohorts of dogs.

Table 3
Factors contributing to clinical severity index as published for canine acute pancreatitis.[3] A higher combined score (>3) is associated with significantly higher mortality. This index has yet to be validated in a larger animal population

Parameter	Point Allocation	Criteria
Cardiac	0	No abnormalities
	1	<60 ventricular premature complexes per 24-h period or heart rate >180 beats per min
	2	Paroxysmal or sustained ventricular tachycardia
Respiratory	0	No abnormalities
	1	Clinical evidence of dyspnea or tachypnea (>40 breaths per min)
	2	Clinical evidence of pneumonia or acute respiratory distress syndrome
Intestinal integrity	0	No abnormalities
	1	Intestinal sounds not detected during >3 auscultations in 24-h period
	2	Hematochezia, melena, or regurgitation
	3	No enteral food intake for >3 d
	4	No enteral food intake for >3 d and at least 2 of the following: hematochezia, melena, and regurgitation
Vascular forces	0	No abnormalities
	1	Systolic arterial blood pressure <60 or >180 mm Hg or serum albumin concentration <18 g/L
	2	Systolic arterial blood pressure <60 or >180 mm Hg and serum albumin concentration <18 g/L

Data from Mansfield CS, James FE, Robertson ID. Development of a clinical severity index for dogs with acute pancreatitis. J Am Vet Med Assoc 2008;233:936–44.

ACUTE PANCREATITIS IN THE CAT

Cats have been increasingly reported to develop acute pancreatitis similar to dogs, with necrosis of the peripancreatic fat region being a predominant feature. A high index of suspicion for acute pancreatitis in the cat is required for a rapid diagnosis because the clinical signs are not pathognomonic (**Table 4**). Additionally, approximately two-thirds of cats with acute pancreatitis have concurrent disease, especially

Table 4
Summary of clinical findings from 3 studies of cats with acute pancreatitis and chronic pancreatitis

Clinical Sign	Hill & Van Winkle,[77] 1993	Kimmel et al,[50] 2001	Ferreri et al,[51] 2003	
Case numbers	n = 40 AP (necropsy based)	n = 46 AP	n = 30 ANP	n = 33 CP
Lethargy (%)	100	83	50	52
Anorexia (%)	97	96	63	70
Dehydration (%)	92	NR	33	51
Hypothermia (%)	68	NR	NR	NR
Vomiting (%)	35	43	43	39
Abdominal pain (%)	25	17	10	
Palpable abdominal mass (%)	23	4	3	
Diarrhea (%)	15	11	NR	NR
Dyspnea (%)	20	NR	16	
Ataxia (%)	15	NR	NR	NR
Weight loss (%)	NR	39	40	21
Jaundice (%)	NR	22	16	24
Pallor (%)	NR	NR	30	30

Abbreviations: ANP, acute necrotizing pancreatitis; AP, acute pancreatitis; CP, chronic pancreatitis; NR, not recorded.
Data from Refs.[50,51,77]

hepatic lipidosis,[49] which makes it likely that there will be nonspecific changes in routine clinical pathology, such as increased bilirubin and other liver enzymes. Cats with large-volume effusion may have hypoalbuminemia and variably increased or decreased white cell counts. Similarly, glucose may be increased either because of concurrent diabetes mellitus/diabetes ketoacidosis or because of stress hyperglycemia. The presence of hypocalcemia has been shown to be a poor prognostic indicator in cats, even in the absence of clinical signs associated with hypocalcemia.[50] However, another study showed no difference in ionized calcium between cats with acute pancreatitis and cats with chronic pancreatitis.[51]

Serum lipase concentration has been shown to increase in cats with experimentally induced acute pancreatitis, although serum amylase remained normal.[52] Unfortunately, serum lipase and amylase are seldom diagnostic in their own right in cats.[53,54]

A feline trypsin-like immunoreactivity (fTLI) assay is also available and has been shown to increase in experimentally induced pancreatitis.[55] There is a range of reported sensitivity for fTLI from 33% to 80% in acute pancreatitis, again sensitivity increasing with disease severity,[53,54,56,57] often dependent on the diagnostic cutoff value used. The concentration of fTLI may also be increased by other diseases, such as renal failure, inflammatory bowel disease, lymphosarcoma, and starvation. Unfortunately, the measurement of trypsinogen activation peptide (a by-product cleaved by trypsin activation) is no more sensitive or specific than the measurement of fTLI; because it is not readily available, it is of little benefit in diagnosing this disease.[57]

A species-specific pancreatic lipase immunoreactivity (fPLI) radioimmunoassay has also been developed, with a reference interval established of 1.2 to 3.8 μg/L.[58] One study showed a very high sensitivity (100%) in 5 cats with acute pancreatitis.[54] Overall, the specificity of fPLI in that study (compared with 8 healthy cats and 3 symptomatic cats with normal pancreatic histopathology) was 91%, which shows there may be minimal effects from other diseases. Once larger studies have been published, the true sensitivity and specificity of this test can be established. However, it does seem as if the sensitivity of fPLI will likely be greater in more severely affected animals.

CHRONIC PANCREATITIS

Chronic pancreatitis is increasingly being recognized in both dogs and cats and is defined as the presence of both fibrosis and active (generally lymphoplasmacytic) inflammation.[59] Chronic pancreatitis may be a prequel to the development of exocrine pancreatic insufficiency or diabetes mellitus.[60] In cats, there is a very high association between chronic pancreatitis and other disease, particularly cholangiohepatitis and inflammatory bowel disease.[51]

In general, all the laboratory tests discussed for acute pancreatitis may be of some use in diagnosing chronic pancreatitis in both dogs and cats. However, the sensitivity of these tests is low for chronic pancreatitis, and so diagnosis generally relies on pancreatic biopsy along with compatible historical and clinical findings. Because of the high incidence of concurrent disease in cats, concurrent histologic assessment of the liver and small intestine as a minimum is recommended.

PANCREATIC NEOPLASIA

Primary pancreatic exocrine neoplasia is rare. Clinical signs in cats are nonspecific and can include anorexia, vomiting, jaundice, and infrequently alopecia; whereas, in dogs, the clinical signs are similar to that of acute pancreatitis albeit extending over a longer period of time.[61] Some dogs with pancreatic neoplasia have been reported with multifocal steatitis.[62] Typical clinicopathologic findings reflect the accompanying pancreatic inflammation or necrosis as well as involvement with other abdominal organs.

Pancreatic Cytology

Fine-needle aspiration of the pancreas is a relatively safe procedure to do, particularly when ultrasound guided.[63] Recent work at the author's institution suggests that 25-G needles are effective for cytologic evaluation and potentially cause fewer traumas than larger-gauge needles. Fine-needle aspirates should be obtained using a 3-mL syringe with some ethylenediaminetetraacetic acid drawn into it and then, with the needle attached, be directed into the area for sampling. The needle should be moved backwards and forwards along the same line several times (but should not be redirected while in the pancreas). No negative pressure is required during sampling, and gentle squash preparation onto glass slides should then be performed. This degree of trauma to the pancreas is minimal and extremely unlikely to cause any direct inflammation.

Cytologic evaluation of the pancreas may be difficult, especially if artifacts occur (**Box 3**). However, pancreatic cytology may be of some benefit in differentiating malignant pancreatic diseases from inflammation[64]; some examples are shown in **Fig. 7**. However, because the characteristics of inflammation (neutrophils, cellular atypia, and anisocytosis) overlap considerably with neoplasia, caution must be exercised regarding overinterpretation.

EXOCRINE PANCREATIC INSUFFICIENCY

The diagnosis of exocrine pancreatic insufficiency (EPI) is usually made once more than 90% of exocrine function has been lost. Animals with EPI typically show signs

---

Box 3
Potential complications or artifacts from pancreatic fine-needle aspiration

- Hemodilution
- Overlap between inflammatory atypia and neoplasia
- Nonrepresentative lesion sampled
- Uneven distribution of disease within the pancreas
- Ruptured cells caused by sampling technique, squash preparation technique, or innate fragility of pancreatic cells
- Inclusion of cells from other abdominal organs
- Contamination with reactive mesothelial cells

---

of weight loss, have fatty, foul-smelling feces (steatorrhea), and polyphagia.[65] EPI is generally caused by pancreatic acinar atrophy but may also be a consequence of end-stage pancreatic inflammation and fibrosis or autoimmune destruction.[60,65] German shepherd dogs and Rough collies seem to be predisposed to EPI,[66] with

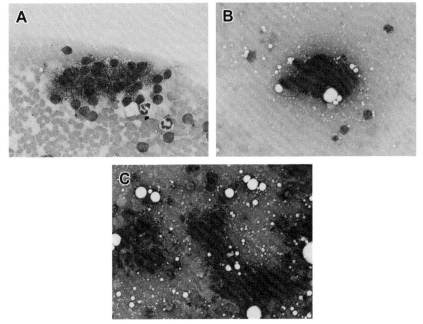

Fig. 7. Pancreatic cytology normal versus neoplasia. (*A*) A fine-needle aspirate obtained from the pancreas of a cat (H&E staining, original magnification ×100). This aspirate shows normal exocrine appearance, with little anisocytosis or anisokaryosis, small round nucleoli, and a single small nucleolus. (*B*) A fine-needle aspirate obtained from a dog (H&E staining, original magnification ×100) that shows features consistent with malignancy: binucleation, nuclear molding, and multiple nuclei. There is abundant granular cytoplasm. (*C*) A fine-needle aspirate (H&E staining, original magnification ×100) from the same dog as in (*B*), showing moderate anisocytosis and anisokaryosis, variability in the nuclear/cytoplasmic ratio, and large nucleoli. There is abundant granular cytoplasm. (*Courtesy of* S Connolly, DVM DACVP, University of Melbourne, Melbourne, Australia.)

inheritance mediated by polygenic autosomal recessive traits.[67] EPI has been considered a rare disease of cats but is being increasingly recognized.[68]

Routine clinical pathology, including total serum amylase and lipase concentration, is not helpful in diagnosing EPI. Animals may have concurrent diabetes mellitus, which can cause hyperglycemia. Because of concurrent dysbiosis in the small intestine, serum cobalamin and folate may be abnormal; but this is not pathognomonic for EPI. However, failure to recognize the potential for hypocobalaminemia may result in suboptimal treatment, particularly in cats.[68] Fecal analysis, assessing proteolytic or fat content, is unreliable and nonspecific.[65]

The most sensitive and specific test for EPI is the measurement of TLI, which is a highly specific indicator of pancreatic mass and function developed as canine or feline specific.[68,69] A serum TLI concentration of less than 2.5 μg/L is considered diagnostic of EPI in dogs, whereas a result of 8 μg/L (as measured by radioimmunoassay at the Gastrointestinal Laboratory, Texas A&M University) is considered diagnostic in cats.[65,70]

In one longitudinal study, Wiberg and colleagues[71] followed dogs that had serum TLI concentrations between 2.5 μg/L and 5.0 μg/L (5 being the lower reference interval for normal dogs). Approximately 50% of these dogs did not develop any signs of EPI, and their TLI rebounded back to more than 5.0 μg/L consistently, whereas the other 50% had repeatedly low TLI concentrations but no clinical signs of EPI. This latter group of dogs were German shepherds or Rough collies, suggesting that there may have been pancreatic acinar atrophy but with enough functional secretory reserves to be perceived as normal. This original study, combined with a later one, demonstrated that a single equivocal result of TLI cannot be used to predict the onset of EPI, that there is large variation in TLI concentrations, and that dogs with persistent results between 2.5 μg/L and 5.0 μg/L likely had a degree of subclinical EPI.[72]

The most widely used application of pancreatic elastase in human medicine is the measurement of the enzyme in feces as a determinant of exocrine pancreatic function.[73] Fecal measurement of cPE-1 seems to be of limited use in dogs for the diagnosis of EPI. A concentration of more than 20 μg/g in feces can be considered a result that excludes EPI, but values less than this are only suggestive of EPI.[74–76]

Unfortunately, no single test seems to be able to diagnose dogs with subclinical EPI or to be able to predict which dog will go on to develop EPI, even with advanced dynamic testing.[65]

REFERENCES

1. Hess RS, Saunders HM, Van Winkle TJ, et al. Clinical, clinicopathologic, radiographic, and ultrasonographic abnormalities in dogs with fatal acute pancreatitis: 70 cases (1986-1995). J Am Vet Med Assoc 1998;213:665–70.
2. Watson P. Pancreatitis in the dog: dealing with a spectrum of disease. In Practice 2004;64–77.
3. Mansfield CS, James FE, Robertson ID. Development of a clinical severity index for dogs with acute pancreatitis. J Am Vet Med Assoc 2008;233:936–44.
4. Mansfield CS. Pathophysiology of acute pancreatitis: potential application from experimental models and human medicine to dogs. J Vet Intern Med 2012;26:875–87.
5. Whitney MS. The laboratory assessment of canine and feline pancreatitis. Vet Med 1993;85:1045–52.
6. Williams DA. Diagnosis and management of pancreatitis. J Small Anim Pract 1994;35:445–54.

7. Holowaychuk MK, Hansen BD, DeFrancesco TC, et al. Ionized hypocalcemia in critically ill dogs. J Vet Intern Med 2009;23:509–13.
8. Jacobs RM, Murtaugh RJ, DeHoff WD. Review of the clinicopathological findings of acute pancreatitis in the dog: use of an experimental model. J Am Anim Hosp Assoc 1985;21:795–800.
9. Akuzawa M, Morizono M, Nagata K, et al. Changes of serum amylase, its isozyme fractions and amylase-creatinine clearance ratio in dogs with experimentally induced acute pancreatitis. J Vet Med Sci 1994;56:269–73.
10. Mansfield CS, Jones BR. Plasma and urinary trypsinogen activation peptide in healthy dogs, dogs with pancreatitis and dogs with other systemic diseases. Aust Vet J 2000;78:416–22.
11. Rallis TS, Koutinas AF, Kritsepi M, et al. Serum lipase activity in young dogs with acute enteritis or gastroenteritis. Vet Clin Pathol 1996;25:65–8.
12. Walter GL, McGraw P, Tvedten HW. Serum lipase determination in the dog: a comparison of a titrimetric method with an automated kinetic method. Vet Clin Pathol 1992;21:23–7.
13. Parent J. Effects of dexamethasone on pancreatic tissue and on serum amylase and lipase activities in dogs. J Am Vet Med Assoc 1982;180:743–6.
14. Stewart AF. Pancreatitis in dogs and cats: cause, pathogenesis, diagnosis, and treatment. Compend Contin Educ Vet 1994;16:1423–30.
15. Hurley PR, Cook A, Jehanli A, et al. Development of radioimmunoassays for free tetra-L-aspartyl-L-lysine trypsinogen activation peptides (TAP). J Immunol Methods 1988;111:195–203.
16. Gudgeon AM, Hurley P, Jehanli A, et al. Trypsinogen activation peptide assay in the early prediction of severity of acute pancreatitis. Lancet 1990; 335:4–8.
17. Neoptolemos JP, Kemppainen E, Mayer JM, et al. Early prediction of severity in acute pancreatitis by urinary trypsinogen activation peptide: a multicentre study. Lancet 2000;355:1955–60.
18. Batt RM. Exocrine pancreatic insufficiency. Vet Clin North Am Small Anim Pract 1993;23:595–608.
19. Simpson KW, Batt RM, McLean L, et al. Circulating concentrations of trypsin-like immunoreactivity and activities of lipase and amylase after pancreatic duct ligation in dogs. Am J Vet Res 1989;50:629–32.
20. Ruaux CG, Atwell RB. Levels of total alpha-macroglobulin and trypsin-like immunoreactivity are poor indicators of clinical severity in spontaneous canine acute pancreatitis. Res Vet Sci 1999;67:83–7.
21. Steiner JM, Williams DA. Purification of classical pancreatic lipase from dog pancreas. Biochimie 2002;84:1245–53.
22. Steiner JM, Berridge BR, Wojcieszyn J, et al. Cellular immunolocalization of gastric and pancreatic lipase in various tissues obtained from dogs. Am J Vet Res 2002;63:722–7.
23. Steiner JM, Rutz GM, Williams DA. Serum lipase activities and pancreatic lipase immunoreactivity concentrations in dogs with exocrine pancreatic insufficiency. Am J Vet Res 2006;67:84–7.
24. Steiner JM, Teague SR, Williams DA. Development and analytic validation of an enzyme-linked immunosorbent assay for the measurement of canine pancreatic lipase immunoreactivity in serum. Can J Vet Res 2003;67:175–82.
25. Steiner JM, Williams DA. Development and validation of a radioimmunoassay for the measurement of canine pancreatic lipase immunoreactivity in serum of dogs. Am J Vet Res 2003;64:1237–41.

26. Huth SP, Relford R, Steiner JM, et al. Analytical validation of an ELISA for measurement of canine pancreas-specific lipase. Vet Clin Pathol 2010;39:346–53.
27. Steiner JM. Diagnosis of pancreatitis. Vet Clin North Am Small Anim Pract 2003; 33:1181–95.
28. Beall MJ, Cahill R, Pigeon K, et al. Performance validation and method comparison of an in-clinic enzyme-linked immunosorbent assay for the detection of canine pancreatic lipase. J Vet Diagn Invest 2011;23:115–9.
29. Steiner JM, Newman S, Xenoulis P, et al. Sensitivity of serum markers for pancreatitis in dogs with macroscopic evidence of pancreatitis. Vet Ther 2008;9: 263–73.
30. Mansfield CS, Anderson GA, O'Hara AJ. Association between canine pancreatic-specific lipase and histologic exocrine pancreatic inflammation in dogs: assessing specificity. J Vet Diagn Invest 2012;24:312–8.
31. Steiner JM, Broussard J, Mansfield CS, et al. Serum canine pancreatic lipase immunoreactivity (cPLI) concentrations in dogs with spontaneous pancreatitis [abstract]. J Vet Intern Med 2001;15:274.
32. McCord K, Morley PS, Armstrong J, et al. A multi-institutional study evaluating the diagnostic utility of the spec cPL™ and SNAP® cPL™ in clinical acute pancreatitis in 84 dogs. J Vet Intern Med 2012;26:888–96.
33. Trivedi S, Marks SL, Kass PH, et al. Sensitivity and specificity of canine pancreas-specific lipase (cPL) and other markers for pancreatitis in 70 dogs with and without histopathologic evidence of pancreatitis. J Vet Intern Med 2011;25:1241–7.
34. Neilson-Carley SC, Robertson JE, Newman S, et al. Specificity of a canine pancreas-specific lipase assay for diagnosing pancreatitis in dogs without clinical or histologic evidence of the disease. Am J Vet Res 2011;72:302–7.
35. Steiner JM, Finco D, Williams DA. Serum lipase activity and canine pancreatic lipase immunoreactivity (cPLI) concentration in dogs with experimentally induced chronic renal failure. Vet Research 2010;3:58–63.
36. Haworth M, Hosgood G, Swindells K, et al. Diagnostic accuracy of the SNAP and spec canine pancreatic lipase (cPL) tests for pancreatitis in privately-owned dogs presenting with clinical signs of acute abdominal disease. J Vet Emerg Crit Care, in press.
37. Newman SJ, Steiner JM, Woosley K, et al. Histologic assessment and grading of the exocrine pancreas in the dog. J Vet Diagn Invest 2006;18:115–8.
38. Hartwig W, Kolvenbach M, Hackert T, et al. Enterokinase induces severe necrosis and rapid mortality in cerulein pancreatitis: characterization of a novel noninvasive rat model of necro-hemorrhagic pancreatitis. Surgery 2007;142:327–36.
39. Malfertheiner P, Buchler M, Stanescu A, et al. Serum elastase 1 in inflammatory pancreatic and gastrointestinal diseases and in renal insufficiency. A comparison with other serum pancreatic enzymes. Int J Pancreatol 1987;2:159–70.
40. Lesi C, Ruffilli E, De Mutiis R, et al. Serum elastase 1 in clinical practice. Pancreas 1988;3:444–9.
41. Millson CE, Charles K, Poon P, et al. A prospective study of serum pancreatic elastase-1 in the diagnosis and assessment of acute pancreatitis. Scand J Gastroenterol 1998;33:664–8.
42. Buchler M, Malfertheiner P, Uhl W, et al. Diagnostic and prognostic value of serum elastase 1 in acute pancreatitis. Klin Wochenschr 1986;64:1186–91.
43. Spillman T, Korrell J, Wittker A, et al. Serum canine pancreatic elastase and canine C-reactive protein for the diagnosis and prognosis of acute pancreatitis in dogs. ECVIM Congress (abstract) 2002.

44. Spillmann T, Happonen I, Sankari S, et al. Evaluation of serum values of pancreatic enzymes after endoscopic retrograde pancreatography in dogs. Am J Vet Res 2004;65:616–9.

45. Mansfield CS. Specificity and sensitivity of serum canine pancreatic elastase-1 concentration in the diagnosis of pancreatitis. J Vet Diagn Invest 2011;23:691–7.

46. Seno T, Harada H, Ochi K, et al. Serum levels of six pancreatic enzymes as related to the degree of renal dysfunction. Am J Gastroenterol 1995;90:2002–5.

47. Al Mofleh I. Severe acute pancreatitis: pathogenic aspects and prognostic factors. World J Gastroenterol 2008;14:675–84.

48. Wu BU, Johannes RS, Sun X, et al. The early prediction of mortality in acute pancreatitis: a large population-based study. Gut 2008;57:1698–703.

49. de Cock HE, Forman MA, Farver T, et al. Prevalence and histopathologic characteristics of pancreatitis in cats. Vet Pathol 2007;44:39–49.

50. Kimmel SE, Washabau RJ, Drobatz KJ. Incidence and prognostic value of low plasma ionized calcium concentration in cats with acute pancreatitis: 46 cases (1996–1998). J Am Vet Med Assoc 2001;219:1105–9.

51. Ferreri JA, Hardam E, Kimmel SE, et al. Clinical differentiation of acute necrotizing from chronic nonsuppurative pancreatitis in cats: 63 cases (1996-2001). J Am Vet Med Assoc 2003;223:469–74.

52. Kitchell BE, Strombeck DR, Cullen J, et al. Clinical and pathologic changes in experimentally induced acute pancreatitis in cats. Am J Vet Res 1986;47: 1170–3.

53. Swift N, Marks SL, MacLachlan NJ, et al. Evaluation of serum feline trypsin-like immunoreactivity for the diagnosis of pancreatitis in cats. J Am Vet Med Assoc 2000;217:37–42.

54. Forman MA, Marks SL, de Cock HE, et al. Evaluation of serum feline pancreatic lipase immunoreactivity and helical computed tomography versus conventional testing for the diagnosis of feline pancreatitis. J Vet Intern Med 2004; 18:807–15.

55. Steiner JM, Williams DA, Moeller EM, et al. Development and validation of an enzyme-linked immunosorbent assay for feline trypsin-like immunoreactivity. Am J Vet Res 2000;61:620–3.

56. Gerhardt A, Steiner JM, Williams DA, et al. Comparison of the sensitivity of different diagnostic tests for pancreatitis in cats. J Vet Intern Med 2001;15: 329–33.

57. Allen HS, Steiner J, Broussard J, et al. Serum and urine concentrations of trypsinogen-activation peptide as markers for acute pancreatitis in cats. Can J Vet Res 2006;70:313–6.

58. Steiner J, Wilson BW, Williams DA. Development and analytical validation of a radioimmunoassay for the measurement of feline pancreatic lipase immunoreactivity in serum. Can J Vet Res 2004;68:309–14.

59. Watson PJ, Archer J, Roulois AJ, et al. Observational study of 14 cases of chronic pancreatitis in dogs. Vet Rec 2010;167:968–76.

60. Watson PJ. Exocrine pancreatic insufficiency as an end stage of pancreatitis in four dogs. J Small Anim Pract 2003;44:306–12.

61. Seaman RL. Exocrine pancreatic neoplasia in the cat: a case series. J Am Anim Hosp Assoc 2004;40:238–45.

62. Brown PJ, Mason KV, Merrett DJ, et al. Multifocal necrotising steatites associated with pancreatic carcinoma in three dogs. J Small Anim Pract 1994;35:129–32.

63. Bjorneby JM, Kari S. Cytology of the pancreas. Vet Clin North Am Small Anim Pract 2002;32:1293–312.

64. Bennett P, Hahn K, Toal R, et al. Ultrasonographic and cytopathological diagnosis of exocrine pancreatic carcinoma in the dog and cat. J Am Anim Hosp Assoc 2001;37:466–73.
65. Westermarck E, Wiberg M. Exocrine pancreatic insufficiency in the dog: historical background, diagnosis and treatment. Top Companion Anim Med 2012;27: 96–103.
66. Batchelor DJ, Noble PJ, Cripps PJ, et al. Breed associations for canine exocrine pancreatic insufficiency. J Vet Intern Med 2007;21:207–14.
67. Westermarck E, Saari SA, Wiberg M. Heritability of exocrine pancreatic insufficiency in German shepherd dogs. J Vet Intern Med 2010;24:450–2.
68. Steiner JM. Exocrine pancreatic insufficiency in the cat. Top Companion Anim Med 2012;27:113–6.
69. Williams DA, Batt RM. Sensitivity and specificity of radioimmunoassay of serum trypsin-like immunoreactivity for the diagnosis of canine exocrine pancreatic insufficiency. J Am Vet Med Assoc 1988;11:191–5.
70. Steiner JM, Williams DA. Serum feline trypsin-like immunoreactivity in cats with exocrine pancreatic insufficiency. J Vet Intern Med 2000;14:627–9.
71. Wiberg M, Nurmi AK, Westermarck E. Serum trypsinlike immunoreactivity measurement for the diagnosis of subclinical exocrine pancreatic insufficiency. J Vet Intern Med 1999;13:426–32.
72. Wiberg ME, Westermarck E. Subclinical exocrine pancreatic insufficiency in dogs. J Am Vet Med Assoc 2002;220:1183–7.
73. Pezzilli R, Talamini G, Gullo L. Behaviour of serum pancreatic enzymes in chronic pancreatitis. Dig Liver Dis 2000;32:233–7.
74. Wiberg ME, Westermarck E, Spillman T, et al. Canine faecal pancreatic elastase (cE1) for the diagnosis of subclinical exocrine pancreatic insufficiency in dogs. Eur J Comp Gastroenterol 2000;5:21–5.
75. Spillmann T, Wittker A, Teigelkamp S, et al. An immunoassay for canine pancreatic elastase 1 as an indicator for exocrine pancreatic insufficiency in dogs. J Vet Diagn Invest 2001;13:468–74.
76. Spillman T, Wiberg M, Teigelkamp S, et al. Canine faecal pancreatic elastase (CE 1) in dogs with clinical exocrine pancreatic insufficiency, normal dogs and dogs with chronic enteropathies. Eur J Comp Gastroenterol 2001;2:5–10.
77. Hill RC, Van Winkle TJ. Acute necrotizing pancreatitis and acute suppurative pancreatitis in the cat. A retrospective study of 40 cases (1976-1989). J Vet Intern Med 1993;7:25–33.

Using Cardiac Biomarkers in Veterinary Practice

Mark A. Oyama, DVM

KEYWORDS

- Natriuretic peptide • BNP • Troponin • Cardiac biomarkers • Heart disease

KEY POINTS

- Blood-based assays for cardiac biomarkers can assist in the diagnosis of heart disease in dogs and cats.
- The most established applications are differentiation of cardiac versus noncardiac causes of respiratory signs and the detection of preclinical cardiomyopathy.
- Cardiac biomarkers are best used as part of the overall clinical cardiac workup that includes the medical history, physical examination, electrocardiogram, thoracic radiographs, and echocardiography.
- The selection of proper patient populations in which to test is key to obtaining reliable results.
- Future applications might include the use of cardiac biomarkers to help guide therapy and improve patient outcomes.

INTRODUCTION: NATURE OF THE PROBLEM

The evaluation of cardiac disease in small animals can be challenging. The patient history is often nonspecific; the presence or intensity of a heart murmur on physical examination is not always a reliable measure of disease severity; concurrent pulmonary disease can confound the interpretation of thoracic radiographs; and other diagnostics, such as echocardiography, are relatively expensive and might not be readily available. For these reasons, blood-based biomarkers that are capable of detecting and staging cardiac disease are a subject of considerable interest.

A biomarker is a substance that is
- Specific to the organ or tissue under study
- Released in proportion to injury or disease

This article originally appeared in Veterinary Clinics of North America: Small Animal Practice, Volume 43, Issue 6, November 2013.

Disclosures: The author consults for and has received funding for clinical trials from IDEXX Laboratories, Westbrook, ME.

Section of Cardiology, Department of Clinical Studies-Philadelphia, School of Veterinary Medicine, University of Pennsylvania, 3900 Delancey Street, Philadelphia, PA 19104, USA

E-mail address: maoyama@vet.upenn.edu

In order to be clinically useful, the biomarker should provide information regarding diagnosis, prognosis, or response to treatment that is otherwise not readily available using conventional testing. The use of blood-based biomarkers for noncardiac organ systems, such as the use of gamma-glutamyl transferase to detect cholestasis or the use of creatinine to detect renal disease, is a familiar concept; cardiac biomarkers act in much the same fashion for the heart. The 2 cardiac biomarkers with the most extensive evaluation in small animals are cardiac troponin-I (cTnI) and 2 forms of B-type natriuretic peptide (BNP), namely, the C-terminal fragment (C-BNP) and the N-terminal fragment (NT-proBNP).

CARDIAC TROPONIN

The cardiac biomarker cTnI, along with troponin-T (cTnT) and troponin-C, form a conglomeration of 3 myocardial proteins that is bound to the actin backbone within myocardiocytes. The troponin complex regulates calcium binding and subsequent interaction between actin and myosin filaments. Damage to the myocardiocyte and to the sarcolemmal membrane dissociates troponin from the actin and allows leakage of troponin into the extracellular space where it then enters into the circulation. The cardiac isoforms of cTnI and cTnT are specific to cardiac tissue and are specific markers of myocardial cell injury or necrosis. In healthy patients, little to no cardiac troponin is detectable blood. Because of its high specificity for cardiac tissue, detection of either circulating cTnI or cTnT is one of the primary diagnostic tools used by emergency department clinicians to diagnose acute myocardial infarction in human patients. Cardiac troponin is also elevated in patients with chronic heart disease, although not to the extent that is seen in acute myocardial infarction; circulating concentrations of cTnI also are a fraction of those seen in acute myocardial infarction. There are 2 commercially available veterinary cardiac troponin assays (i-Stat Cardiac Troponin assay, Abaxis, Union City, CA; Troponin-I, IDEXX Laboratories, Westbrook, ME), both of which test for cTnI. Current veterinary tests are plagued by a relatively low limit of detection of approximately 0.2 ng/mL, whereas circulating cTnI concentrations in dogs with mild to moderate myxomatous mitral valve disease (MMVD) are often less than 0.03 ng/mL and can be detected only using newer high-sensitivity assays.[1] Despite these relatively modest elevations, cTnI concentrations are predictive of the outcome in human patients with chronic heart failure as well as in dogs with MMVD.[2] The troponin molecules are highly conserved across species, and many high-sensitivity assays designed for human testing can be used to detect canine and feline cTnI. Thus, cardiac troponin assays have the potential to provide both diagnostic and prognostic information. In a meta-analysis of more than 6800 human patients with stable chronic heart failure, patients with elevated cTnI or cTnT were 2.9 times more likely to die during the study follow-up period than those patients with lower values.[3] Acute myocardial infarction in dogs and cats is rare. However, chronic heart diseases, such as MMVD and dilated cardiomyopathy (DCM) in dogs and hypertrophic cardiomyopathy (HCM) in cats, are relatively common; the diagnostic and prognostic value of cardiac troponin is a subject of interest. There are several factors that potentially limit the usefulness of cardiac troponin in veterinary patients. Although elevated cardiac troponin is sensitive for the presence of myocardial injury, it is not specific to any one underlying cause. Moreover, animals with mild disease can have normal cTnI concentrations. Thus, the utility of the test to screen for specific heart diseases in various populations is limited. Cardiac troponin is partially excreted through renal mechanisms, and cardiac injury in the presence of chronic or acute kidney disease can result in false elevations.[4] Finally, cTnI concentrations increase slightly but significantly with age; additional studies establishing age-related reference ranges are needed (**Box 1**).[5]

NATRIURETIC PEPTIDES

BNP and its parent protein proBNP along with A-type natriuretic peptide (ANP) and its parent protein proANP are the main natriuretic hormones produced by myocardial tissue. Both proBNP and proANP are constitutively produced by atrial and to a lesser extent ventricular myocardiocytes. Stress or stretch of the myocardium (for instance, in response to volume overload) increases the production of proBNP and proANP, particularly within ventricular myocardiocytes. On release, these substances are quickly cleaved into separate N-terminal and C-terminal fragments. C-BNP and C-terminal ANP (C-ANP) elicit vasodilation and diuresis through binding of specific natriuretic receptors found in vascular and renal tissue. Their actions provide a counterbalance to those of the renin-angiotensin-aldosterone system. In humans, C-BNP and NT-proBNP assays are primarily used to help discriminate between cardiac causes (ie, congestive heart failure [CHF]) and noncardiac causes of respiratory clinical signs as well as to help estimate the risk of morbidity and mortality in patients with chronic heart disease. C-BNP and C-ANP have short half-lives, whereas NT-proBNP and NT-proANP are more stable and make more attractive targets for assay detection. There are 3 commercially available assays in the United States for natriuretic peptides, all involving various plasma forms of BNP: one for C-BNP in dogs (Cardio-BNP, Antech Diagnostics, Chesterfield, MO) and 2 for NT-proBNP, one each for dogs (CardioPet proBNP-Canine, IDEXX Laboratories, Westbrook, ME) and cats (CardioPet proBNP-Feline, IDEXX Laboratories, Westbrook, ME). Both the C-BNP and NT-proBNP assays require special blood-collection techniques to slow degradation during collection and transport to the reference laboratory. C-BNP and NT-proBNP are elevated in a variety of cardiac conditions, including MMVD, DCM, and HCM.[6–8] Increased concentrations also are present in noncardiac disease conditions that secondarily affect the heart, such as hyperthyroidism and systemic and pulmonary hypertension.[9,10] In both dogs and cats, concentrations are positively correlated with radiographic and echocardiographic measures of disease severity, and the ability of C-BNP and NT-proBNP assays to provide diagnostic and prognostic information is a subject of considerable interest. Most of the studies investigating the clinical utility of BNP in veterinary patients involve testing for NT-proBNP, and comparatively little is known about specific guidelines and cut points using the C-BNP assay (**Box 2**).

INDICATIONS FOR C-BNP AND NT-PROBNP TESTING

There are several indications for C-BNP or NT-proBNP testing, including differentiating cardiac versus noncardiac causes of respiratory signs, detection of occult

---

Box 1
Key points regarding cTnI

- Marker of myocardial cell injury and necrosis.
- Specific for cardiac muscle injury but not specific as to the underlying cause.
- Elevated in dogs and cats with a variety of heart and systemic diseases.

Box 2
Key points regarding C-BNP and NT-proBNP

- Parent molecule, proBNP, is produced in myocardiocytes in response to mechanical stress.
- Both are formed from the cleavage of the parent molecule proBNP.
- Both are released into circulation in a variety of heart diseases in dogs and cats.
- Both are positively correlated to clinical, radiographic, and echocardiographic measures of disease severity.

DCM in Doberman pinschers and occult HCM in cats, and as a prognostic tool in dogs with MMVD or DCM.

Differentiation of Cardiac Versus Noncardiac Causes of Respiratory Signs

Dogs and cats with respiratory signs represent a considerable diagnostic challenge because, for many cases, the cause of the clinical signs is not immediately clear. Most potential causes can be classified as either cardiac in origin (ie, CHF) or noncardiac (primary airway or parenchymal diseases, such as asthma, chronic bronchitis, pneumonia, and so forth). Studies have demonstrated the utility of C-BNP and NT-proBNP assay in distinguishing the cause of respiratory signs in dogs[6,11,12] and the utility of the NT-proBNP assay in distinguishing the cause of respiratory signs in cats.[13,14] A low NT-proBNP concentration is most consistent of a noncardiac cause, whereas an elevated concentration is more suggestive of CHF. In human medicine, NT-proBNP is best used as a test to help rule out CHF because patients with low or normal NT-proBNP are highly unlikely to have CHF. The diagnostic value of an elevated NT-proBNP concentration is less than that of a low concentration because patients with symptomatic respiratory disease and concurrent asymptomatic heart disease could have elevated concentrations. For this reason, the recommended cutoff values suggestive of a cardiac cause of respiratory signs in dogs and cats are more than the upper reference value for healthy animals. NT-proBNP and C-BNP assays are not stand-alone tests; their results should be evaluated in the context of the medical history, physical examination, and other diagnostic testing, such as radiography and echocardiography. In cases for which traditional diagnostic testing reveals the cause of the respiratory signs, BNP testing adds little additional value to the already apparent diagnosis. In cases for which the diagnosis is uncertain, the addition of the NT-proBNP assay to the diagnostic workup improved the accuracy and confidence of diagnosis in cats with respiratory signs (**Box 3**).[15]

Box 3
Guidelines for differentiation of cardiac versus noncardiac causes of respiratory signs in dogs and cats using NT-proBNP assay

- Low or normal NT-proBNP concentration is most consistent with a noncardiac cause of the current signs, whereas elevated NT-proBNP is more suggestive of a cardiac cause, such as CHF.
- In animals with asymptomatic heart disease, an increased NT-proBNP concentration can confound the diagnosis of a noncardiac cause of the respiratory signs.
- Results should be viewed in context of the medical history, physical examination, and traditional diagnostics, such as thoracic radiography.

Detection of Occult Cardiomyopathy in Doberman Pinschers and in Cats

Cardiomyopathy is common in particular breeds of dogs and cats. For instance, the lifetime incidence of DCM in Doberman pinschers is as high as 60%, and the Maine coon, ragdoll, and Persian breeds of cats, among others, are highly predisposed to HCM.[16,17] Both DCM and HCM are characterized by a long preclinical (occult) phase during which clinical signs of disease are absent despite the presence of underlying cardiac dysfunction. In animals with occult cardiomyopathy, the first clinical sign of disease can be sudden death or life-threatening CHF; thus, the detection of preclinical disease using preliminary tests is a subject of interest. The gold standard for the diagnosis of occult DCM in Doberman pinschers is the detection of ventricular premature beats via in-hospital electrocardiogram (ECG) or Holter monitoring and/or the detection of left ventricular systolic dysfunction via echocardiography. Some dogs with occult DCM will demonstrate both abnormalities, whereas others will have only one or the other. Three studies have investigated the ability to detect occult DCM in Doberman pinschers, 2 involving NT-proBNP[18,19] and one involving C-BNP.[20] C-BNP has a high sensitivity (95.2%) but a low specificity (61.9%), resulting in a high number of false-positive results. The studies involving NT-proBNP yielded similar results; the NT-proBNP assay was good at detecting dogs with systolic dysfunction whether or not they also had arrhythmias, but was poor at detecting dogs whose sole criterion for occult DCM was ventricular arrhythmias. Thus, NT-proBNP cannot be used as a stand-alone test to detect occult DCM. However, the combination of an NT-proBNP assay with Holter monitoring was 94.5% sensitive and 87.8% specific for detecting all dogs with occult disease.[19] From these studies, NT-proBNP assay does not replace the current gold standards for diagnosis. In instances when echocardiography is not immediately accessible, an elevated NT-proBNP or C-BNP concentration would support the pursuit of echocardiographic examination. Thus, BNP assesses the likelihood of finding significant abnormalities on gold standard testing rather than being a diagnostic test in and of itself. This distinction is subtle but important if the number of false-positive and negative results inherent in the BNP assays are to be avoided.

Feline cardiomyopathy has a long preclinical phase similar to canine DCM, and detection of underlying heart disease in apparently healthy cats can be challenging. Unlike the situation in the dog, wherein the presence of a heart murmur is a reliable sign of underlying heart disease, cats commonly have heart murmurs of benign origin. Moreover, not all cats with cardiomyopathy will have a heart murmur; this further confounds the ability to readily detect heart disease on physical examination. The gold standard for the diagnosis of feline cardiomyopathy is echocardiography. In instances when heart disease is suspected because of a murmur, gallop, or arrhythmia, NT-proBNP has a sensitivity of 70% to 100% and a specificity of 67% to 100% to indicate the presence of significant echocardiographic abnormalities.[8,21–23] The exact sensitivity and specificity depends on the cutoff values used, with lower cutoff values resulting in higher sensitivity but lower specificity, and higher cutoff values resulting in lower sensitivity but higher specificity (**Table 1**). The NT-proBNP assay is best suited to identify cats with moderate to severe echocardiographic changes, and it is these cats that likely benefit from additional monitoring or treatment. NT-proBNP testing has been studied only in cats that have risk factors for cardiomyopathy (ie, murmur, gallop, arrhythmia, and so forth), and the clinical usefulness of NT-proBNP assay to detect cardiomyopathy in the general population is unknown (**Box 4**). For this reason, indiscriminate testing of cats is not recommended, particularly in instances when the likelihood of significant disease is very low (ie, young cats undergoing neutering). The

Table 1
Diagnostic uses of cardiac biomarker tests in dogs and cats

Indication	Marker	Cutoff Values	Sensitivity (%)	Specificity (%)	Comments
Differentiating cardiac vs noncardiac causes of respiratory signs in cats	NT-proBNP[13,14]	220, 265 (pmol/L)	90–94	88	Low values indicate cardiac causes are unlikely, high values suggest CHF
Differentiating cardiac vs noncardiac causes of respiratory signs in dogs	NT-proBNP[12,38]	1158, 1400 (pmol/L)	86–92	81	Low values indicate cardiac causes are unlikely, high values suggest CHF
	C-BNP[6,11]	17.4, 6.0 (pg/mL)	86–90	78–81	Low values indicate cardiac causes are unlikely, high values suggest CHF
Detection of cardiomyopathy in at-risk cats	cTnI[33,34]	0.157, 0.20 (ng/mL)	85–87	84–97	Elevated values not specific for primary heart disease
	NT-proBNP[21–23]	95, 99, 100 (pmol/L)	71–92	94–100	Studies were performed in populations with clinical suspicion for heart disease (ie, those with murmur, gallop, arrhythmias, and so forth)
Detection of cardiomyopathy in Doberman pinschers	NT-proBNP[18,19]	457, 550 (pmol/L)	70–79	81–90	NT-proBNP poor at detecting dogs with arrhythmias only, sensitivity and specificity improved if used in tandem with Holter monitoring
	C-BNP[20]	6.2 (pg/mL)	95	62	Low specificity results in large number of false positives

The reported cutoff values and range of respective sensitivities and specificities for various indications are presented. Cardiac biomarker assays indicate risk of a particular condition being present, and additional diagnostics are often needed to obtain a definitive diagnosis. Cardiac biomarker assays are not stand-alone diagnostic assays. When interpreting results, values that far exceed cutoff values provide more reliable information than those at or near the cutoff value.

> **Box 4**
> **Guidelines for detection of occult cardiomyopathy in Doberman pinschers and in cats using NT-proBNP assay**
>
> - Testing should be done on selected patients that are at high risk for cardiac disease, such as adult Doberman pinschers and Maine coon cats and cats with a heart murmur or arrhythmia.
> - Elevated concentrations increase the likelihood of clinically significant echocardiographic abnormalities, and further diagnostics should be pursued.
> - Elevated concentrations could help assess the need or urgency to pursue more costly or time-consuming diagnostic tests if the presence of clinically significant disease is initially unclear.
> - Elevated concentrations are not diagnostic of any one particular disease, and results should be interpreted in the context of the medical history, physical examination, and traditional diagnostic testing.

likelihood of a test result being either false positive or false negative is partly dependent on the prevalence of the disease condition in the population being tested. The less prevalent the disease, the less likely a patient has the disease, even if a test result is positive. As an example, in a dog living in Alaska, there is a high likelihood that a positive heartworm antigen test is actually a false-positive result simply because of the very low prevalence of disease in this region, whereas a positive heartworm antigen test from a dog living in the Mississippi River Valley is almost certainly a true positive. Thus, clinicians must select the appropriate patient population in which to test in order to optimize the reliability of the assay.

Predicting Morbidity and Mortality in Dogs with Heart Disease

Aside from their role in the diagnosis of heart disease, whether BNP assays can predict the risk of CHF in dogs with preclinical disease or predict the risk of cardiovascular mortality is a subject of interest. The use of the NT-proBNP assay to predict the first-onset of CHF in dogs with preclinical MMVD has been studied. In one study, baseline NT-proBNP concentration was 80% sensitive and 76% specific for identifying dogs that developed CHF within the subsequent 12 months.[24] Another study in dogs with preclinical MMVD reported that those with NT-proBNP greater than 1500 pmol/L were approximately 6 times more likely to develop CHF over the subsequent 3 to 6 months than dogs with lower values.[25] The predictive value of NT-proBNP was best when combined with measures of radiographic or echocardiographic left side of the heart size, and NT-proBNP should be used alongside traditional diagnostic methods.

Several studies have revealed an association between NT-proBNP and survival in dogs with MMVD.[2,24,26] In the most recent studies, increases in NT-proBNP, high sensitivity cTnI, and echocardiographic heart size were negatively associated with survival.[2] For each incremental increase of 100 pmol/L in NT-proBNP, the risk of death caused by cardiac disease increased by 7%. Two studies have investigated NT-proBNP and the survival of dogs with DCM. In one study, Doberman pinschers with DCM and elevated NT-proBNP had a median survival time that was 6 times shorter than those with lower values[19]; in another study, NT-proBNP predicted the survival of dogs with DCM 60 days after the initial examination.[27]

The use of the NT-proBNP assay to help predict the risk of either CHF or survival has several important limitations, and further studies are needed before the assay becomes part of the standard workup for dogs with MMVD (**Box 5**). Firstly, sensitivity and specificity are performance indices that apply to populations of individuals; the

> **Box 5**
> **Guidelines for stratification of risk in dogs with MMVD**
>
> - Dogs with preclinical MMVD, radiographic or echocardiographic heart enlargement, and NT-proBNP greater than 1500 pmol/L are likely at an increased risk for the development of CHF.
> - In dogs at an increased risk of morbidity or mortality, increased vigilance for subtle signs of heart failure and more frequent monitoring is recommended.
> - There are no clinical studies assessing the value of treatment decisions based on NT-proBNP concentrations.

accuracy of the diagnostic test in any one individual is not 100%. Secondly, elevated NT-proBNP concentrations specify the risk, not the certainty, of morbidity or mortality. Elevated NT-proBNP, especially in dogs with radiographic or echocardiographic cardiomegaly, likely warrants heightened vigilance for early signs of CHF. In animals at high risk for CHF, owners can be counseled about how to obtain the animal's resting respiratory rate. In healthy dogs, the average sleeping respiratory rate is 13 breaths per minute and rarely exceeds 30 breaths per minute.[28] Respiratory rates of more than 41 breaths per minute have been shown to be a sensitive indicator for the detection of CHF.[29] Finally, there are no data indicating that NT-proBNP concentrations can be used to guide therapy decisions, such as when to initiate or alter existing drugs, such as diuretics or angiotensin converting enzyme inhibitor. In human patients with heart failure, 2 meta-analyses[30,31] indicated that BNP-guided therapy resulted in better outcomes, although these results are controversial. In one study of dogs being treated for CHF, dogs with NT-proBNP less than 965 pmol/L following therapy survived longer than those dogs with NT-proBNP concentrations more than 965 pmol/L,[32] suggesting the possibility that therapeutic targets of NT-proBNP could be useful. These data require specifically designed prospective studies for validation.

INDICATIONS FOR CARDIAC TROPONIN TESTING

Specific guidelines for cardiac troponin testing are not well established. Circumstances that might warrant testing include suspected myocarditis or cardiomyopathy or as a prognostic tool in dogs with MMVD or DCM. Troponin testing has also been used to detect myocardial injury in babesiosis, gastric dilatation and volvulus, brachycephalic airway syndrome, sepsis, racing and sled-dog athletes, heartworm disease, dogs receiving doxorubicin, and cases of respiratory distress with unknown cause. In general, cardiac troponin concentrations reflect the severity of cardiac injury and are inversely associated with morbidity and mortality[1,2,5]; however, more studies are needed before specific treatment guidelines can be made using specific concentrations.

Cats with HCM have higher cTnI concentrations than healthy cats; in 2 small studies, elevated cTnI was 85% to 87% sensitive and 84% to 97% specific for the detection of disease.[33,34] Comparatively, the diagnostic ability of cTnI to detect preclinical (occult) DCM in dogs is poor.[20] The cTnI concentrations are higher in cats and dogs with respiratory signs secondary to CHF, but the overlap between these animals and animals with respiratory signs caused by noncardiac causes is wide enough to limit clinical usefulness.[11,35] Elevated cTnI is not specific to primary cardiac disease because any systemic condition that causes hypoxemia and myocardial ischemia could result in elevated cTnI. In the author's experience, some of the highest cTnI concentrations observed have been from dogs with severe pulmonary parenchymal disease and resultant hypoxemia.

In dogs with MMVD, a serum cTnI concentration more than 0.025 ng/mL was associated with a 1.9 times risk for death compared with lower concentrations.[2] Animals with elevated troponin concentrations might benefit from further diagnostic tests, such as ECG, thoracic radiography, and echocardiography (**Box 6**). Whether cardiac troponin concentrations can be used to help guide therapy is an intriguing possibility but requires well-designed prospective trials. In the author's experience, serial troponin measurements in dogs with suspected myocarditis offer some prognostic information; declining values often signify a one-time insult and myocardial recovery, whereas persistently elevated or increasing concentrations are a poor prognostic indicator.

LIMITATIONS OF CARDIAC BIOMARKERS

There are important limitations to the use of cardiac biomarkers in veterinary patients. These limitations involve technical issues, such as failure to properly collect and transport samples, as well as biologic issues, such as the effect of systemic disease on the production or excretion of cTnI and NT-proBNP. Both NT-proBNP and C-BNP assays require special sample collection procedures using manufacturer-supplied blood-collection tubes designed to prevent degradation of BNP during shipping. Improper collection techniques, extended storage at room temperature, or multiple freeze-thaw cycles likely produce inaccurate results. Both NT-proBNP and C-BNP are excreted via renal filtration and can be elevated in animals with acute or chronic kidney disease.[36,37] These elevations are relatively modest in patients with mild disease but increase as renal function worsens. Many clinical studies of NT-proBNP excluded patients with renal disease, highlighting the need to interpret cutoff values in these patients with caution. Other conditions associated with increased NT-proBNP include pulmonary hypertension[10] and feline hyperthyroidism,[9] and results from animals with these diseases should be interpreted with similar caution. Since the introduction of the canine NT-proBNP assay in 2006, there have been several revisions to the assay, the most recent involving the introduction of special blood-collection tubes in 2008. Earlier clinical studies, including those investigating the detection of occult DCM in Doberman pinschers and the discrimination of cardiac versus noncardiac causes of respiratory signs in dogs were performed using the pre-2008 version of the canine assay. Ideally, these studies should be repeated using the most current version of the assay.

Box 6
Guidelines for cardiac troponin testing

- Consider testing in animals with suspected myocarditis or myocardial injury.
- Concentrations generally reflect the magnitude of myocardial injury.
- Serial evaluations that reveal declining values suggest a one-time insult and myocardial recovery, whereas persistently elevated or increasing values suggest ongoing myocardial injury.
- Consider testing as an adjunctive diagnostic test to detect cats with a high likelihood for HCM.
- It is not useful as a test to differentiate cardiac versus noncardiac causes of respiratory signs in dogs and cats.

SUMMARY

Cardiac biomarkers are an exciting and growing science. Much data regarding their clinical use in dogs and cats have been generated; however, many questions remain unanswered. The most established applications involve use of cTnI to help detect myocarditis and feline cardiomyopathy and the use of NT-proBNP to help detect occult cardiomyopathy and differentiate cardiac versus noncardiac causes of respiratory signs. Compared with NT-proBNP, there is relatively little data regarding C-BNP. However, applications of the C-BNP assay are likely similar to those involving NT-proBNP. Both cTnI and NT-proBNP assays help predict the risk of cardiovascular mortality in dogs with MMVD, but additional study is needed to better understand how to use these data in everyday clinical practice. Cardiac biomarker tests are complementary to existing cardiac diagnostic testing and should be interpreted in the context of the overall clinical picture rather than being used as a stand-alone test. Future studies will help determine whether cardiac biomarker assays can help guide therapy and lead to improved outcomes in dogs and cats with cardiac disease.

REFERENCES

1. Ljungvall I, Hoglund K, Tidholm A, et al. Cardiac troponin I is associated with severity of myxomatous mitral valve disease, age, and C-reactive protein in dogs. J Vet Intern Med 2010;24(1):153–9.
2. Hezzell MJ, Boswood A, Chang YM, et al. The combined prognostic potential of serum high-sensitivity cardiac troponin I and N-terminal pro-B-type natriuretic peptide concentrations in dogs with degenerative mitral valve disease. J Vet Intern Med 2012;26(2):302–11.
3. Nagarajan V, Hernandez AV, Tang WH. Prognostic value of cardiac troponin in chronic stable heart failure: a systematic review. Heart 2012;98(24):1778–86.
4. Sharkey LC, Berzina I, Ferasin L, et al. Evaluation of serum cardiac troponin I concentration in dogs with renal failure. J Am Vet Med Assoc 2009;234(6):767–70.
5. Oyama MA, Sisson DD. Cardiac troponin-I concentration in dogs with cardiac disease. J Vet Intern Med 2004;18(6):831–9.
6. DeFrancesco TC, Rush JE, Rozanski EA, et al. Prospective clinical evaluation of an ELISA B-type natriuretic peptide assay in the diagnosis of congestive heart failure in dogs presenting with cough or dyspnea. J Vet Intern Med 2007;21(2):243–50.
7. Oyama MA, Fox PR, Rush JE, et al. Clinical utility of serum N-terminal pro-B-type natriuretic peptide concentration for identifying cardiac disease in dogs and assessing disease severity. J Am Vet Med Assoc 2008;232(10):1496–503.
8. Connolly DJ, Magalhaes RJ, Syme HM, et al. Circulating natriuretic peptides in cats with heart disease. J Vet Intern Med 2008;22(1):96–105.
9. Menaut P, Connolly DJ, Volk A, et al. Circulating natriuretic peptide concentrations in hyperthyroid cats. J Small Anim Pract 2012;53(12):673–8.
10. Kellihan HB, Mackie BA, Stepien RL. NT-proBNP, NT-proANP and cTnI concentrations in dogs with pre-capillary pulmonary hypertension. J Vet Cardiol 2011;13(3):171–82.
11. Prosek R, Sisson DD, Oyama MA, et al. Distinguishing cardiac and noncardiac dyspnea in 48 dogs using plasma atrial natriuretic factor, B-type natriuretic factor, endothelin, and cardiac troponin-I. J Vet Intern Med 2007;21(2):238–42.
12. Oyama MA, Rush JE, Rozanski EA, et al. Assessment of serum N-terminal pro-B-type natriuretic peptide concentration for differentiation of congestive heart failure

from primary respiratory tract disease as the cause of respiratory signs in dogs. J Am Vet Med Assoc 2009;235(11):1319–25.

13. Connolly DJ, Soares Magalhaes RJ, Fuentes VL, et al. Assessment of the diagnostic accuracy of circulating natriuretic peptide concentrations to distinguish between cats with cardiac and non-cardiac causes of respiratory distress. J Vet Cardiol 2009;11(Suppl 1):S41–50.

14. Fox PR, Oyama MA, Reynolds C, et al. Utility of plasma N-terminal pro-brain natriuretic peptide (NT-proBNP) to distinguish between congestive heart failure and non-cardiac causes of acute dyspnea in cats. J Vet Cardiol 2009;11(Suppl 1): S51–61.

15. Singletary GE, Rush JE, Fox PR, et al. Effect of NT-pro-BNP assay on accuracy and confidence of general practitioners in diagnosing heart failure or respiratory disease in cats with respiratory signs. J Vet Intern Med 2012;26(3):542–6.

16. O'Grady MR, O'Sullivan ML. Dilated cardiomyopathy: an update. Vet Clin North Am Small Anim Pract 2004;34(5):1187–207.

17. Trehiou-Sechi E, Tissier R, Gouni V, et al. Comparative echocardiographic and clinical features of hypertrophic cardiomyopathy in 5 breeds of cats: a retrospective analysis of 344 cases (2001-2011). J Vet Intern Med 2012;26(3):532–41.

18. Wess G, Butz V, Mahling M, et al. Evaluation of N-terminal pro-B-type natriuretic peptide as a diagnostic marker of various stages of cardiomyopathy in Doberman pinschers. Am J Vet Res 2011;72(5):642–9.

19. Singletary GE, Morris NA, O'Sullivan ML, et al. Prospective evaluation of NT-proBNP assay to detect occult dilated cardiomyopathy and predict survival in Doberman pinschers. J Vet Intern Med 2012;26:1330–6.

20. Oyama MA, Sisson DD, Solter PF. Prospective screening for occult cardiomyopathy in dogs by measurement of plasma atrial natriuretic peptide, B-type natriuretic peptide, and cardiac troponin-I concentrations. Am J Vet Res 2007;68(1):42–7.

21. Fox PR, Rush JE, Reynolds CA, et al. Multicenter evaluation of plasma N-terminal probrain natriuretic peptide (NT-pro BNP) as a biochemical screening test for asymptomatic (occult) cardiomyopathy in cats. J Vet Intern Med 2011;25(5): 1010–6.

22. Wess G, Daisenberger P, Mahling M, et al. Utility of measuring plasma N-terminal pro-brain natriuretic peptide in detecting hypertrophic cardiomyopathy and differentiating grades of severity in cats. Vet Clin Pathol 2011;40(2):237–44.

23. Tominaga Y, Miyagawa Y, Toda N, et al. The diagnostic significance of the plasma N-terminal pro-B-type natriuretic peptide concentration in asymptomatic cats with cardiac enlargement. J Vet Med Sci 2011;73(8):971–5.

24. Chetboul V, Serres F, Tissier R, et al. Association of plasma N-terminal pro-B-type natriuretic peptide concentration with mitral regurgitation severity and outcome in dogs with asymptomatic degenerative mitral valve disease. J Vet Intern Med 2009;23(5):984–94.

25. Reynolds CA, Brown DC, Rush JE, et al. Prediction of first onset of congestive heart failure in dogs with degenerative mitral valve disease: the PREDICT cohort study. J Vet Cardiol 2012;14(1):193–202.

26. Moonarmart W, Boswood A, Luis F, et al. N-terminal pro B-type natriuretic peptide and left ventricular diameter independently predict mortality in dogs with mitral valve disease. J Small Anim Pract 2010;51(2):84–96.

27. Noszczyk-Nowak A. NT-pro-BNP and troponin I as predictors of mortality in dogs with heart failure. Pol J Vet Sci 2011;14(4):551–6.

28. Rishniw M, Ljungvall I, Porciello F, et al. Sleeping respiratory rates in apparently healthy adult dogs. Res Vet Sci 2012;93(2):965–9.

29. Schober KE, Hart TM, Stern JA, et al. Detection of congestive heart failure in dogs by Doppler echocardiography. J Vet Intern Med 2010;24(6):1358–68.
30. Porapakkham P, Porapakkham P, Zimmet H, et al. B-type natriuretic peptide-guided heart failure therapy: a meta-analysis. Arch Intern Med 2010;170(6):507–14.
31. Felker GM, Hasselblad V, Hernandez AF, et al. Biomarker-guided therapy in chronic heart failure: a meta-analysis of randomized controlled trials. Am Heart J 2009;158(3):422–30.
32. Wolf J, Gerlach N, Weber K, et al. Lowered N-terminal pro-B-type natriuretic peptide levels in response to treatment predict survival in dogs with symptomatic mitral valve disease. J Vet Cardiol 2012;14(3):399–408.
33. Herndon WE, Kittleson MD, Sanderson K, et al. Cardiac troponin I in feline hypertrophic cardiomyopathy. J Vet Intern Med 2002;16(5):558–64.
34. Connolly DJ, Cannata J, Boswood A, et al. Cardiac troponin I in cats with hypertrophic cardiomyopathy. J Feline Med Surg 2003;5(4):209–16.
35. Herndon WE, Rishniw M, Schrope D, et al. Assessment of plasma cardiac troponin I concentration as a means to differentiate cardiac and noncardiac causes of dyspnea in cats. J Am Vet Med Assoc 2008;233(8):1261–4.
36. Miyagawa Y, Tominaga Y, Toda N, et al. Relationship between glomerular filtration rate and plasma N-terminal pro B-type natriuretic peptide concentrations in dogs with chronic kidney disease. Vet J 2013, in press.
37. Lalor SM, Connolly DJ, Elliott J, et al. Plasma concentrations of natriuretic peptides in normal cats and normotensive and hypertensive cats with chronic kidney disease. J Vet Cardiol 2009;11(Suppl 1):S71–9.
38. Fine DM, Declue AE, Reinero CR. Evaluation of circulating amino-terminal-pro-B-type natriuretic peptide concentration in dogs with respiratory distress attributable to congestive heart failure or primary pulmonary disease. J Am Vet Med Assoc 2008;232(11):1674–9.

Use of Lactate in Small Animal Clinical Practice

Leslie C. Sharkey, DVM, PhD[a],*, Maxey L. Wellman, DVM, MS, PhD[b]

KEYWORDS

- Lactate • L-Lactate • D-Lactate • Lactic acidosis • Hypoxia • Hypoperfusion
- Metabolic acidosis

KEY POINTS

- Lactate concentration is used as an indicator of tissue hypoperfusion and hypoxia, particularly in critical care or perioperative settings.
- Lactate concentration is used to determine the severity of an underlying disorder, assess response to therapy, and predict outcome, especially if serial lactate levels are measured.
- Decreasing levels of lactate suggest improvement, whereas prolonged increases in lactate concentration imply deterioration with a poor prognosis.
- Repeated lactate concentrations should be determined on the same instrument with close attention to sample collection and processing and adherence to recommendations for instrument quality control.

INTRODUCTION

Lactate is formed primarily as the end product of anaerobic glycolysis, although small amounts are produced during aerobic metabolism. Hyperlactatemia refers to mildly increased lactate concentration without concurrent metabolic acidosis. Lactic acidosis occurs when hyperlactatemia is more severe and is accompanied by a decrease in blood pH.[1–3] Lactic acidosis occurs most commonly with tissue hypoperfusion and hypoxia, often as a consequence of systemic or regional hypoperfusion, severe anemia, or hypermetabolic states. Liver disease, kidney disease, diabetes mellitus, sepsis, drugs and toxins, and uncommon mitochondrial defects can cause lactic acidosis from various mechanisms including decreased aerobic metabolism and lactate consumption.[4]

In healthy adult dogs, serum lactate measures 0.3 to 2.5 mmol/L.[5] Puppies have higher lactate concentrations that decrease to adult values by 2 to 3 months of age.[6]

This article originally appeared in Veterinary Clinics of North America: Small Animal Practice, Volume 43, Issue 6, November 2013.
Disclosures: Dr M.L. Wellman is a paid consultant for IDEXX Laboratories and Marshfield Labs.
[a] Veterinary Clinical Sciences Department, University of Minnesota College of Veterinary Medicine, 1352 Boyd Avenue, St Paul, MN 55108, USA; [b] Department of Veterinary Biosciences, The Ohio State University, 1925 Coffey Road, Columbus, OH 43210, USA
* Corresponding author.
E-mail address: Shark009@umn.edu

Serum lactate in healthy adult cats is 0.5 to 2.0 mmol/L.[7] Indications for measuring serum lactate include assessment of tissue perfusion and oxygenation, predicting outcome or response to therapy in critically ill patients, and evaluation of metabolic acidosis. In people, serum lactate concentration has been used as a risk stratification biomarker.[8] Several studies in veterinary medicine indicate that lactate concentration may have similar implications for prognosis.[4,9–11] In dogs, 3 to 5 mmol/L is considered a mild increase; 5 to 8 mmol/L is considered a moderate increase, and greater than 8 mmol/L is considered a marked increase in blood lactate concentration.[12]

LACTATE PHYSIOLOGY AND METABOLISM

Under aerobic conditions, glucose is metabolized to pyruvic acid, which diffuses into mitochondria to enter the Krebs cycle and undergo oxidative phosphorylation for energy production or transformation in glucose via gluconeogenesis (**Fig. 1**). However, in red blood cells (RBC) and other cells that lack mitochondria, and in other tissues during periods of hypoxia, glucose is metabolized to pyruvic acid by anaerobic glycolysis. In the final step of anaerobic glycolysis, lactic acid dehydrogenase cata-lyzes the conversion of pyruvic acid to lactic acid, a reaction that favors lactic acid formation by a ratio of 10:1 during normal metabolism (**Fig. 2**).[8]

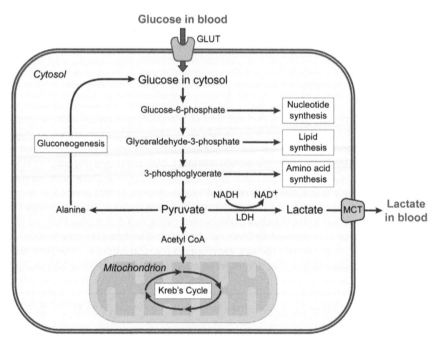

Fig. 1. Glucose metabolism. Glucose enters the cell via the GLUT family of membrane pro-teins. Glucose is metabolized through several steps (only some of which are shown in the diagram) to pyruvate. Pyruvate can be oxidized via the Kreb's cycle in the mitochondrion or transformed to glucose via the gluconeogenesis pathway. Pyruvate also can be converted to lactate via the enzyme lactate dehydrogenase (LDH), which generates nicotine adenine dinucleotide (NAD). This reaction occurs more readily when there is tissue hypoxia. Lactate in the cytoplasm crosses the cell membrane into the blood via a monocarboxylate-proton cotransporter (MCT), an anion exchange system, and simple diffusion.

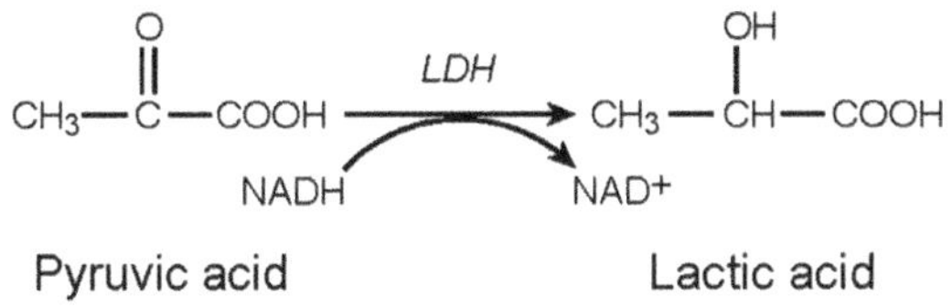

Fig. 2. The final step of anaerobic glycolysis.

Lactic acid ($C_3H_6O_3$) is a nonvolatile (fixed) acid that readily dissociates into a lactate ion [$C_3CH(OH)COO^-$] and a hydrogen ion (H^+) in body fluids at physiologic pH. Lactate ion most often is referred to simply as lactate. A monocarboxylate-proton cotransporter, an anion exchange system, and simple diffusion allow lactate to cross the cell membrane into the blood. The H^+ ions are titrated by various body buffers, but when lactate production is increased, the buffers are depleted and acidemia develops. Lactate and H^+ are metabolized to glucose or oxidized to H_2O and CO_2 when aerobic conditions are restored.[4]

The concentration of lactate in blood depends on the balance between formation and clearance. Daily lactate production is generated primarily by skeletal muscle, skin, brain, heart, intestine, renal medulla, and RBC, but lactate production occurs in many other tissues during illness.[1,4,8] For example, large amounts of lactate are produced by the lungs during acute lung injury and by leukocytes during phagocytosis or from leukocyte activation associated with sepsis. Lactate is metabolized primarily by the liver (60%–70%) and kidney (20%–30%) via the Cori cycle, in which lactate produced in other tissues is converted back to pyruvate and then to glucose through gluconeogenesis.[8,13] Lactate is freely filtered by the glomerulus and most is reabsorbed in the proximal tubules, with only minimal amounts being excreted in urine.[1,8,14] In chronic liver disease like cirrhosis, lactate clearance is maintained, but in acute liver disease and impaired renal function can contribute to increased blood levels of lactate due to decreased clearance. Acidosis decreases hepatic clearance and may cause increased hepatic lactate production, whereas renal clearance is increased with acidosis.[4,15] In marked hypoperfusion associated with shock, the liver and kidney may switch from lactate consumption to lactate production, emphasizing the importance of reinstating adequate perfusion and oxygen delivery.[1]

Lactate has 2 optical isomers, L-lactate, and its mirror image, D-lactate. L-Lactate is produced almost exclusively in healthy monogastric animals. D-Lactate can come from bacterial fermentation of carbohydrates in the intestinal tract or from alternate metabolic pathways that occur with some toxins or in certain diseases. Increases in D-lactate have been reported in diabetes mellitus and propylene glycol toxicity, or from intestinal bacterial overgrowth (small intestinal dysbiosis).[4,16,17] Routine testing measures only L-lactate concentration. D-Lactic acidosis is sometimes suspected when there is unexplained metabolic acidosis with an increased anion gap and normal L-lactate concentration. D-Lactate can be measured by high-pressure liquid chromatography or mass spectrometry in select laboratories.[17]

CLASSIFICATION OF LACTIC ACIDOSIS

There are 3 types of lactic acidosis. Type A lactic acidosis is more common and occurs when there is tissue hypoperfusion and hypoxia from either decreased oxygen delivery or increased oxygen demand. Shock is an example of hypoperfusion; anemia is an example of decreased oxygen delivery, and seizures are an example of increased oxygen demand (**Box 1**). Type B lactic acidosis occurs when oxygen delivery

Box 1
Causes of lactic acidosis

Type A lactic acidosis

Decreased oxygen delivery

    Hypovolemic, cardiogenic, or septic shock

    Severe anemia (PCV <10%) or severe hypoxemia (Po_2 <30 mm Hg)

    Global or regional hypoperfusion

    Carbon monoxide toxicity

Increased oxygen demand

    Exercise, seizures, uncontrolled shivering

Type B lactic acidosis

Type B_1 (underlying disease)

    Acute liver disease

    Chronic kidney disease (renal failure)

    Hyperthyroidism

    Diabetes mellitus

    Neoplasia

    Sepsis

    Systemic inflammatory response syndrome

    Alkalosis

Type B_2 (drugs or toxins)

    Aceteminophen, salicylates

    Ethylene glycol, propylene glycol

    Catecholamines

    Carbon monoxide

    Bicarbonate

    Others: cyanide, strychnine, nitroprusside, halothane, terbutaline, activated charcoal

Type B_3 (mitochondrial diseases)

    Mitochondrial myopathies

    Mitochondrial encephalomyopathy with lactic acidosis and stroke syndrome (MELAS)

D-Lactic acidosis

Diabetes mellitus

Intestinal bacterial overgrowth (small intestinal dysbiosis)

Exocrine pancreatic insufficiency

Propylene glycol toxicity

Data from Pang DS, Boysen S. Lactate in veterinary critical care: pathophysiology and management. J Am Anim Hosp Assoc 2007;43:273–4; and Allen SE, Holm JL. Lactate: physiology and clinical utility. J Vet Emerg Crit Care 2008;18:125.

is adequate but there is altered carbohydrate metabolism or mitochondrial function. Type B_1 lactic acidosis occurs in acute hepatitis, chronic kidney disease (see **Box 1**), and other diseases associated with decreased lactate clearance. Type B_2 lactic acidosis occurs with some toxins or medications that inhibit oxidative phosphorylation. Type B_3 is the least common form of lactic acidosis and occurs when there are inborn errors of mitochondrial metabolism.[4,8,18–20] As mentioned above, type D-lactic acidosis has been reported in diabetes mellitus, intestinal bacterial overgrowth (small intestinal dysbiosis), exocrine pancreatic insufficiency, and propylene glycol toxicity.[4,16,17]

During classic type A lactic acidosis, there is increased anaerobic glycolysis and accumulation of pyruvate, which cannot enter the mitochondrion for oxidative phosphorylation because of low levels of oxygen. Hypoxia also inhibits the enzyme that converts pyruvate to acetyl coenzyme A for entry into the Krebs cycle and the enzyme that converts pyruvate into oxaloacetate, both of which contribute to an accumulation of pyruvate and the shift of pyruvate metabolism to form lactate. Intracellular lactate concentration increases and is shuttled to the bloodstream via the monocarboxylate transporter.[8,21] There may be features of both type A and type B lactic acidosis in critically ill patients. For example, in sepsis, there may be tissue hypoperfusion, increased metabolism associated with inflammation, diminished lactate clearance, decreased entry of pyruvate into the Krebs cycle, and abnormal mitochondrial function.[1,4]

SAMPLE COLLECTION AND LACTATE ANALYSIS

Lactate is measured in plasma by automated chemistry analyzers or in whole blood by point-of-care (POC) instruments. Although sampling site affects lactate concentration, differences are not clinically relevant.[5] For plasma samples, anti-coagulated blood should be centrifuged and the plasma removed from the RBCs to avoid false increases in lactate concentration because of in vitro metabolism. Plasma samples should be kept at $4°C$ if analysis is delayed for more than 30 minutes for samples collected in heparin.[22] Plasma can be stored longer at $-20°C$, although immediate analysis is useful for most clinical patients. For POC instruments using whole blood, 0.5 to 1.0 mL of venous or arterial blood should be collected in lithium heparin (preferred) or sodium fluoride and samples should be processed immediately.[1,12,23] Recent exercise, seizures, stress, excitement, food intake, and prolonged venous stasis during sample collection can increase lactate concentration 2.5 to 10.0 mmol/L.[1,22] One study showed a transient 10-fold increase in lactate in healthy cats that were stressed before sample collection.[24] However, a more recent study found that struggling during venipuncture caused no statistical differences in lactate concentrations in cats.[25] Increases from exercise, restraint, and seizures typically return to normal within 2 hours.

Lactate can be measured by enzymatic colorimetry or enzymatic amperometry.[1,4] In automated chemistry analyzers, which use enzymatic colorimetry, oxidation of L-lactate is catalyzed by lactic acid dehydrogenase to produce the reduced form of nicotinamide adenine dinucleotide, which is detected by spectrophotometry and is proportional to the sample lactate concentration. Enzymatic amperometry is used in POC instruments because results are available in minutes. The enzymatic activity of lactate oxidase on lactate generates H_2O_2, an electroactive analyte that is oxidized by an electrical potential to generate an electrical current on a platinum electrode that is proportional to the sample lactate concentration.[1,4] POC instruments are useful in critical care and intraoperative settings during which serial lactate measurements guide patient management. Recent studies in people have shown that more rapid turnaround time for lactate results in improved clinical outcomes for critically ill patients.[23] Comparison of lactate values obtained from POC instruments with those determined by automated chemistry analyzers indicate that POC performance is acceptable as long as there is close attention to sample collection and processing and adherence to recommendations for quality control of the instrument.[26,27] However, using the same instrument for repeated measurements is recommended because of differences in methodology and sample requirements.

ANALYTICAL INTERFERENCES

Ethylene glycol exposure may falsely increase plasma lactate concentration measured by some instruments that use enzymatic amperometry, likely because glycolate, a major metabolite of ethylene glycol, is chemically similar to lactate,[28] which is different from propylene glycol intoxication, in which L-lactate and D-lactate are metabolites of propylene glycol.[16] Lactate is one of the main components of lactated Ringer's solution (LRS). The lactate in LRS is metabolized to glucose or is oxidized to water and CO_2, both of which consume H^+ ions and contribute to an overall alkalinizing effect. Administration of LRS does not typically cause an increase in lactate.[1,29–31] Although increased lactate associated with LRS administration has been described in dogs with lymphoma, recent studies are less convincing.[32,33] However, small amounts of LRS in catheters that are not appropriately flushed before sample collection can cause a falsely increased lactate concentration.[4,34] Solutions that do not contain lactate can cause a dilutional effect if the sample is collected from a catheter that is inadequately cleared.

DIAGNOSTIC APPLICATION OF LACTATE CONCENTRATION

Metabolic acidosis is a common disorder in small animal patients, particularly in dogs, and increased lactate concentration causes a significant proportion of high anion gap metabolic acidoses in dogs and cats.[35,36] A study of serial lactate concentrations in systemically ill dogs found that although increases in initial lactate concentrations were not related to outcome, failure of lactate concentration to improve by ≥50% was associated with increased mortality.[11] More targeted studies have evaluated lactate concentrations in specific conditions that cause type A, type B, or D-lactic acidosis in dogs and cats.

Type A Lactic Acidosis

Although tissue hypoperfusion from hypovolemic or cardiogenic shock likely is a common cause of lactic acidosis in dogs and cats, there are few studies in specific subpopulations of animals that show the consistent occurrence of hyperlactatemia and lactic acidosis that has been shown in human patients with shock.[1,10] Lactate levels have been used as a prognostic indicator in people, but prognostic implications may vary with the cause of lactic acidosis. Human patients with hemorrhagic shock and high lactate levels may have a better prognosis than patients with cardiogenic shock and similar lactate levels.[1,37] Lactic acidosis has been used as a prognostic indicator in critically ill human patients with septic shock, and lactate concentration has been used to determine efficacy of interventions in canine models of septic shock.[38] However, evaluation of blood lactate in a cohort of dogs with pyometra failed to demonstrate differences in plasma lactate between affected and control dogs, or between dogs with pyometra with or without evidence of systemic inflammatory response syndrome.[39]

Several studies have evaluated the prognostic value of lactate in dogs with gastric dilatation volvulus, which could cause lactic acidosis because of either regional or systemic hypoperfusion.[40,41] One study found that survival was significantly higher in dogs with an initial lactate concentration ≤9.0 mmol/L. In dogs with a lactate concentration greater than 9.0 mmol/L, there was no difference in mean lactate values between survivors and nonsurvivors, although posttreatment lactate of greater than 6.4 mmol/L or a reduction of ≤4 mmol/L or ≤42.5% was a negative prognostic indicator.[41] In another study, an initial plasma lactate of greater than 6.0 mmol/L failed to predict macroscopic gastric wall necrosis or a negative outcome consistently. However, a greater than 50% reduction in plasma lactate was a positive prognostic indicator.[40] Similarly, a more recent study found that an initial plasma lactate concentration of 7.4 mmol/L was a strong prognostic indicator of gastric necrosis and outcome.[42]

Hypoxemia associated with severe anemia causes type A lactic acidosis. A large retrospective study of dogs with immune-mediated hemolytic anemia found that blood lactate was inversely correlated with PCV and nonsurvivors had higher median blood lactate concentrations at presentation than survivors (4.8 mmol/L vs 2.9). All dogs in which blood lactate normalized by 6 hours survived, whereas 71% of dogs with persistent hyperlactatemia survived, implying that serial monitoring may improve the predictive value of lactate evaluation.[43] Canine babesiosis is another cause of anemia associated with hyperlactatemia. However, the pathophysiology is complex and includes neurologic and respiratory abnormalities as other potential causes of increased lactate. In one cohort of 90 dogs with babesiosis, 50% had increased blood lactate and persistent hyperlactatemia despite therapy as a negative prognostic indicator.[11]

Hypoxemia due to exercise-induced increases in oxygen demand can cause increased blood lactate, and this is a potential source of preanalytical error. However, in a study of healthy Labrador retrievers exercised to exhaustion, there was no significant increase in blood lactate.[44] In another study, lactate levels in agility dogs evaluated immediately, within 2 minutes after, and 4 hours after completing an agility course increased incrementally more in dogs with higher agility immediately after course completion, were close to baseline at the final time point, and all values remained within the reference interval.[45]

Type B Lactic Acidosis

The most common type B lactic acidosis in veterinary species is type B_1 associated with underlying disease. Proposed mechanisms for lactic acidosis in the presence of other diseases include decreased clearance, as in acute hepatic failure or chronic kidney disease, or dysfunctional carbohydrate metabolism, as in hyperthyroidism and sepsis, but multiple mechanisms likely occur, including combinations of type B and type A lactic acidosis. Serum lactate concentrations were higher in hyperthyroid cats compared with diabetic or control cats, possibly related to increased rates of glucose use.[46] Neoplasia has been implicated as a cause of hyperlactatemia, but the veterinary medical literature does not support a strong association. In a retrospective study of dogs with intracranial disease or intervertebral disc disease anesthetized for advanced imaging or surgery revealed that dogs with meningioma or hydrocephalus had higher lactate concentrations than dogs with intervertebral disc disease. However, only one dog with meningioma had clinically significant hyperlactatemia.[47] One prospective study of 37 dogs with various hematopoietic or solid tumors failed to identify increased lactate concentrations and concluded that neoplasia is associated with an increase in lactate only in rare or complicated cases.[48] A more focused retrospective study of 55 dogs with lymphoma observed hyperlactatemia in 40%, but the authors concluded that only 5 had cancer-related increases, and the authors reported that the mean blood lactate concentration in dogs with lymphoma was not statistically different from their normal value of 2.5 mmol/L.[49]

As discussed previously, exposure to exogenous compounds such as ethylene and propylene glycol may be associated with type B_2 hyperlactatemia. A prospective cross-over study of healthy adult Beagles demonstrated significantly increased blood lactate levels 4 and 14 days after receiving daily anti-inflammatory (1 mg/kg) and immunosuppressive (4 mg/kg) oral prednisone.[49] Although not directly evaluated, corticosteroid-mediated increases in gluconeogenesis from protein and enhanced use of glucose were implicated as mechanisms for the modest but significant increase greater than 2.5 mmol/L. Type B_3 hyperlactatemia seems to be rare in dogs and cats.[50] However, increased lactate was reported in a Sussex spaniel with pyruvate dehydrogenase deficiency.[51]

D-Lactic Acidosis

Marked increases in blood and urine D-lactic acid with normal blood L-lactate were reported in a cat with exocrine pancreatic insufficiency.[7] Cats with gastrointestinal disease have increased blood D-lactate compared with healthy control cats, whereas L-lactate levels were not significantly different in sick cats.[17] In cats with gastrointestinal disease, D-lactate concentrations were not correlated with the presence of neurologic abnormalities or the results of other gastrointestinal function tests, such as pancreatic lipase immunoreactivity, trypsin-like immunoreactivity, or serum cobalamin and folate levels.[17] In propylene glycol intoxication, the L-lactate metabolite is metabolized much faster than the D-lactate metabolite, which may result in persistent metabolic acidosis from D-lactate, which typically is not measured.[16]

LACTATE CONCENTRATION IN OTHER BODY FLUIDS

Lactate concentration has been evaluated in other body fluids as an indication of sepsis or neoplasia. Lactate concentrations are higher in abdominal fluid in dogs and cats with septic peritonitis than in those with nonseptic or nonneoplastic effusions.[52–54] In dogs, fluid lactate levels of greater than 5.5 mmol/L or a difference of greater than 2 mmol/L between fluid and peripheral blood lactate are suggestive of bacterial peritonitis.[52] Dogs with neoplastic effusions have higher abdominal fluid lactate concentrations than dogs with nonneoplastic effusions but lactate levels in pericardial fluid are not as helpful in differentiating neoplastic from nonneoplastic effusions.[55,56]

SUMMARY

Lactate forms primarily during anaerobic glycolysis. Lactate concentration is used clinically as an indicator of tissue hypoperfusion and hypoxia, particularly in critical care or perioperative settings, to determine the severity of an underlying disorder, assess response to therapy, and predict outcome. Serial determination of lactate levels may be more helpful than a single lactate concentration. Decreasing levels of lactate suggest improvement, whereas prolonged increases in lactate concentration imply deterioration with a poor prognosis. Repeated lactate concentrations should be determined on the same instrument with close attention to sample collection and processing and adherence to recommendations for instrument quality control.

REFERENCES

1. Pang DS, Boysen S. Lactate in veterinary critical care: pathophysiology and management. J Am Anim Hosp Assoc 2007;43:270–9.

2. Shapiro BA, Peruzzi WT. Interpretation of blood gases. In: Ayres SM, Grenvik A, Holbrook PR, et al, editors. Textbook of critical care. 3rd edition. Philadelphia: WB Saunders; 1995. p. 278–94.
3. Tonnessen TI. Intracellular pH and electrolyte regulation. In: Ayres SM, Grenvik A, Holbrook PR, et al, editors. Textbook of critical care. 3rd edition. Philadelphia: WB Saunders; 1995. p. 172–87.
4. Allen SE, Holm JL. Lactate: physiology and clinical utility. J Vet Emerg Crit Care 2008;18:123–32.
5. Hughes D, Rozanski ER, Shofer FS, et al. Effect of sampling site, repeated sampling, pH, and PCO2 on plasma lactate concentrations in healthy dogs. Am J Vet Res 1999;60:521–4.
6. McMichael MA, Lees GE, Hennessey J, et al. Serial plasma lactate concentrations in 68 puppies aged 4 to 80 days. J Vet Emerg Crit Care 2005;15: 17–21.
7. Packer RA, Cohn LA, Wohlstadter DR, et al. D-Lactic acidosis secondary to exocrine pancreatic insufficiency in a cat. J Vet Intern Med 2005;19:106–10.
8. Vernon C, LeTourneau JL. Lactic acidosis: recognition, kinetics, and associated prognosis. Crit Care Clin 2010;26:255–83.
9. dePapp E, Drobatz KJ, Hughes D. Plasma lactate concentration as a predictor of gastric necrosis and survival among dogs with gastric dilatation-volvulus: 102 cases (1995–1998). J Am Vet Med Assoc 1999;215(1):49–52.
10. Lagutchik MS, Ogilvie GK, Hackett TB, et al. Increased lactate concentrations in ill and injured dogs. J Vet Emerg Crit Care 1998;8:117–27.
11. Nel M, Lobetti RG, Keller N, et al. Prognostic value of blood lactate, blood glucose, and hematocrit in canine babesiosis. J Vet Intern Med 2004;18: 471–6.
12. Mathews KA. Monitoring fluid therapy and complications of fluid therapy. In: DiBartola SP, editor. Fluid, electrolyte, and acid-base disorders in small animal practice. 4th edition. St Louis (MO): Elsevier Saunders; 2012. p. 386–404.
13. Madias NE. Lactic acidosis. Kidney Int 1986;29:752–74.
14. Yudkin J, Cohen RD. The contribution of the kidney to the removal of a lactic acid load under normal and acidotic conditions in the conscious rat. Clin Sci Mol Med 1975;48:121–31.
15. Record CO, Iles RA, Cohen RD, et al. Acid-base and metabolic disturbances in fulminant hepatic failure. Gut 1975;16(2):144–9.
16. Claus MA, Jandrey KE, Poppenga RH. Propylene glycol intoxication in a dog. J Vet Emerg Crit Care 2011;21:679–83.
17. Packer RA, Moore GE, Chang CY, et al. Serum D-lactate concentrations in cats with gastrointestinal disease. J Vet Intern Med 2012;26:905–10.
18. Kruse JA, Carlson RW. Lactate metabolism. Crit Care Clin 1987;5(4):725–46.
19. Luft FC. Lactic acidosis update for critical care clinicians. J Am Soc Nephrol 2001;12:S15–9.
20. Mizock BA, Falk JL. Lactic acidosis in critical illness. Crit Care Med 1992;20(1): 80–93.
21. Stryer L. Oxidative phosphorylation. In: Stryer L, editor. Biochemistry. 4th edition. New York: WH Freeman and Company; 1995. p. 529–58.
22. Lagutchik MS. Lactate. In: Vade SL, Knoll JS, Smith FW, et al, editors. Blackwell's five-minute veterinary consult: laboratory tests and diagnostic procedures. Ames (IA): Wiley-Blackwell Publishing; 2009. p. 388–9.
23. Karon BS, Scott R, Burritt MF, et al. Comparison of lactate values between point-of care and central laboratory analyzers. Am J Clin Pathol 2007;128:168–71.

24. Rand JS, Kinnaird E, Baglioni A, et al. Acute stress hyperglycemia in cats is associated with struggling and increased concentrations of lactate and norepinephrine. J Vet Intern Med 2002;16:123–32.

25. Redavid LA, Sharp CR, Mitchell MA, et al. Plasma lactate measurement in healthy cats. J Vet Emerg Crit Care 2012;22:580–7.

26. Karagiannis MH, Mann FA, Madsen RW, et al. Comparison of two portable lactate meters in dogs. J Am Anim Hosp Assoc 2013;49:8–15.

27. Thorneloe C, Bedard C, Boysen S. Evaluation of a hand held lactate analyzer in dogs. Can Vet J 2007;48:283–7.

28. Hopper K. Falsely increased plasma lactate concentration due to ethylene glycol poisoning in 2 dogs. J Vet Emerg Crit Care 2013;23:63–7.

29. Didwania A, Miller J, Kassel D, et al. Effect of intravenous lactated ringer's solution infusion on the circulating lactate concentration: part 3. Results of a prospective, randomized, double-blind, placebo-controlled trial. Crit Care Med 1997;25(11):1851–4.

30. Pascoe PJ. Perioperative management of fluid therapy. In: DiBartola SP, editor. Fluid, electrolyte, and acid-base disorders in small animal practice. 3rd edition. St Louis (MO): Elsevier; 2006. p. 391–419.

31. Us MH, Ozcan S, Oral L, et al. Comparison of the effects of hypertonic saline and crystalloid infusions on haemodynamic parameters during haemorrhagic shock in dogs. J Int Med Res 2001;29:508–15.

32. Vail DM, Ogilvie GK, Fettman MJ, et al. Exacerbation of hyperlactemia by infusion of lactated ringer's solution in dogs with lymphoma. J Vet Intern Med 1990; 4(5):228–32.

33. Touret M, Boysen SR, Nadeau ME. Retrospective evaluation of potential causes associated with clinically relevant hyperlactatemia in dogs with lymphoma. Can Vet J 2012;53:511–7.

34. Jackson EV, Wiese J, Sigal B, et al. Effects of crystalloid solutions on circulating lactate concentrations: part I. Implications for the proper handling of blood specimens obtained from critically ill patients. Crit Care Med 1997;25(11): 1840–6.

35. Hopper K, Epstein SE. Incidence, nature, and etiology of metabolic acidosis in dogs and cats. J Vet Intern Med 2012;26:1107–14.

36. Stevenson CK, Kidney BA, Duke T, et al. Serial blood lactate concentrations in systemically ill dogs. Vet Clin Pathol 2007;36:234–9.

37. Vitek V, Cowle RA. Blood lactate in the prognosis of various forms of shock. Ann Surg 1971;173:308–13.

38. Hicks CW, Sweeney DA, Danner RL, et al. Efficacy of selective mineralocorticoid and glucocorticoid agonists in canine septic shock. Crit Care Med 2012;40: 199–207.

39. Hagman R, Reezigt BJ, Ledin HB, et al. Blood lactate levels in 31 female dogs with pyometra. Acta Vet Scand 2009;51:2–9.

40. Green TI, Tonozzi CC, Kirby R, et al. Evaluation of initial plasma lactate values as a predictor of gastric necrosis and initial and subsequent plasma lactate values as a predictor of survival in dogs with gastric dilatation-volvulus: 84 dogs (2003-2007). J Vet Emerg Crit Care 2011;21:36–44.

41. Zacher LA, Berg J, Shaw SP, et al. Association between outcome and changes in plasma lactate concentration during presurgical treatment in dogs with gastric dilatation-volvulus; 64 cases. J Am Vet Med Assoc 2010;236:892–7.

42. Beer KA, Syring RS, Drobatz KJ. Evaluation of plasma lactate concentration and base excess at the time of hospital admission as predictors of gastric necrosis

and outcome and correlation between those variables in dogs with gastric dilatation-volvulus: 78 cases (2004-2009). J Am Vet Med Assoc 2013;242:54–8.

43. Holahan ML, Brown AJ, Drobatz KJ. The association of blood lactate concentration with outcome in dogs with idiopathic immune-mediated hemolytic anemia: 173 cases. J Vet Emerg Crit Care 2010;20:413–20.

44. Ferasin L, Marcora S. Reliability of an incremental exercise test to evaluate acute blood lactate, heart rate, and body temperature responses in Labrador Retrievers. J Comp Physiol B 2009;179:839–45.

45. Baltzer WI, Firshman AM, Stang B, et al. The effect of agility exercise on eicosanoid excretion, oxidant status, and plasma lactate in dogs. BMC Vet Res 2012; 8:249–59.

46. Christopher MM, O'Neill S. Effect of specimen collection and storage on blood glucose and lactate concentrations in healthy, hyperthyroid and diabetic cats. Vet Clin Pathol 2000;29:22–8.

47. Sullivan LA, Campbell VL, Klopp LS, et al. Blood lactate concentrations in anesthetized dogs with intracranial disease. J Vet Intern Med 2009;23:488–92.

48. Touret M, Boysen SR, Nadeau ME. Prospective evaluation of clinically relevant type B hyperlactatemia in dogs with cancer. J Vet Intern Med 2010;24:1458–61.

49. Boysen SR, Bozzetti M, Rose L, et al. Effects of prednisone on blood lactate concentrations in healthy dogs. J Vet Intern Med 2009;23:1123–5.

50. Shelton GD. Routine and specialized laboratory testing for the diagnosis of neuromuscular diseases in dogs and cats. Vet Clin Pathol 2010;39:278–95.

51. Abramson CJ, Platt SR, Shelton GD. Pyruvate dehydrogenase deficiency in a Sussex spaniel. J Small Anim Pract 2004;45:162–5.

52. Bonczynski JJ, Ludwig LL, Tarton LF, et al. Comparison of peritoneal fluid and peripheral blood pH, bicarbonate, glucose and lactate concentrations a diagnostic tool for septic peritonitis in dogs and cats. Vet Surg 2003;32:161–6.

53. Levin GM, Bonczynski JJ, Ludwig LL, et al. Lactate as a diagnostic test for septic peritoneal effusions in dogs and cats. J Am Anim Hosp Assoc 2004; 40:364–71.

54. Swann H, Hughes D. Use of abdominal fluid pH, pO2, [glucose], and [lactate] to differentiate bacterial peritonitis from non-bacterial causes of abdominal effusion in dogs and cats. Proceed International Veterinary Emergency and Critical Care Society Meeting. San Antonio (TX): 1996. p. 884.

55. Nestor DD, McCullough SM, Schaeffer DJ. Biochemical analysis of neoplastic versus nonneoplastic abdominal effusions in dogs. J Am Anim Hosp Assoc 2004;40:372–5.

56. de Laforcade AM, Freeman LM, Rozanski EA, et al. Biochemical analysis of pericardial fluid and whole blood in dogs with pericardial effusion. J Vet Intern Med 2005;19:833–6.

Diagnosis of Disorders of Iron Metabolism in Dogs and Cats

Andrea A. Bohn, DVM, PhD

KEYWORDS

- Anemia of chronic disease • Ferritin • Hemochromatosis • Inflammation
- Iron deficiency • Percent saturation • Transferrin

KEY POINTS

- Serum iron concentration is often not an accurate reflection of body iron stores.
- Serum iron concentration decreases with inflammation and iron deficiency.
- Ferritin is currently the best assay for body iron stores.
- Low ferritin indicates iron deficiency; normal ferritin does not rule it out.
- Care must be taken when interpreting levels of ferritin and transferrin because they are acute-phase proteins and inflammation can affect results.
- On a hemogram, MCV_{retic} and CH_{retic} may indicate iron deficiency before MCV and mean cell hemoglobin concentration.

REVIEW OF NORMAL IRON METABOLISM

Function

Iron is an essential element and is used by every cell in the body. Although iron is instrumental in oxygen transport and erythropoiesis, it is also necessary for numerous enzymatic reactions and is important in energy metabolism, DNA synthesis, and cellular immune responses.[1] Contrary to its importance, iron can also cause cell damage with the formation of reactive oxygen species; therefore, its regulation is tightly controlled.[2]

Location

Most total body iron is found within heme, predominantly as hemoglobin of erythroid cells and myoglobin of muscle with lesser amounts within enzymatic hemoproteins. A significant amount of total body iron can also be in storage. Within cells, the most important iron storage protein is ferritin. Much of stored iron is present within

This article originally appeared in Veterinary Clinics of North America: Small Animal Practice, Volume 43, Issue 6, November 2013.
Disclosures: The author has nothing to disclose.
Department of Microbiology, Immunology, and Pathology, College of Veterinary Medicine and Biomedical Sciences, Colorado State University, 1619 Campus Delivery, Fort Collins, CO 80523, USA
E-mail address: andrea.bohn@colostate.edu

hepatocytes. Macrophages in the spleen, liver, and bone marrow can also store large quantities of iron. Hemosiderin, formed by partial degradation of ferritin, is less soluble and may become more abundant than ferritin when iron stores are high.[3]

Plasma Iron

Very little iron (<0.1% of total body iron) is actually in circulation. This iron is mostly bound to the iron transport protein, transferrin, and is turned over multiple times each day. Iron circulating in plasma is predominantly recycled iron from senescent erythrocytes that have been phagocytized by reticuloendothelial macrophages. Only a small amount of plasma iron comes from ingestion, which is the only natural route for taking iron into the body.[1] Small amounts of iron are routinely lost with the shedding of enterocytes, uroepithelial cells, and skin cells and can also occur with blood loss and sweating. Normally, the amount of iron loss about equals the amount absorbed from diet.[2]

Regulation

The regulation of body iron content occurs at the level of absorption by enterocytes because there are no known significant routes of excretion. The amount of iron that is absorbed from diet is controlled by the iron regulatory hormone hepcidin, which works as a negative regulator. It has recently been shown that the acute effect of increased hepcidin concentration is proteosomal-mediated degradation of DMT1, the apical transporter, which normally allows inorganic iron to enter the enterocyte from the intestinal lumen (**Fig. 1**).[4] Therefore, when hepcidin concentrations are elevated, less iron is able to enter the enterocyte, whereas at low hepcidin concentrations, DMT1 is available for transport.

After iron is absorbed by enterocytes from the intestinal lumen, this iron cannot be released to the systemic circulation without a different membrane transport protein on the basolateral membrane of the enterocyte, called ferroportin (see **Fig. 1**). How much ferroportin is available for transport is also dependent on hepcidin concentrations; more ferroportin is available with low hepcidin concentrations and less ferroportin with high hepcidin.

Hephaestin is a ferroxidase expressed on the basolateral membrane of duodenal enterocytes and associated with ferroportin (see **Fig. 1**). Its only known function is to mediate the reoxidation of Fe^{2+} to Fe^{3+} as iron leaves the enterocyte. Exported iron is immediately bound to transferrin for transport through the circulation. Transferrin is a glycoprotein with high affinity for one to two Fe^{3+} ions.

The general mechanism by which hepcidin has been shown to decrease ferroportin numbers has been by binding to ferroportin, which results in internalization and degradation of the membrane transport protein, although new data suggest that hepcidin may influence ferroportin expression on enterocytes by an alternative route, possibly at the level of translation.[4] In addition to enterocytes, ferroportin is also present in the membranes of hepatocytes and macrophages. Ferroportin is the only known membrane protein that exports inorganic iron from mammalian cells and hepcidin seems to be the principal factor in determining ferroportin numbers. Hepcidin, therefore, not only affects serum iron concentration through its effects on enterocytes, but also causes sequestration of iron within macrophages and hepatocytes, preventing efflux of iron into plasma (**Fig. 2**).

The factors that influence the concentration of hepcidin (and, therefore, the extracellular movement of iron) include iron status and the amount of body iron stores, tissue hypoxia, erythropoiesis, and inflammation.[5] Plentiful iron and inflammation result in increased hepcidin transcription, whereas anemia, hypoxia, and iron deficiency suppress its expression. An excellent review of hepcidin has recently been published.[5]

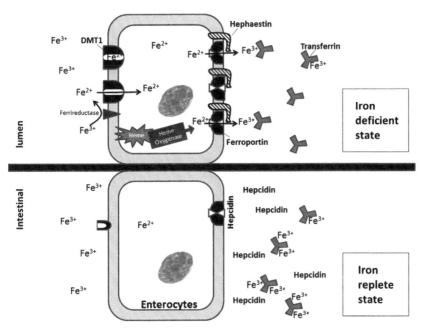

Fig. 1. In the small intestine, iron is absorbed into enterocytes through the apical transmembrane transporter, DMT-1 (*top*). Ferric iron is reduced to the ferrous state before transport. Iron is transported from the cell into circulation through a different transmembrane protein on the basolateral membrane of the enterocyte, called ferroportin. Immediately, ferrous iron is reoxidized to the ferric state by hephaestin, a multicopper feroxidase, and then bound to transferrin. In the presence of hepcidin, degradation and decreased expression of DMT-1 and ferroportin result in decreased ability of iron to enter the enterocyte and systemic circulation (*bottom*). Modifying the amount of iron absorbed by enterocytes is the primary mechanism for regulation of body iron content because no excretory pathways are known.

Understanding the homeostatic regulation of iron is important to understand the pathogenesis of diseases associated with iron metabolism and the limitations on different assays of iron status.

ASSAYS USED IN THE ASSESSMENT OF IRON STATUS

Assays to directly assess iron status include the measurement of serum iron concentration, ferritin concentration, and transferrin.

Serum Iron Concentration

In general, serum iron concentration is not an accurate indication of whole body iron status because it represents such a small fraction of total body iron (<0.1%) and is influenced by numerous other factors. This transport component of iron can increase with hemolysis, iron supplementation, recent blood transfusions, a decrease in erythropoietic uptake during hypoplastic or aplastic anemia, exogenous administration of corticosteroids, and liver disease.[3] In addition to iron deficiency, serum iron concentration can decrease with inflammation, hypoproteinemia, hypothyroidism, and renal disease.

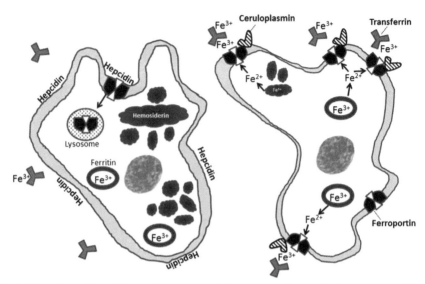

Fig. 2. The effect of hepcidin on iron transport from macrophages. In the presence of hepcidin (*left*) ferroportin is internalized and degraded by lysosomes, resulting in the sequestration of stored iron within the cell. At low concentrations of hepcidin, ferroportin is present in the cell membrane, allowing the exportation of iron (*right*). Immediately after leaving the cell, ferrous iron is reoxidized to the ferric state by ceruloplasmin, a multicopper feroxidase, and then bound to transferrin.

Ferritin

Ferritin is considered to be a better indication of total body iron content and is accurate in health. Unfortunately, it is also an acute-phase reactant and therefore levels increase with inflammation. A serum ferritin concentration below the reference interval indicates iron deficiency. Not all cases of iron deficiency, however, have a low ferritin concentration, especially if inflammation is present. Serum ferritin concentrations above the reference interval may be associated with either iron overload or with inflammation. One should consider measuring the concentration of other acute phase proteins concurrently to help with the interpretation of ferritin concentration. The ferritin assay is an enzyme-linked immunosorbent assay that is species specific; it is offered commercially by the Kansas State Veterinary Diagnostic Laboratory.

Transferrin

Transferrin is indirectly measured and reported as total iron binding capacity (TIBC). Transferrin may increase in the face of iron deficiency but is often normal. Elevated levels have been associated with iron overload and dogs with chronic liver disease.[3] Transferrin is a negative-phase reactant, so changes associated with iron deficiency can potentially be masked by inflammation. Inflammation is typically associated with decreased or low normal transferrin concentrations.

Percent Saturation

The ratio of serum iron concentration to TIBC is reported as percent saturation (%sat), which is the percentage of the TIBC that is actually occupied by iron. Normal %sat is typically between 20% and 50%. Factors that affect serum iron concentration and

TIBC also affect %sat. A %sat less than 20% is suggestive of iron deficiency. Hemochromatosis patients typically have a %sat greater than 50%.

Tissue Iron Concentration

Tissue iron concentration can be subjectively or quantitatively determined by collecting tissue from the bone marrow, liver, or spleen for cytologic or histologic examination or it can be quantitatively determined by submitting tissue to a laboratory for measurement of iron, typically on a dry-weight basis. These techniques are more invasive and are therefore less commonly performed. Cytology and histology preparations can be stained with Prussian blue stain, which highlights iron that is in the form of hemosiderin. It must be remembered that cats normally do not contain hemosiderin in their bone marrow and therefore a lack of staining is not significant in this species.

Other Assays Not Yet Available in Veterinary Medicine

In people, measuring the soluble form of the transferrin receptor 1 (sTfR1) has been very helpful in differentiating iron deficiency anemia from anemia of chronic disease. sTfR1 increases with the increased iron demand of erythropoiesis and is not affected by inflammation. It is typically used in a ratio with log serum ferritin for analysis.[2] Unfortunately, the ability to make an assay for sTfR1 for veterinary species has been elusive.

Serum hepcidin has not replaced any of the other measures of iron status in people, but its measurement in blood and urine has helped the investigation of disease pathogenesis and its central role in iron regulation could be a target for treatment of anemia and iron-overload disorders in the future.[6] Along with the other measures of iron status, hepcidin may still prove to be useful in guiding therapeutic decisions. Although hepcidin and ferritin typically respond similarly to inflammation and iron availability, changes in hepcidin concentrations occur faster than those of ferritin. In addition, aberrant response patterns may occur if an abnormality in hepcidin concentration is the cause of a disorder.[5]

ASSESSMENT OF IRON STATUS IN DISEASES ASSOCIATED WITH IRON METABOLISM

Diseases associated with iron metabolism are associated with either excess or insufficient iron availability. This could be caused by alterations in either total iron body content or in the physiologic availability of iron despite total iron body content.

Iron Deficiency

Causation
Lack of adequate body iron content (iron depletion) is uncommon, especially in cats, but can be seen in young, nursing animals that deplete their body iron stores as they grow because of the low iron content of milk.[3] Typically, the only way an adult animal on a commercial diet becomes iron depleted is because of chronic blood loss. This is most often associated with gastrointestinal bleeding (eg, bleeding tumors, such as leiomyoma, leiomyosarcoma, and carcinoma; or gastric ulceration, often from ulcerogenic drugs including corticosteroids and nonsteroidal anti-inflammatory drugs). Ectoparasites (fleas) and endoparasites (hookworms, whipworms) can also cause iron deficiency, especially in puppies and kittens. The urinary tract is another possible location for occult blood loss. Rarely, coagulopathies may lead to chronic blood loss from these sites. When iron becomes depleted, less is available for erythropoiesis, eventually resulting in anemia.

Iron assays

Expected findings associated with iron deficiency include decreased serum iron concentration, decreased ferritin concentration, normal or possibly elevated TIBC, and low %sat (**Table 1**). Results of assays for iron status must be interpreted with a patient's history, clinical findings, and other laboratory results given the potential confounding factors that can influence these values. Serum iron is often low in animals without iron deficiency, especially when inflammation is present. Ferritin concentration may be within normal limits in the face of iron deficiency if an inflammatory process is present.

Hematology

Iron deficiency anemia is often not recognized until a complete blood count reveals microcytosis or hypochromasia (**Table 2**). As a note, red blood cells from kittens and puppies are normally macrocytic or normocytic, not microcytic, at birth. Given the long half-life of erythrocytes, it takes weeks to months to accumulate a sufficient number of microcytes to shift the average erythrocyte size (mean corpuscular volume [MCV]) below the normal reference interval.[3] Red cell distribution width (RDW) is often increased because of the combination of microcytic and normocytic erythrocytes in circulation. Mean cell hemoglobin concentration (MCHC) may be normal or decreased. The overall amount of hemoglobin an erythrocyte contains may be decreased, but its concentration may be within normal limits given the cell's smaller size.

The evaluation of histograms or scattergrams from hematology analyzers can also be useful in providing evidence of iron deficiency, possibly detecting a shift toward microcytosis before the MCV becomes abnormal. Two instrument printouts demonstrating this shift are shown in **Fig. 3**.

Blood film review may also detect erythrocyte morphology that has been associated with iron deficiency anemia. Hypochromasia is caused by decreased hemoglobin concentration and is recognized when an erythrocyte contains a thin, pale red rim around an enlarged area of central pallor (**Fig. 4**). Be careful not to misinterpret "punched out" cells as hypochromic; these cells have had their hemoglobin pushed peripherally,

Table 1								
Expected results in disorders of iron metabolism								
Disorder	Serum Iron	TIBC	%sat	Ferritin	Bone Marrow Iron	MCV	MCHC	Hepcidin
Iron deficiency anemia	Low	N/high	Low	Low	Low	Low	N/low	Low
Anemia of chronic disease	Low	N/low	N/low	N/high	High	N	N	High
Acute inflammation	Low	N/low	N/low	N/high	N	N	N	High
Hemolytic anemia	High	N/low	High	High	N	N/high	N/low	Low
Portosystemic shunt	Low	N/low	N/low	N/high	N	Low	Low	?
Acute iron poisoning	High	N	High	N	N	N	N	High
Hemochromatosis	High	Low	High	High	High	N	N	High

Abbreviations: MCHC, mean cell hemoglobin concentration; MCV, mean corpuscular volume; N, normal (within reference interval); TIBC, total iron binding capacity; ?, unknown.

Table 2
Erythrogram from an 8-week-old Bernese mountain dog that presented with respiratory distress and anorexia[a]

Hemogram	Patient		Reference Interval
PCV	23	Low	40%–55%
RDW	18.6	High	12–15
MCV	50	Low	62–73 fl
MCHC	25	Low	33–36 g/dL
Reticulocytes	234,500	High	0–60,000/ul
CH_{retic}	15.8	Low	22.3–27.9 pg
MCV_{retic}	61	Low	77.8–100.2 fl

Hemopathology consists of hypochromasia, polychromasia, keratocytes, and schistocytes (see **Fig. 4**).

Abbreviations: MCHC, mean cell hemoglobin concentration; MCV, mean corpuscular volume; PCV, packed cell volume; RDW, red cell distribution width.

[a] The abnormalities present indicate iron deficiency anemia.

creating a larger central pallor, but with a thick, dark red rim of hemoglobin. Poikilocytosis has also been associated with iron deficiency anemia, especially keratocytes and schistocytes in dogs (see **Fig. 4**).

Reticulocyte indices
Evaluation of reticulocyte indices is known to be useful in detection of iron deficiency in people and may provide earlier recognition of iron deficiency anemia in dogs and cats. Because reticulocytes have a short life span in circulation of only approximately 2 days (compared with the life span of erythrocytes of 70 days [cats] or 120 days [dogs]), their hemoglobin content better reflects the recent functional availability of iron for erythropoiesis.[7,8] These indices are determined by the larger hematology analyzers used at reference laboratories and have shown likely value in veterinary medicine.[9–11] The hemoglobin content of reticulocytes (CH_{retic}) and average size of reticulocytes (MCV_{retic}) were associated with other indications of iron deficiency in these studies. In people, CH_{retic} seems to be the most sensitive indicator of iron deficiency.[7] Using receiver operating characteristic curve analysis, Prins and colleagues[11] found cut-off points (1.22 fmol in dogs and 0.88 fmol in cats) at which CH_{retic} was 95.2% and 93.8% sensitive and 90.5% and 76.9% specific for iron deficiency in dogs and cats, respectively. Specificity of low MCV_{retic} and CH_{retic} for iron deficiency has not been fully evaluated but observations by the author suggest that, not surprisingly, inflammatory processes can also result in decreased reticulocyte indices. Although more studies are needed to assess the use of CH_{retic} and MCV_{retic} in cats and dogs, their ability to reflect "real-time" iron availability is likely valuable and, when available in a complete blood count panel, CH_{retic} and MCV_{retic} should be monitored for possible iron-deficient states in veterinary patients (see **Table 2**).

Iron-refractory iron deficiency
Iron deficiency that is refractory to iron supplementation has been reported in humans with genetic defects in hepcidin or ferroportin. There was a recent mention of an unpublished case of a cocker spaniel with iron-refractory iron deficiency.[12] This case involved a defect in a regulatory protein (*Tmprss6*) that normally responds to iron deficiency by downregulating hepcidin.

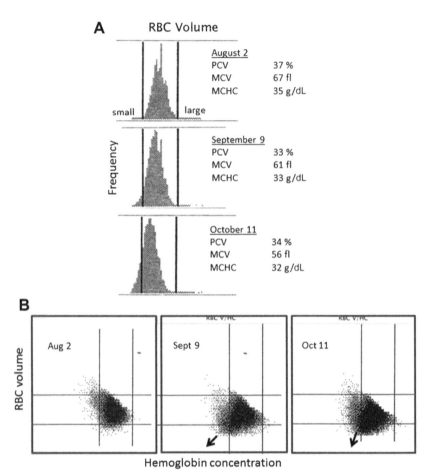

Fig. 3. Print-outs from an Advia 120 hematology analyzer showing the frequency histograms (*A*) and volume/HC scattergrams (*B*) for erythrocytes from the blood of a dog that developed iron deficiency. Samples were drawn approximately 1 month apart; values for packed cell volume (PCV), mean corpuscular volume (MCV), and mean cell hemoglobin concentration (MCHC) on each date are shown in (*A*). In (*A*), the *dark vertical lines* depict the lower and upper limits of normal erythrocyte size. As the dog becomes iron deficient, the histogram shifts to the left, indicating the presence of smaller erythrocytes. In (*B*), the *vertical lines* depict the lower and upper limits of normal hemoglobin concentration and the *horizontal lines* depict normal erythrocyte volume. As cells become smaller and contain less hemoglobin, the erythrocyte population shifts down and to the left, respectively. RBC, red blood cell.

Anemia of Inflammation (Anemia of Chronic Disease)

Causation

Lack of available iron despite adequate body stores is commonly associated with inflammation. This has been associated with the hepcidin hormone, which is increased by inflammatory cytokines. It is thought to be a protective mechanism by denying essential nutrients to infectious organisms. The increase in hepcidin causes degradation of ferroportin, which results in poor absorption of enteric iron and sequestration of stored iron within macrophages, which lead to low circulating iron concentrations (see

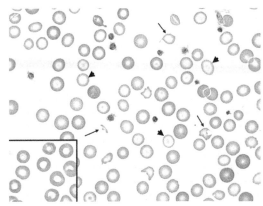

Fig. 4. Blood film from an 8-week-old Bernese mountain dog that presented with respiratory distress (probable distemper), anorexia, and diarrhea. The hemogram is indicative of iron deficiency; microcytosis is present (see **Table 2**). Hypochromasia is evident (*arrowheads*) and poikilocytosis is present, including keratocytes and schistocytes (*arrows*). The inset is blood from a dog that is not iron deficient and has "punched out" erythrocytes rather than hypochromatic cells. Note the thick, dark rim of hemoglobin with a crisp line surrounding the pale central area where hemoglobin has been pushed peripherally rather than decreased in content. The iron deficiency anemia was likely multifactorial, including poor stores caused by the dog's young age, decreased intake, and decreased gastrointestinal absorption or gastrointestinal hemorrhage caused by concurrent gastrointestinal disease.

Fig. 2, left). This gives rise to functional iron deficiency and contributes to the development of anemia.

Iron assays
Whether acute or chronic, inflammation results in low serum iron concentrations (see **Table 2**). In addition, as acute-phase proteins, transferrin decreases and ferritin increases with inflammation. Therefore, differentiating anemia of inflammation and iron deficiency anemia is often challenging because inflammation masks some of the changes typically seen with iron deficiency.

Classically, anemia of inflammation is characterized by increased iron stores, in contrast to iron deficiency anemia, which has decreased stores. Anemia of inflammation is therefore expected to have increased ferritin concentrations. TIBC and %sat are typically within normal limits or may be low.

Hemochromatosis

Causation
Iron overload can result in increased iron stores. Hemosiderosis is an increase in tissue iron stores without associated tissue damage, whereas hemochromatosis is defined as tissue damage and dysfunction from the deposition of hemosiderin in parenchymal cells.[13] Iron overload is not a common problem in small animals, but is possible with multiple blood transfusions or excess dietary iron. One case of hemochromatosis has been reported in a dog after several years of blood transfusions.[14] Hemochromatosis has also been recognized as a sequela to pyruvate kinase deficiency, likely caused by increased intestinal iron absorption associated with active hemolytic anemia.[15–17] There is a similar sequela in cats with chronic intermittent severe hemolytic anemia in which pathologic liver changes have been described.[18] Although

dogs and cats seem relatively resistant to developing iron overload, the point at which too much iron causes a problem is unknown.

Iron assays
In people at risk for hemochromatosis, the standard way to monitor total iron body stores has been biopsy of the liver for iron quantification. Imaging modalities have more recently been developed to estimate liver iron concentration.[19] Ferritin has been used as a screening test for clinically significant iron overload in people, although ferritin concentrations do not correlate well with liver iron concentration and causes of elevated levels are nonspecific.[20] It has been determined, however, that cirrhosis of the liver generally does not occur in people with ferritin concentrations less than 1000 µg/L.[21] Unfortunately, ferritin concentrations have not been reported in small animal species with hemochromatosis and therefore no guidelines or cut-off values exist. It is recommended that %sat be taken into account when interpreting ferritin concentrations because %sat should also be elevated with hemochromatosis.[22] Expected abnormalities associated with hemochromatosis are shown in **Table 1**.

Portosystemic Shunt Microcytosis

Causation
The microcytosis associated with congenital or acquired portosystemic shunt is attributed to altered iron metabolism, although the exact mechanism is unknown.

Iron assays
In general, serum iron concentration is decreased, ferritin is normal to high, and TIBC is normal to low, similar to anemia of inflammation (see **Table 1**).

Copper Deficiency
Copper deficiency is associated with anemia in mammals. Typically, the anemia has been described as either microcytic or normocytic.

Causation
Copper deficiency is more of a problem in large animals, but there is one case report of suspected deficiency caused by long-term copper chelation in a dog.[23] In addition, puppies developed copper deficiency after being fed a copper-restricted diet for several months.[24] These dogs had a decrease in serum copper concentration, in ceruloplasmin oxidase activity, in hemoglobin concentration, and in PCV. Copper deficiency is thought to result in functional iron deficiency with or without iron depletion because of the importance of the copper-containing proteins hephaestin and ceruloplasmin for iron transport. Copper deficiency has been shown to result in decreased release of iron from enterocytes to plasma and from tissue iron stores.[3]

Iron assays
Presumably serum iron concentration is low as a result of copper deficiency in dogs and cats. It may be difficult to predict expected changes in iron stores because species variation exists.[3]

REFERENCES

1. Pantopoulos K, Porwal SK, Tartakoff A, et al. Mechanisms of mammalian iron homeostasis. Biochemistry 2012;51:5705–24.
2. Lawen A, Lane DJ. Mammalian iron homeostasis in health and disease: uptake, storage, transport, and molecular mechanisms of action. Antioxid Redox Signal 2013;18(18):2473–507.

3. Harvey JW. Iron metabolism and its disorders. In: Kaneko JJ, Harvey JW, Bruss ML, editors. Clinical biochemistry of domestic animals. 6th edition. Burlington (MA): Elsevier, Inc; 2008. p. 259–85.

4. Brasse-Lagnel C, Karim Z, Letteron P, et al. Intestinal DMT1 cotransporter is down-regulated by hepcidin via proteasome internalization and degradation. Gastroenterology 2011;140:1261–71.

5. Grimes CN, Giori L, Fry MM. Role of hepcidin in iron metabolism and potential clinical applications. Vet Clin North Am Small Anim Pract 2012;42:85–96.

6. Ganz T, Nemeth E. The hepcidin-ferroportin system as a therapeutic target in anemias and iron overload disorders. Hematology Am Soc Hematol Educ Program 2011;2011:538–42.

7. Urrechaga E, Borque L, Escanero JF. Erythrocyte and reticulocyte indices in the assessment of erythropoiesis activity and iron availability. Int J Lab Hematol 2013; 35:144–9.

8. Mast AE, Blinder MA, Dietzen DJ. Reticulocyte hemoglobin content. Am J Hematol 2008;83:307–10.

9. Fry MM, Kirk CA. Reticulocyte indices in a canine model of nutritional iron deficiency. Vet Clin Pathol 2006;35:172–81.

10. Steinberg JD, Olver CS. Hematologic and biochemical abnormalities indicating iron deficiency are associated with decreased reticulocyte hemoglobin content (CHr) and reticulocyte volume (rMCV) in dogs. Vet Clin Pathol 2005; 34:23–7.

11. Prins M, van Leeuwen MW, Teske E. Stability and reproducibility of ADVIA 120-measured red blood cell and platelet parameters in dogs, cats, and horses, and the use of reticulocyte haemoglobin content (CH(R)) in the diagnosis of iron deficiency. Tijdschr Diergeneeskd 2009;134:272–8.

12. Naigamwalla DZ, Webb JA, Giger U. Iron deficiency anemia. Can Vet J 2012;53: 250–6.

13. Dorland's illustrated medical dictionary. 27th edition. Philadelphia: W.B. Saunders Co; 1988. p. 747–51.

14. Sprague WS, Hackett TB, Johnson JS, et al. Hemochromatosis secondary to repeated blood transfusions in a dog. Vet Pathol 2003;40:334–7.

15. Gultekin GI, Raj K, Foreman P, et al. Erythrocytic pyruvate kinase mutations causing hemolytic anemia, osteosclerosis, and secondary hemochromatosis in dogs. J Vet Intern Med 2012;26:935–44.

16. Weiden PL, Hackman RC, Deeg HJ, et al. Long-term survival and reversal of iron overload after marrow transplantation in dogs with congenital hemolytic anemia. Blood 1981;57:66–70.

17. Zaucha JA, Yu C, Lothrop CD Jr, et al. Severe canine hereditary hemolytic anemia treated by nonmyeloablative marrow transplantation. Biol Blood Marrow Transplant 2001;7:14–24.

18. Kohn B, Goldschmidt MH, Hohenhaus AE, et al. Anemia, splenomegaly, and increased osmotic fragility of erythrocytes in Abyssinian and Somali cats. J Am Vet Med Assoc 2000;217:1483–91.

19. Joe E, Kim SH, Lee KB, et al. Feasibility and accuracy of dual-source dual-energy CT for noninvasive determination of hepatic iron accumulation. Radiology 2012; 262:126–35.

20. Majhail NS, Lazarus HM, Burns LJ. Iron overload in hematopoietic cell transplantation. Bone Marrow Transplant 2008;41:997–1003.

21. Waalen J, Felitti VJ, Gelbart T. Screening for hemochromatosis by measuring ferritin levels: a more effective approach. Blood 2008;111:3373–6.

22. Ferraro S, Mozzi R, Panteghini M. Revaluating serum ferritin as a marker of body iron stores in the traceability era. Clin Chem Lab Med 2012;50:1911–6.

23. Seguin MA, Bunch SE. Iatrogenic copper deficiency associated with long-term copper chelation for treatment of copper storage disease in a Bedlington terrier. J Am Vet Med Assoc 2001;218:1593–7.

24. Zentek J, Meyer H. Investigations on copper deficiency in growing dogs. J Nutr 1991;121:S83–4.

Making Sense of Lymphoma Diagnostics in Small Animal Patients

 CrossMark

Mary Jo Burkhard, DVM, PhD[a],*, Dorothee Bienzle, DVM, PhD[b]

KEYWORDS

- Lymphoma • Cytology • Immunophenotyping • Flow cytometry
- PCR for clonal antigen receptor gene rearrangement (PARR)
- Immunohistochemistry/immunocytochemistry

KEY POINTS

- Cytologic assessment is diagnostic in most cases of diffuse large B-cell and diffuse lymphoblastic lymphoma in dogs.
- The cytologic diagnosis of lymphoma is more challenging in cats than in dogs.
- Although cytology is useful for staging lymphoma, histopathology is necessary for classification and grading.
- Immunophenotyping by flow cytometry allows evaluation of lymphocyte populations using a panel of antibodies, and serves as an adjunctive tool for both diagnosis and prognosis.
- Polymerase chain reaction (PCR) to detect clonal antigen receptor gene rearrangement (PARR) is a relatively new test in veterinary medicine that has strong potential for supporting the diagnosis of lymphoma. However, false-positive and false-negative results may confound the diagnosis, and PARR is less sensitive in cats than in dogs.
- Immunohistochemistry and immunocytochemistry should not be used as stand-alone diagnostic techniques, nor should an interpretation be based on a single antibody label.

INTRODUCTION

Lymphoma is the most common hemolymphatic malignancy in dogs and cats and, similar to lymphoma in people, is a heterogeneous disease with variable clinical signs and response to therapy.[1] Patient genetics, immunocompetence, location, and morphologic subtype all contribute to the heterogeneity of the disease and prognosis (**Box 1**).

This article originally appeared in Veterinary Clinics of North America: Small Animal Practice, Volume 43, Issue 6, November 2013.
Funding Sources: None.
Conflict of Interest: None.
[a] Department of Veterinary Biosciences, College of Veterinary Medicine, The Ohio State University, 1925 Coffey Road, Columbus, OH 43210, USA; [b] Department of Pathobiology, University of Guelph, 50 Stone Road East, Guelph, Ontario N1G 2W1, Canada
* Corresponding author.
E-mail address: burkhard.19@osu.edu

Clin Lab Med 35 (2015) 591–607
http://dx.doi.org/10.1016/j.cll.2015.05.008
0272-2712/15/$ – see front matter © 2015 Elsevier Inc. All rights reserved.
labmed.theclinics.com

> **Box 1**
> **Clinical evaluation of lymphoma**
>
> Several options are available for the diagnosis and characterization of lymphoma. This review helps in choosing the best test or tests for the patient.

Anatomically, lymphoma can be characterized as multicentric, alimentary, mediastinal, or extranodal. In dogs, multicentric lymphoma accounts for 80% to 85% of reported cases, and diffuse large B-cell lymphoma is the most common histomorphologic variant.[2] However, other types of B-cell lymphomas as well as T-cell lymphomas also are frequently diagnosed. The prognosis of lymphoma variants in dogs depends not only on the type of neoplastic lymphocyte but also on the location, characteristics of the cells, and the stage of disease. In cats, the diagnosis is more challenging because lymphoma more commonly affects extranodal sites, particularly the alimentary and upper respiratory tract.[3,4] Lymphoma affecting the gastrointestinal tract is common but particularly challenging to diagnose, owing to the relative inaccessibility for sampling and potential progression from lymphocytic inflammation to neoplasia. Other types of lymphoma in cats often contain a heterogeneous population of neoplastic lymphocytes plus reactive lymphocytes, plasma cells, and other inflammatory cells.

The diagnosis of lymphoma classically depended on morphologic characteristics identified by cytology and/or histopathology. In recent years, additional assays such as immunocytochemistry (ICC), immunohistochemistry (IHC), immunophenotyping by flow cytometry, and polymerase chain reaction (PCR) to detect clonal antigen receptor gene rearrangement (PARR) have been used to assist in the diagnosis of lymphoma and to classify lymphoma for prognostic purposes. Diagnostic tests are not perfectly sensitive or specific; therefore multiple assays are often used in conjunction or in sequence to enhance the accuracy of diagnosis and assist with prognosis. This article considers the utility and pitfalls of each diagnostic tool (**Box 2**).

CYTOLOGY

Cytologic examination of blood films and samples obtained by fine-needle aspiration (FNA) of tissues or fluids is commonly used in the diagnosis of lymphoma in dogs and cats. Advantages of cytology are that sample collection and slide examination are rapid and can be performed in-house with the minimal resources of glass slides, a Romanowsky stain such as Diff Quick or Wright Giemsa, and a high-quality microscope. Limitations of FNA in comparison with an incisional or excisional biopsy are that FNA does not allow assessment of tissue architecture, and material for additional studies (eg, IHC) is unavailable. Blood sampling and aspiration of superficial masses

> **Box 2**
> **Tools available for the diagnosis and characterization of lymphoma**
>
> Cytology
>
> Histopathology
>
> Immunocytochemistry and immunohistochemistry
>
> Phenotyping by flow cytometry
>
> Polymerase chain reaction to detect clonal antigen receptor gene rearrangement (PARR)

and peripheral lymph nodes are safe and simple techniques for most patients. FNA of internal organs such as the liver or spleen or abdominal or thoracic masses is more challenging, but is still commonly performed and often is diagnostically rewarding.

Lymphocyte Morphology

Lymphocyte cytomorphology is characterized by cell size, nuclear features, and cytoplasmic features (**Fig. 1**). It is important when using cytomorphology to examine only those cells that are both intact and adequately spread out on the slide.

Diagnosis of Lymphoma by Cytology

The cytologic diagnosis of lymphoma is the most straightforward if the tumor is diffuse and the entire node is replaced by a uniform population of large neoplastic lymphocytes; this is the most common type of lymphoma in dogs. Most diffuse lymphomas yield FNA that consist entirely or predominantly of large neoplastic cells. However, diffuse lymphomas composed of small or intermediate cells can be difficult to diagnose by cytology, because the cells more closely resemble benign lymphocytes. In contrast to diffuse lymphoma, follicular lymphoma, which is uncommon in dogs, may yield a heterogeneous population of benign and malignant cells of variable size and morphology, which is challenging to interpret by cytology.

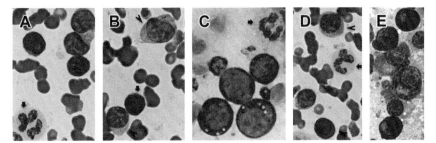

Fig. 1. Lymphocyte cytomorphology. Fine-needle aspiration (FNA) of lymph node from a dog (Wright Giemsa stain, original magnification ×1000). (*A*) One neutrophil (*lower left*) and 4 small lymphocytes: these lymphocytes are smaller than a neutrophil (*arrow*) and have a dense round nucleus that comprises the majority of the cell. Nucleoli are not seen. Cytoplasm is scant (sometimes only a very thin rim is visible). (*B*) One intermediate lymphocyte (*arrow*) and 2 small lymphocytes (*arrowheads*): intermediate lymphocytes are similar in size to neutrophils, have more abundant cytoplasm that is typically lightly basophilic, and may contain small azurophilic granules. Nuclei are often slightly eccentric within the cell and have less condensed chromatin. Indistinct nucleoli may be seen. (*C*) Four large lymphocytes and one neutrophil (*arrow*): large lymphocytes, also called lymphoblasts, are equal to or greater in size than neutrophils and contain round to oval nuclei with fine or stippled chromatin. Nucleoli are commonly seen. A rim of deeply basophilic cytoplasm surrounds the nucleus. Occasionally (especially in cats) the cytoplasm may contain punctate vacuoles, as shown in the 2 large lymphocytes at the bottom of this panel. (*D*) One reactive lymphocyte (*arrow*), 2 small lymphocytes (*arrowheads*), and 1 neutrophil: reactive lymphocytes are similar in morphology to small lymphocytes but slightly larger, and have more abundant, more deeply basophilic cytoplasm. (*E*) Several plasma cells: plasma cells are medium to large cells that contain small, round, eccentrically placed nuclei with coarsely clumped chromatin. Cytoplasm is abundant, deeply basophilic, and often contains a prominent perinuclear, clear zone that corresponds to the Golgi apparatus. The Golgi apparatus is clearly shown in the 2 plasma cells in the center.

Lymphoma in cats less commonly affects lymph nodes, and more commonly affects other tissues such as the intestine, nasal cavity, kidneys, liver, stomach, thymus, and spinal cord. In addition, those feline lymphomas that involve 1 or several peripheral lymph nodes often comprise a heterogeneous population of small and large lymphocytes as well as plasma cells and macrophages, making the diagnosis of lymphoma in cats by cytology more challenging than in dogs.

Hence, when lymph node FNA from either dogs or cats yield heterogeneous cell populations, reactive hyperplasia must be considered as a differential diagnosis (**Table 1**). Histopathology, in conjunction with ancillary diagnostic tests, should be used for additional characterization of the cell population.

Supporting Cytologic Features

There are several cytologic features (**Fig. 2**) that are more often associated with lymphoma than with benign lymphocyte proliferations, and these may be helpful in establishing a diagnosis. However, these features may be seen in both neoplastic and reactive populations and are not pathognomonic.

Staging of Lymphoma by Cytology

The World Health Organization staging scheme is based on the degree of metastasis, invasiveness, and presence of clinical signs. Cytology is useful in the staging of lymphoma by helping to identify the degree of metastasis (**Box 3**).

Limitations of Cytology

Diagnosis of small-cell and intermediate-cell lymphoma by cytology is challenging. Diagnosis in these cases may require additional supportive evidence such as generalized lymphadenopathy, identification of cells with similar cytologic features in multiple tissues, and lack of detection of infectious agents. Additional diagnostic tests such as histopathologic evaluation, flow-cytometric analysis, or PARR may be required for diagnosis.

Another cytologic diagnostic challenge is differentiating early lymphoma and reactive hyperplasia. In both processes, the percentage of lymphoblasts (large lymphocytes) will be increased within an overall heterogeneous population of lymphocytes. In these cases, examination by flow cytometry may also reveal a heterogeneous lymphocyte population, and therefore may be less specific than histopathology or PARR. Many lymphomas in cats are composed of such heterogeneous cell populations, and are therefore challenging to diagnose by cytology.

Sample Requirements

Sample collection and processing for FNA cytology of lymphoid tissue is relatively straightforward, and has been described in numerous texts and continuing education

Table 1 Differentiating lymphoma and reactive hyperplasia	
Lymphoma	**Hyperplasia**
≥50%, often >80/90% of cells are composed of homogeneous lymphoblasts or atypical lymphocytes	<50%, usually <20% lymphoblasts A heterogeneous lymphoid population that includes small lymphocytes, intermediate lymphocytes, and lymphoblasts. Plasma cells and other inflammatory cells are usually also present
Plasma cells and other inflammatory cells are rare	

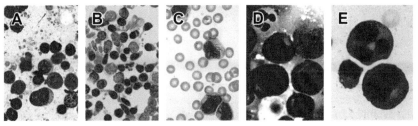

Fig. 2. Common cytologic features of lymphoma. FNA of enlarged lymph nodes from dogs with lymphoma. (*A*) Cytoplasmic fragments ("lymphoglandular bodies") are small, round, homogeneous, basophilic structures around and between cells. The presence of such fragments in cytologic preparations of lymphoid tissue is often associated with increased numbers of lymphoblasts resulting from neoplasia or hyperplasia (Wright Giemsa stain, original magnification ×1000). (*B*) Cytoplasmic pseudopodia ("uropods") may be present in some neoplastic T cells, but pseudopodia also may be present in activated T cells associated with reactive lymphoid hyperplasia (Wright Giemsa stain, original magnification ×200). (*C*) Cytoplasmic granulation is often a feature of CD8$^+$ T cells (cytotoxic T cells or CTLs) and natural killer (NK) cells. An increased proportion of granulated lymphocytes is commonly seen in rickettsial infections as well as in T-cell chronic lymphocytic leukemia (CLL) of dogs (Wright Giemsa stain, original magnification ×1000). (*D*) The Golgi apparatus is an eccentric, perinuclear clear zone often suggested as a feature of B cells and plasma cells, both reactive and neoplastic. However, the Golgi apparatus is an organelle found in most cells, including T cells and myeloid cells (Wright Giemsa stain, original magnification ×1000). (*E*) Irregular nuclear shapes such as cerebriform and flower-shaped nuclei often are present with T-cell diseases such as Sézary syndrome (a type of cutaneous lymphoma) and epitheliotropic lymphoma (a type of lymphoma that preferentially targets the cutaneous or gastrointestinal epithelium). In cats and dogs with CLL, more subtle nuclear irregularities such as small indentations and nuclear cleaves are commonly noted, and tend to be more obvious in formalin-fixed tissues. However, irregular nuclear morphology has also been described in B-cell lymphoma and leukemia (Wright Giemsa stain, original magnification ×1000).

seminars. Accurate interpretation, however, requires a representative and cellular sample of the lesion, and well-prepared and stained slides with adequate numbers of intact, spread-out, and well-stained cells for cytologic evaluation. Interpretation should always be made in the context of the signalment, history, clinical signs, and any additional diagnostic data from the patient. Samples that do not have a homogeneous population of large lymphocytes, or contain lymphocytes with cytologic atypia, should be evaluated by additional diagnostic methods.

Box 3
World Health Organization staging criteria for canine lymphoma

Stage I: Disease restricted to a single lymph node

Stage II: Regional lymphadenopathy (restricted to one side of diaphragm)

Stage III: Generalized lymphadenopathy

Stage IV: Hepatosplenomegaly (with or without lymphadenopathy)

Stage V: Bone marrow, central nervous system, or involvement of other extranodal sites

    Substage a: no clinical signs

    Substage b: clinical signs of illness

HISTOPATHOLOGY
Overview

Although both cytology and histopathology may be adequate for the diagnosis of lymphoma, histologic examination provides additional information about tissue architecture, cell distribution, and mitotic figures, and allows assessment of certain nuclear features important in the classification of lymphoma. Classification into morphologic subtypes allows comparison with published data and can provide prognostic information. Availability of paraffin-embedded tissue also allows additional studies such as IHC to be performed, and may provide a source of DNA for PARR. Histologic classification criteria include tissue involvement, the pattern of distribution of neoplastic cells within the tissue, neoplastic cell type, nuclear size, nuclear shape (cleaved vs noncleaved), presence of nucleoli, frequency of mitotic figures, presence and location of nonneoplastic cell types, and expression of surface markers (**Table 2**).[1,2]

Sample Requirements

The majority of dogs with lymphoma present with lymphadenopathy associated with diffuse effacement of lymph node parenchyma by a homogeneous population of large lymphocytes. In these cases, fine-needle biopsy typically yields sufficient numbers of cells for diagnosis. However, in the dogs with small-cell lymphoma or follicular lymphoma, and for many cats with lymphoma, excisional or Tru-Cut biopsy samples often are necessary for a definitive diagnosis. Biopsies should be placed in formalin for adequate fixation, and submitted to a veterinary diagnostic laboratory for processing and interpretation.

IMMUNOPHENOTYPING BY FLOW CYTOMETRY
Overview

One of the goals of immunophenotyping by flow-cytometric analysis is to define the types of lymphocyte in fluid samples by light-scatter characteristics and expression of phenotypic markers, thereby providing a more objective characterization of lymphocyte populations. Lymphocyte phenotyping by flow-cytometric analysis has become a relatively widely available assay to aid in the classification of benign and neoplastic lymphocytes, and in the differentiation of hematopoietic cell populations, in small animal patients.[5,6]

Flow-Cytometric Panels

Neoplastic lymphocytes often fail to express the same phenotype as their nonneoplastic counterparts, and may express antigens inappropriate for their level of differentiation. Neoplastic lymphocytes may also upregulate additional markers not typically expressed on nonneoplastic cells. Therefore, it is recommended that a panel of antibodies be used to characterize the neoplastic cell population. In both dogs and cats, several well-characterized antibodies are available for evaluation of lymphoid populations, with fewer antibodies available for examination of histiocytic, granulocytic, monocytic, erythroid, and megakaryocytic cells (**Table 3**).

Certain phenotypes, patterns of expression, or specific markers have prognostic or diagnostic utility (**Table 4**).[7–10]

Sample Requirements

Blood and nonhemorrhagic fluid samples (cerebrospinal fluid, peritoneal fluid, pleural effusion fluid, and so forth) can be placed in ethylenediaminetetraacetic acid or serum tubes, respectively, and readily processed for flow cytometry. Solid tissue aspirates

Table 2
Classification of common canine lymphoma types

Category	Typical Location and Clinical Features	Histopathologic Pattern	Cell Features	Immunophenotypic Features
Diffuse large B-cell lymphoma, NOS	LN, often generalized	Diffuse	Large cells, round nuclei, central single nucleolus, high MR	CD1, CD20, CD21, CD79, MHC II; CD18^{low}
Marginal-zone lymphoma	Nodal, splenic white pulp, or extranodal mucosal origin	Follicular	Small to intermediate cells, low MR	CD20, CD21, CD79, MHC II; CD18^{intermed}
Follicular lymphoma	LN, single to multiple	Follicular	Variable cell size, low MR	CD20, CD79
Mantle-cell lymphoma	Splenic white pulp	Follicular	Small cells, round to irregular nuclei, low MR	CD20, CD79
Peripheral T-cell lymphoma, NOS	LN, often generalized, hypercalcemia possible	Diffuse	Variable cell morphology and MR	CD3, TCRαβ, CD4 or CD8 single or dual positive or negative, CD18^{high}
Small T-cell lymphoma	LN	Paracortical, progressing to diffuse	Small to intermediate cells with variable morphology	CD3
Primary cutaneous epitheliotropic lymphoma	Mucocutaneous sites	Epitheliotropic, may form plaques	Variable cell size and morphology	CD3, CD8, TCRαβ or TCRγδ
Hepatosplenic lymphoma	Splenic red pulp origin with diffuse spread to liver and marrow. Cytopenia common	Diffuse	Cytoplasmic granulation and high MR	CD3, CD8, CD11d, CD18, TCRγδ

Abbreviations: LN, lymph node; MR, mitotic rate; NOS, not otherwise specific.

Table 3
Cell-surface markers commonly detected by flow cytometry on canine and feline leukocytes

Marker	Primary Cell Type	Additional Notes
CD1	Dendritic cells	Subpopulations of B cells and monocytes also express CD1 molecules
CD3	T cells	
CD4	Helper T cells	Canine neutrophils constitutively express CD4. Monocytes, macrophages, and dendritic cells can upregulate CD4
CD4/CD8 dual positive	Thymocytes	
CD5	T cells	In some species, CD5 is also expressed on the B-1 subset of B cells
CD8	Cytotoxic T cells	Also on a subset of natural killer cells
CD14	Monocytes	Also on some types of macrophages
CD18	All leukocytes	Greater expression intensity on granulocytes and monocytes than on lymphocytes; variable expression on different types of lymphocytes
CD21, CD22	Mature B cells	Absent on plasma cells
CD34	Hematopoietic stem cells	Present on cells in some cases of acute leukemia of either lymphoid or myeloid origin
CD45	All hematopoietic cells (except erythroid cells)	CD45 intensity varies among cell types and can be used to help differentiate cells. CD45 may be absent or reduced on neoplastic lymphocytes
CD79a or CD79b	B cells of all stages	Intracellular antigen; detection requires a directly conjugated antibody and an additional permeabilization step to allow the antibody to enter the cell. Expression is absent in plasma cells
MHC II	Antigen-presenting cells, most canine and feline lymphocytes	
Surface IgM	Immature B cells	
Light-chain expression	Antibody-producing B cells, plasma cells	λ-Light-chain expression far outweighs κ-chain expression in dogs and cats in both benign and neoplastic disorders

Abbreviation: IgM, immunoglobulin M.

also can be analyzed as long as they are processed to yield cell suspensions. FNA samples from solid tissue (eg, lymph node) should be placed into a tube containing buffered saline and a small amount of serum (bovine serum is often used) to help stabilize the cells before analysis. As there is some variation between laboratories, the collaborating laboratory should be contacted to confirm the specific submission guidelines. In general, at least 2 million cells are needed to apply a complete immunophenotyping panel for flow cytometry. Samples from different sites should not be mixed together. Samples should be shipped by express delivery, cold but not frozen,

Table 4
Flow-cytometric diagnostic and prognostic patterns

Diagnostic Patterns		
Type of Neoplasm	**Morphologic Features**	**Common Phenotype**
Canine CLL: T-cell subtype	Small to intermediate lymphocytes often with granules	CD3$^+$ CD5$^+$ CD8$^+$
Canine CLL: B-cell subtype	Small lymphocytes	CD21$^+$ CD79$^+$, may have monoclonal gammopathy
Feline CLL	Small lymphocytes	CD5$^+$ CD4$^+$
Acute lymphoblastic leukemia	Large cells	Some are CD45$^+$ CD34$^+$
Diffuse large B-cell lymphoma	Large lymphocytes, effacement of node	CD21$^+$ CD79$^+$ CD1$^+$ CD18^{low}
Marginal-zone lymphoma	Small to intermediate lymphocytes	CD21$^+$ CD79$^+$ CD1$^-$, CD18^{intermed}
Prognostic Patterns		
Type of Neoplasm	**Change**	**Suggested Prognostic Impact**
B-cell lymphoma	Loss of MHC II	Reduced survivability
Canine CLL	B-cell subtype	Reduced survivability compared with T-cell CLL
Canine CLL	Atypical subtype (null T cell, dual CD4$^+$/CD8$^+$, dual T/B lineage)	Markedly reduced survivability
ALL vs stage V lymphoma	CD34 expression	CD34 expression supports ALL rather than stage V lymphoma

Abbreviations: ALL, acute lymphoblastic leukemia; CLL, chronic lymphocytic leukemia; MHC, major histocompatibility complex.

to a laboratory that performs immunophenotyping by flow cytometry. A delay between sampling and processing can result in degradation of the cells and/or loss of marker expression or marker intensity. In general, 3 days at refrigeration temperature is the maximum period for retaining diagnostically useful samples.

An informal survey among veterinary laboratories in North America, Europe, and Asia determined that all laboratories used panels of antibodies for characterization of leukocytes. The antibody panels, fluorochromes, and instruments were variable, but similar markers were detected for classification of lymphocytes and other leukocytes. Laboratories also varied regarding the preferred anticoagulant for blood samples, the preferred additive for stabilizing cells, and the duration that samples were considered suitable for analysis after collection. Therefore, clinicians should contact individual laboratories regarding their protocols before submission of samples for flow cytometry.

PARR

Although neoplastic lymphocytes are clonal in origin, not all clonal populations of lymphocytes are neoplastic. Certain inflammatory and infectious diseases such as rickettsial infections can result in clonal lymphocyte expansions. There are no cell-surface markers that identify clonal T-cell populations in humans or veterinary species. In humans, expression of κ or λ light chain can identify clonal B-cell populations when there is uniform expression of one light chain. However, antibodies for detection of canine or feline light chains by flow cytometry are unavailable, and λ light-chain expression far outweighs κ-chain expression in dogs and cats in both benign and neoplastic disorders.[11] Therefore, the utility of light-chain expression for the diagnosis of clonal B-cell populations is limited for dogs and cats with lymphoma.

Identification of T-cell or B-cell clonality in dogs and cats requires detection of clonal receptor gene rearrangement. This detection is most typically done by PCR, and is referred to as PCR for antigen receptor gene rearrangement (PARR).[12–14] As part of their development, T cells undergo rearrangement of genes encoding the T-cell receptor (TCR), whereas B cells undergo rearrangement of genes encoding the immunoglobulin (Ig) receptor. The result is that nearly every lymphocyte has a slightly different TCR or Ig receptor. However, small stretches in the DNA coding for each receptor are similar in all lymphocytes, and allow use of primers that will amplify most receptors and yield PCR products that vary slightly in size and composition.[15] Therefore, PARR of benign lymphoid tissue detects a smear or ladder of PCR products representing the diversity of benign receptors (**Fig. 3**). Because neoplastic transformation of lymphocytes typically occurs after the cells have undergone receptor rearrangement, malignant daughter cells will have the same antigen receptor gene, which is detected on PCR as a single product and represents a monoclonal population (see **Fig. 3**). Occasionally biclonal or triclonal neoplastic populations may also be detected. Nonlymphoid neoplasms will not produce discrete PCR products, called amplicons, because gene segments for lymphocyte receptors are located too distantly from each other in nonlymphoid cells.

One of the strengths of PARR is the ability to detect a clonal population within a larger reactive process, such as might occur in early lymphoma arising amid a reactive population.

Caveats for PARR

PARR has potential to be very sensitive and specific; however, false-positive and false-negative results occur for a variety of reasons. PARR may detect lymphocytes with clonally rearranged receptor DNA, but lymphoid clonality does not always correspond to neoplasia. Oligoclonal or monoclonal expansions of reactive lymphocytes with identical gene rearrangements can be seen in chronic infections, such as with the causative agents of ehrlichiosis, anaplasmosis, Rocky Mountain spotted fever, or Lyme disease. Factors inherent to PCR amplification of DNA templates with very small sequence variation may also yield nonspecific amplicons. False-negative results can occur when the sample does not contain sufficient numbers of cells with clonal antigen receptor genes to create a visible discrete amplicon in PCR amplification, or when primers do not anneal to the particular clonal receptor genes.

In addition, PARR is substantially less sensitive in cats than it is in dogs. In dogs, the assay detects 75% to 80% of confirmed cases of lymphoma or lymphocytic leukemia. In cats, currently available protocols detect 60% to 65% of neoplastic lymphocyte samples.[14] Although a positive result is diagnostically supportive for lymphoma, a negative result in either species does not rule out lymphoma.

Sample Requirements

DNA for PCR can be harvested from blood, fluid samples, air-dried (stained or unstained) cytology slides, and histology slides or sections. The minimum number of cells needed for the assay is approximately 50,000. A unique feature of this diagnostic modality is that slides can be examined cytologically and then submitted for cell removal, DNA extraction, and PCR analysis. This process facilitates the clinical diagnosis because it ensures that the cells in question are present on the slide in adequate

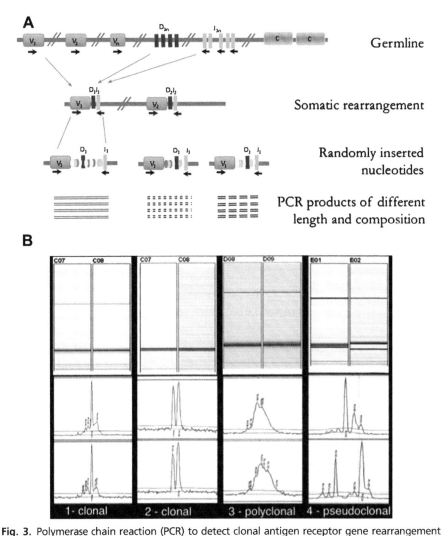

Fig. 3. Polymerase chain reaction (PCR) to detect clonal antigen receptor gene rearrangement (PARR). (*A*) Lymphocyte antigen receptor gene rearrangement. In **germline** configuration, different gene segments (V = variable; D = diversity; J = joining; C = constant) of lymphocyte antigen receptors are located distant from each other, and yield no PCR product with primers (*black arrows*) to conserved regions in different segments. During **somatic recombination** different V, D, and J regions are brought into proximity. Additional diversity is generated by **random insertion of nucleotides** (*yellow-orange*) at the joining regions. Amplification with primers to conserved regions in the V and J segment yields a **range of PCR products**. (*B*) High-resolution electrophoresis detects size variability among amplicons. Heteroduplex analysis (not shown) involves melting and reannealing of double-stranded amplicons before electrophoresis to detect sequence variability in addition to size variability. Capillary electrophoresis (*top panel*) and BioCalculator (Qiagen, Valencia, CA, USA) software analysis plots (*bottom panel*) of antigen receptor gene arrangement PCR on DNA extracted from 4 different dogs (*1–4*). Major peaks reflect homogeneous amplicons, minor small peaks at the baseline reflect background DNA, and markers are size indicators. Dog 1 is a 7-year-old mixed breed with peripheral T-cell lymphoma, not otherwise specified (PTCL-NOS), and PARR shows a single sharp peak from a homogeneous amplicon, which confirmed clonal lymphocyte gene receptors. Dog 2 is a 1.5-year-old Dachshund with diffuse large B-cell lymphoma (DLBCL), also confirmed by detection of 2 clonal amplicons with this assay. The PCR result from dog 3 shows a range of different-sized amplicons indicating a polyclonal (reactive) result. The PCR result from dog 4 shows amplicons consisting of multiple peaks that differ in size in replicate assays, which is termed pseudoclonal, because primers likely annealed nonspecifically and the result does not reflect a clonal population. ([*B*] *Courtesy of* Dr Bill Vernau, University of California at Davis, Davis, CA.)

numbers. In addition, samples can be archived while owners consider additional diagnostic or therapeutic decisions. Fluid and blood samples should be shipped by express delivery, cold but not frozen, to a laboratory that performs PARR. Glass slides can be shipped by a variety of methods, but should be placed in a shipping container.

PARR is a relatively new test in veterinary medicine, and fewer than 10 veterinary laboratories throughout the world currently perform PARR for diagnostic purposes. There is much variation in the number and nature of primers used by different laboratories, whether amplifications are performed in single, duplicate, or quadruplicate format, whether the analysis of amplicons involves heating and reannealing of double-stranded products to increase specificity, and other test aspects. Some laboratories interpret PARR results only in conjunction with review of other laboratory data such as cytologic or histologic slides, IHC, flow cytometry, and other data, whereas other laboratories interpret PARR results as a stand-alone-test. For these reasons, until PARR becomes a more standardized test across laboratories it is best for clinicians to contact individual laboratories regarding the types of sample accepted and the nature of test interpretation.

IMMUNOHISTOCHEMISTRY AND IMMUNOCYTOCHEMISTRY
Diagnostic Utility

IHC and ICC are used to demonstrate cell antigens in tissue sections (IHC) or cytology preparations (ICC) (**Fig. 4**). In both IHC and ICC, antibodies are used to bind to specific antigens, and the binding of these antibodies is detected by a histochemical reaction

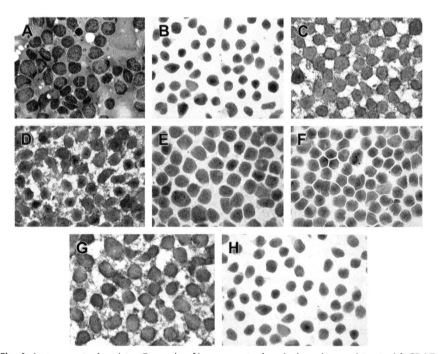

Fig. 4. Immunocytochemistry. Example of immunocytochemical results consistent with CD4 T-cell ($\alpha\beta$ TCR) lymphoma from a 5-year-old Boxer with generalized lymphadenopathy. All images were photographed at 75× and labeled as follows: (A) Wright stain; (B) negative control; (C) CD3; (D) CD4; (E) CD8α; (F) CD79a; (G) TCR$\alpha\beta$; (H). TCR$\gamma\delta$. (*Courtesy of* Dr Bill Vernau, University of California at Davis, Davis, CA.)

to produce a color change in positive cells. As in a cytology slide or histologic section, the location of this color change in cells can then be precisely determined by microscopy. Antibodies are often species specific or species limited; therefore, not all antibodies are equally suitable for dog and cat tissues.

Key Considerations for Clinical Application

When considering IHC and ICC results, diagnostic and prognostic interpretation is performed in a manner similar to that for antibody detection by flow cytometry.[16,17] In fact, some of the same antibodies (albeit with different detection labels) may be used for both flow cytometry and IHC/ICC. However, there is more often the opportunity to request a single antibody in IHC/ICC, whereas a diagnostic panel is typically performed for flow-cytometric analysis. Moreover, tissues fixed in formalin have altered expression of antigens, and are no longer suitable for evaluation with the range of antibodies that bind to unfixed cells. Given the variability of neoplastic cells to upregulate or downregulate gene expression, a single antibody label should not be considered sufficient for diagnosis. For example, confirmation of a T-cell lymphoma by CD3 expression should, at minimum, also include exclusion of B-cell type by the lack of labeling for CD79 or another B-cell antigen. IHC or ICC should never be considered stand-alone diagnostic techniques because interpretation requires expert evaluation within the context of each tumor type.[16]

In addition to classification of lymphoma type, immunostaining can be very useful for the differentiation of lymphoma from other neoplasms composed of nonlymphoid round cells. Nasal carcinomas, particularly in cats, may be morphologically similar to some lymphomas, and IHC for CD3, CD79, and cytokeratin assists in their distinction.[17]

Sample Requirements

IHC is typically performed on formalin-fixed and paraffin-embedded samples. Proper fixation is critical for consistent antigen detection, and either underfixation or overfixation may alter the ability to detect antigens. Before IHC, sections are deparaffinized and subjected to antigen retrieval. Different methods for antigen retrieval may be applied for different antibodies.

ICC may be performed on air-dried unstained, air-dried previously stained, or wet-fixed slides. Use of air-dried previously stained slides, however, is least preferred because of the potential for loss of cells, disruption of cells and cell membranes, or loss of signal detection. Cells on cytology slides progressively lose reactivity with antibodies during storage; therefore, it is best to analyze freshly prepared slides by ICC.

TUMOR BIOMARKERS

Tumor biomarkers are substances released from neoplastic cells into blood, urine, or other fluids that can be measured through specific assays. In human medicine, assessment of tumor biomarkers is increasingly performed to aid in establishing both the diagnosis and prognosis of lymphoma.

Thymidine kinase is an enzyme highly expressed by rapidly dividing cells. In both dogs and cats, serum thymidine kinase activity is increased in patients with lymphoma, and in dogs, activity was inversely associated with survival time.[18,19] However, the overall sensitivity for the test is low, owing to the lack of increased serum activity in a proportion of small animal patients with lymphoma. Therefore, as with any diagnostic test, serum thymidine kinase activity should be considered a supporting tool to be used in context with other diagnostic methods. The greatest value for serum thymidine kinase activity and other biomarkers may be for their roles in monitoring the response to treatment.

CASE STUDIES

Case 1

A 12-year-old female spayed domestic short-haired cat, presented for recheck of inflammatory bowel disease.

Numerical complete blood count results were within reference limits; however, the lymphocyte count was higher than normal (3.7 × 10⁹/L), and evaluation of the lymphocyte morphology revealed uniform cells with mild nuclear irregularities commonly seen in feline patients with chronic lymphocytic leukemia (CLL) (**Fig. 5**A). Flow cytometry (**Fig. 5**B) revealed that the lymphocyte population was composed of a heterogeneous population of T cells and B cells. However, the T cells had an abnormal phenotype and were primarily negative for both CD4 and CD8. In healthy cats, 30% to 50% of blood lymphocytes are CD4⁺ and 15% to 25% are CD8⁺. A blood sample evaluated by PARR identified a clonal T-cell receptor gene rearrangement.

Summary: Early CLL in a cat. Most feline CLL is CD4 T-cell in origin. However, null (CD4⁻ CD8⁻) as well as CD8 CLL also has been reported.

Case 2

An 8-year-old male neutered Golden Retriever with generalized massive lymph node enlargement and weight loss.

Lymph node aspirate and biopsy are shown in (**Fig. 6**A and B). The histopathologic classification was "diffuse large B-cell lymphoma of immunoblastic type."

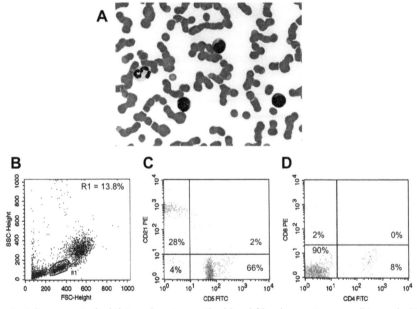

Fig. 5. Feline case study. (*A*) Lymphocytes on the blood film demonstrate small irregularities in the nuclear membrane including indentations and small nuclear cleaves (Wright stain, original magnification ×100). (*B*) Flow-cytometric analysis of blood leukocytes. The lymphocyte population (R1) was 13.8% of the total population and was gated for analysis. (*C*) Sixty-six percent of the lymphocytes were CD5⁺ T cells and 28% were CD21⁺ B cells. (*D*) The majority (90%) of lymphocytes were negative for both CD4 and CD8. Quadrant lines are set at the isotype control and the percentages of cells beyond background are listed in each quadrant.

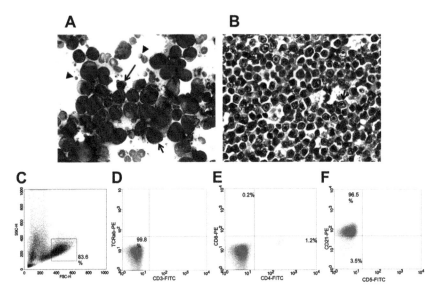

Fig. 6. Canine case study. (A) The cytology preparation from an FNA of an enlarged lymph node consists of numerous very large lymphocytes, many cytoplasmic fragments (*arrowheads*), occasional plasma cells (*short arrow*) and small lymphocytes (*long arrow*), and scattered red blood cells (Wright stain, original magnification ×100). (B) On histopathology, the lymph node architecture was replaced by a diffuse infiltrate of large lymphocytes with a single prominent central nucleolus (*arrow*) (hematoxylin-eosin stain, original magnification ×400). (C) Flow-cytometric evaluation of a lymph node aspirate showed a prominent population of cells with high forward and side scatter, and a few other cells with light-scatter properties of neutrophils, small lymphocytes, and red blood cells. Large gated cells lacked CD3 and TCRα/β expression (D) and contained a few CD4+ cells (likely neutrophils, E), and the majority expressed CD21 but not CD5 (F). These findings are consistent with diffuse large B-cell lymphoma.

Flow-cytometric analysis (**Fig. 6**C–F) was also consistent with a diffuse large B-cell lymphoma. The dog was treated with combination chemotherapy, achieved remission at 3 weeks, and remained in remission for 11 months.

SUMMARY

There is no single stand-alone assay for the diagnosis, characterization, and staging of lymphoma in small animal patients. In addition to cytology and histopathology, immunophenotyping by flow cytometry, PARR, and immunohistochemistry or immunocytochemistry all provide important diagnostic and prognostic information. However, for accurate diagnosis and staging the findings must be evaluated in concert with the clinical history, physical examination, and other ancillary data.

ACKNOWLEDGMENTS

Figs. 3B and 4 were graciously provided by Dr Bill Vernau, University of California at Davis. The following collaborators shared their protocols and provided input regarding preferred samples, standards for interpretation, and important controls for flow cytometric and PARR assays performed in their laboratories: Anne Avery (Fort Collins, Colorado); Mary Jo Burkhard (Columbus, Ohio); Stefano Comazzi (Milan,

Italy); Dorothee Bienzle (Guelph, Ontario); Jonathan Fogle, Mary Tompkins, Hiroyuki Mochizuki (Raleigh, North Carolina); Beverly Kidney (Saskatoon, Saskatchewan); Matti Kiupel (Lansing, Michigan); Casey LeBlanc (Knoxville, Tennessee); Jaime Modiano, Daisuke Ito (Minneapolis, Minnesota); Masahiko Sato, Hajime Tsujimoto (Tokyo, Japan); Tracy Stokol, Deanna Schaefer (Ithaca, New York); Masamine Takanosu (Asaka, Ohtawara, Japan); Bill Vernau, Peter Moore (Davis, California); and Melinda Wilkerson (Manhattan, Kansas).

REFERENCES

1. Bienzle D, Vernau W. The diagnostic assessment of canine lymphoma: implications for treatment. Clin Lab Med 2011;31:21–39. Available at: http://www.ncbi.nlm.nih.gov/pubmed/21295720. Accessed March 15, 2013.
2. Valli VE, San Myint M, Barthel A, et al. Classification of canine malignant lymphomas according to the World Health Organization criteria. Vet Pathol 2011;48:198–211. Available at: http://vet.sagepub.com/content/48/1/198. Accessed March 15, 2013.
3. Chino J, Fujino Y, Kobayashi T, et al. Cytomorphological and immunological classification of feline lymphomas: clinicopathological features of 76 cases. J Vet Med Sci 2013;75(6):701–7. Available at: https://www.jstage.jst.go.jp/article/jvms/advpub/0/advpub_12-0246/_pdf. Accessed March 15, 2013.
4. Little L, Patel R, Goldschmidt M. Nasal and nasopharyngeal lymphoma in cats: 50 cases (1989-2005). Vet Pathol 2007;44:885–92. Available at: http://vet.sagepub.com/content/44/6/885.full.pdf+html. Accessed March 15, 2013.
5. Sözmen M, Tasca S, Carli E, et al. Use of fine needle aspirates and flow cytometry for the diagnosis, classification, and immunophenotyping of canine lymphomas. J Vet Diagn Invest 2005;17:323–9. Available at: http://vdi.sagepub.com/content/17/4/323.long. Accessed March 15, 2013.
6. Wilkerson MJ, Dolce K, Koopman T, et al. Lineage differentiation of canine lymphoma/leukemias and aberrant expression of CD molecules. Vet Immunol Immunopathol 2005;106:179–96. Available at: http://www.sciencedirect.com/science/article/pii/S0165242705000681. Accessed March 15, 2013.
7. Williams MJ, Avery AC, Lana SE, et al. Canine lymphoproliferative disease characterized by lymphocytosis: immunophenotypic markers of prognosis. J Vet Intern Med 2008;22:596–601.http://onlinelibrary.wiley.com/store/10.1111/j.1939-1676.2008.0041.x/asset/j.1939-1676.2008.0041.x.pdf?v=1&t=hesqsixk&s=fea778825eef6f313b93d655433bb6f3381b6a6e. Accessed March 15, 2013.
8. Campbell MW, Hess PR, Williams LE. Chronic lymphocytic leukaemia in the cat: 18 cases (2000-2010). Vet Comp Oncol 2012. http://dx.doi.org/10.1111/j.1476-5829.2011.00315.x. Available at: http://www.ncbi.nlm.nih.gov/pubmed/22372648. Accessed March 15, 2013.
9. Comazzi S, Gelain ME, Martini V, et al. Immunophenotype predicts survival time in dogs with chronic lymphocytic leukemia. J Vet Intern Med 2011;25:100–6. Available at: http://onlinelibrary.wiley.com/store/10.1111/j.1939-1676.2010.0640.x/asset/j.1939-1676.2010.0640.x.pdf?v=1&t=hesqx3gu&s=43f36e809bfb6e49a5a92cbd14d320f7a42f3bf1. Accessed March 15, 2013.
10. Rao S, Lana S, Eickhoff J, et al. Class II Major histocompatibility complex expression and cell size independently predict survival in canine B-cell lymphoma. J Vet Intern Med 2011;25:1097–105. Available at: http://onlinelibrary.wiley.com/store/10.1111/j.1939-1676.2011.0767.x/asset/jvim767.pdf?v=1&t=hesqtx53&s=ea850c4b936160f27a4115195e5e86a12efa9f25. Accessed March 15, 2013.

11. Klotz FW, Gathings WE, Cooper MD. Development and distribution of B lineage cells in the domestic cat: analysis with monoclonal antibodies to cat mu-, gamma-, kappa-, and lambda-chains and heterologous anti-alpha antibodies. J Immunol 1985;134:95–100. Available at: http://www.ncbi.nlm.nih.gov/pubmed/3917286. Accessed March 15, 2013.

12. Vernau W, Moore PF. An immunophenotypic study of canine leukemias and preliminary assessment of clonality by polymerase chain reaction. Vet Immunol Immunopathol 1999;69:145–64. Available at: http://www.sciencedirect.com/science/article/pii/S0165242799000513. Accessed March 15, 2013.

13. Burnett RC, Vernau W, Modiano JF, et al. Diagnosis of canine lymphoid neoplasia using clonal rearrangements of antigen receptor genes. Vet Pathol 2003;40:32–41. Available at: http://vet.sagepub.com/content/40/1/32.full.pdf+html. Accessed March 15, 2013.

14. Moore PF, Woo JC, Vernau W, et al. Characterization of feline T cell receptor gamma (TCRG) variable region genes for the molecular diagnosis of feline intestinal lymphoma. Vet Immunol Immunopathol 2005;106:167–78. Available at: http://www.sciencedirect.com/science/article/pii/S0165242705000632#. Accessed March 15, 2013.

15. Dongen JJ, Langerak AW, Bruggemann M, et al. Design and standardization of PCR primers and protocols for detection of clonal immunoglobulin and T-cell receptor gene recombinations in suspect lymphoproliferations: Report of the BIOMED-2 Concerted Action BMH4-CT98-3936. Leukemia 2003;17:2257–317. Available at: http://www.nature.com/leu/journal/v17/n12/full/2403202a.html. Accessed March 15, 2013.

16. Sato H, Fujino Y, Uchida K, et al. Comparison between immunohistochemistry and genetic clonality analysis for cellular lineage determination in feline lymphomas. J Vet Med Sci 2011;73:945–7. Available at: https://www.jstage.jst.go.jp/article/jvms/73/7/73_10-0528/_article. Accessed March 15, 2013.

17. Nagata K, Lamb M, Goldschmidt MH, et al. The usefulness of immunohistochemistry to differentiate between nasal carcinoma and lymphoma in cats: 140 cases (1986-2000). Vet Comp Oncol 2012. http://dx.doi.org/10.1111/j.1476-5829.2012.00330.x. Available at: http://www.ncbi.nlm.nih.gov/pubmed/22520498. Accessed March 15, 2013.

18. Von Euler H, Einarsson R, Olsson U, et al. Serum thymidine kinase activity in dogs with malignant lymphoma: a potent marker for prognosis and monitoring the disease. J Vet Intern Med 2004;18:696–702. Available at: http://www.ncbi.nlm.nih.gov/pubmed/15515587. Accessed March 15, 2013.

19. Taylor SS, Dodkin S, Papasouliotis K, et al. Serum thymidine kinase activity in clinically healthy and diseased cats: a potential biomarker for lymphoma. J Feline Med Surg 2013;15:142–7. Available at: http://jfm.sagepub.com/content/15/2/142.long. Accessed March 15, 2013.

Hematology of the Domestic Ferret (*Mustela putorius furo*)

Stephen A. Smith, MS, DVM, PhD[a],*,
Kurt Zimmerman, DVM, PhD, DACVP[a],
David M. Moore, MS, DVM, DACLAM[b]

KEYWORDS

• Ferret • Blood collection • Hematology • Hemogram • White blood cells

KEY POINTS

• Today, the ferret is an important laboratory animal used in biomedical research as a model for a number of important human clinical syndromes and disease processes, such as Reye syndrome, *Helicobacter* gastritis, and antiemetic drug screening.
• Pet ferrets are presented to veterinary clinics for routine care and treatment of clinical diseases and female reproductive problems.
• In addition to obtaining clinical history, additional diagnostic testing may be required, including hematological assessments. This article describes common blood collection methods, including venipuncture sites, volume of blood that can be safely collected, and handling of the blood.

The domestic ferret (*Mustela putorius furo*) belongs to the family Mustelidae in the order Carnivora. They have been domesticated for more than a thousand years and were historically used for hunting of animals that lived in burrows. Today, the ferret is an important laboratory animal used in biomedical research as a model for a number of important human clinical syndromes and disease processes, such as Reye syndrome, *Helicobacter* gastritis, and antiemetic drug screening. There are 2 basic color types, the fitch and albino, but there are more than 30 recognized color combinations. Ferrets may live up to 12 years, but more commonly have a life span of 5 to 8 years. Males (hobs) may weigh 1 to 2 kg, and the smaller females (jills) may weigh 500 to 900 g.

This article originally appeared in Veterinary Clinics of North America: Exotic Animal Practice, Volume 18, Issue 1, January 2015.
[a] Department of Biomedical Sciences and Pathobiology, Virginia-Maryland Regional College of Veterinary Medicine, Virginia Tech, 245 Duck Pond Drive, Blacksburg, VA 24061, USA; [b] North End Center, Virginia Tech, 300 Turner Street Northwest, Suite 4120, Blacksburg, VA 24061, USA
* Corresponding author.
E-mail address: stsmith7@vt.edu

In 2012, approximately 748,000 ferrets were maintained as pets in approximately 334,000 households in the United States.[1] As a resource for veterinarians and their technicians, this article describes the methods for collection of blood and identification of blood cells in ferrets.

METHODOLOGY FOR BLOOD COLLECTION
Restraint

Proper techniques for handling and restraint of ferrets have been described in a number of publications.[2–5] A brief description of standard handling and restraint methods for ferrets is provided in the following sections.

Manual restraint
Specific manual restraint techniques are described in the section on venipuncture techniques.

Chemical restraint
Doses of anesthetics and tranquilizers used in ferrets are provided in other publications.[6,7] In general, anesthesia is not required for most blood collection procedures, and based on the clinical status of the patient at the time of presentation, the clinician should determine whether an animal should or should not be anesthetized. For sedation, midazolam (midazolam 0.25–1.0 mg/kg intramuscularly) may be used, or general anesthesia, using isoflurane or sevoflurane, can be used if the handler or phlebotomist is relatively inexperienced. Isoflurane may adversely affect the results of blood parameters in ferrets, and this should be considered when interpreting the results.[8,9] Total red cell, white cell, and platelet numbers can be significantly lower in anesthetized ferrets.[9,10]

Blood Collection Sites: Location and Preparation, and Venipuncture Techniques

Blood collection techniques in a ferret are comparable to those in the cat. Common sites used for blood collection are the lateral saphenous vein, the cephalic vein, the jugular vein, dorsal metatarsal vein, and the cranial vena cava.[2,11–15] Less common sites, not recommended in a private practice setting, are the caudal artery of the tail, and the orbital sinus. Depending on the vessel selected, a 22-gauge to 30-gauge needle should be used. For smaller veins, a 1-mL syringe should be used to prevent collapse of the vessel during aspiration of the blood sample.

The jugular vein is the most accessible site for the collection of blood in the domestic ferret. A variety of restraint techniques may be used. The ferret may be placed in dorsal or lateral recumbency with the head extended and the front legs pulled/restrained in a caudal direction. The fur should be clipped over the venipuncture site, and the area swabbed with an appropriate disinfectant solution. The ferret jugular vein, as compared with that in the cat, runs in a more lateral position. A 22-gauge to 25-gauge needle is inserted into the vein in a cranial direction, and the blood aspirated into the syringe. After the needle is withdrawn, firm pressure should be applied to prevent hematoma formation. A second method involves placing the animal in sternal recumbency, pulling the front legs downward over the edge of the examination table, and flexing the head in a caudal direction. A third method involves having the animal held by the scruff of the neck by one individual, suspended perpendicular to the floor or examination table, while the phlebotomist performs the venipuncture. In this technique, the needle and syringe are parallel to the floor, and the needle is inserted perpendicular to the ferret. A fourth method involves wrapping the animal securely in a towel, with the head and neck exposed.

The cranial vena cava[16] also can be used to obtain blood; however, the ferret should be sedated to reduce the risk of laceration of the vessel by the needle (should the animal move), resulting in significant internal hemorrhage. In the unanesthetized ferret, 2 handlers should provide restraint of the animal. The animal is placed in dorsal recumbency on the examination table, one individual restraining and stabilizing the head, and the other individual restraining the lower body and drawing the front legs in a caudal direction. The fur should be clipped over the venipuncture site, and the area swabbed with an appropriate disinfectant solution. The needle is inserted in the right thoracic notch (the animal's right side), the space between the manubrium and the first rib. A 25-gauge to 27-gauge 0.5-inch needle, held at a 30° angle with respect to the plane of the body, is inserted in a caudolateral direction, "aiming" it toward the left hip. As the needle is inserted, the phlebotomist should draw back on the plunger of the syringe to create negative pressure. Once blood is seen to flow into the needle hub or syringe, the phlebotomist will stop insertion of the needle, and stabilize the needle and syringe to complete the collection of the sample. After the needle is withdrawn, pressure should be applied to the site, but this will only prevent flow of blood from the puncture in the skin, but not stop any flow that might occur within the thoracic cavity.

The lateral saphenous may be used for collecting small amounts of blood for packed cell volume (PCV) or complete blood count. As with the vena cava collection, 2 persons should manually restrain the unanesthetized ferret for blood collection by the phlebotomist. The fur over the venipuncture site, on the lateral aspect below the stifle, should be clipped, and the area swabbed with an appropriate disinfectant solution. One individual restrains the animal's upper body, and the second individual restrains the lower body, and restrains the leg and applies pressure over the vessel at a point above the stifle. Alternatively, a Penrose drain may be used as a tourniquet. A 25-gauge to 27-gauge needle on a 0.5-mL to 1.0-mL syringe is inserted in a proximal direction in the vessel, with the phlebotomist applying slow, gentle aspiration to prevent the vein from collapsing. After the needle is withdrawn, firm pressure should be applied to prevent hematoma formation.

The procedure for cephalic vein venipuncture and blood collection is similar to that in cats. However, because this vein is ideal for intravenous catheter placement, it should perhaps be preserved by selecting an alternate venipuncture site. Manual restraint can be accomplished by wrapping the animal in a towel, with the limb exposed. The animal also can be restrained by the scruff of the neck, and the limb extended, with digital pressure or a tourniquet applied proximal to the venipuncture site.

By outward appearance, blood collection via the caudal tail artery is painful or distressing to the animal. Additionally, hematological parameters can vary greatly when blood is collected by this method.[2] One individual restrains the animal in dorsal recumbency. The phlebotomist, using a 20-gauge to 21-gauge needle on a 1-mL to 3-mL syringe, inserts the needle into the groove on the midline of the ventral surface of the tail, beginning about 1 to 2 inches (2–5 cm) from the base of the tail, and inserting the needle at a 45° angle in a proximal direction. Because of the arterial pressure, the arteriopuncture site should be held off for 3 minutes or longer to ensure adequate hemostasis, and to prevent hematoma formation.

Volume Collected

The estimated whole blood volume, based on body weight, and the recommended maximum safe blood volume that should be considered, are provided in **Table 1**. It would be prudent to collect a smaller volume of blood (0.5% of body weight) from geriatric, anemic, hypoproteinemic, or otherwise clinically ill patients.

Table 1
Determining maximum safe blood sample volumes in ferrets based on body weight

Body Weight (kg)	Whole Blood Volume (mL) (5%–6% of Body Weight)	Draw No More than 7.5%–10% of WBV (Safe Volume to Collect - mL)
0.5	25–30	1.88–3
0.75	37.5–45	2.8–4.5
1.0	50–60	3.75–6
1.25	62.5–75	4.7–7.5
1.50	75–90	5.6–9
1.75	87.5–105	6.6–10.5
2.0	100–120	7.5–12

Abbreviation: WBV, whole blood volume.

MORPHOLOGY AND NUMBERS OF PERIPHERAL BLOOD CELLS

Anesthesia, sex, age, reproductive cycle, circadian rhythm, restraint, stress, and the site of blood sampling can affect hemogram results. A generalized reference range for normal hematological values reported for the domestic ferret is listed in **Table 2**.[17–20] More complete hematologic reference intervals or individual-specific values may be found scattered throughout the ferret literature.[21–26]

Most values are similar to values reported for other domestic carnivores; however, the hematocrit, hemoglobin, and total erythrocyte and reticulocyte counts in ferrets are generally higher than in the dog or cat.[27] Additionally, ferrets have no detectable blood groups and therefore no naturally occurring antibodies against unmatched erythrocyte antigens. Therefore, repeated transfusions without the development of antibodies are possible in the ferret.[27]

Table 2
Referenced ranges of normal hematological parameters in the ferret (*Mustela putorius furo*)

Parameter	Adult Male	Adult Female	Age 2–3 mo
RBC ($\times 10^6/\mu L$)	6.5–13.2	6.7–9.34	4.8–7.8
PCV (%)	33.6–49.8	35.6–55	27.0–38.5
Hgb (g/dL)	12.0–18.2	12.9–17.4	9.6–13.8
MCV (fL)	44.1–52.5	44.4–53.7	47.8–57.6
MCH (pg)	16.5–19.7	16.4–19.4	17.5–22.8
MCHC (%)	33.7–42.2	33.2–35.3	34.7–37.0
Platelets ($\times 10^3/\mu L$)	297–730	310–910	—
WBC ($\times 10^3/\mu L$)	4.4–15.4	2.5–18.2	5.3–12.6
Neutrophils (%)	24–76	43–78	46.1–76.6
Lymphocytes (%)	12–66.6	12–67	42.2–68.2
Eosinophils (%)	0–8.5	0–8.5	2.1–6.9
Basophils (%)	0–3	0–2.9	0–1.3
Monocytes (%)	0–8.2	1–6.3	0.7–4.7

Abbreviations: Hgb, hemoglobin; MCH, mean corpuscular hemoglobin; MCHC, mean corpuscular hemoglobin concentration; MCV, mean corpuscular volume; PCV, packed cell volume; RBC, red blood cell; WBC, white blood cell.
Data from Refs.[17–20]

Erythrocytes (Red Blood Cell)

The mean red blood cell (RBC) diameter for ferrets is reported to be 5.94 μm (range of 4.6–7.7 μm) in males and 6.32 μm (range of 4.6–7.7 μm) in females.[19,27–29] The hematocrit of ferrets ranges between 30% and 61%, but usually averages between 40% and 50% for adult ferrets and between 32% and 39% for juvenile ferrets. The mean percentage of reticulocytes is reported to be 4% (range of 1%–12%) in male ferrets and 5.3% (range of 2%–14%) in female ferrets.[19] Low numbers of Howell-Jolly bodies have been reported in a small percentage of both male and female ferrets. Other red blood cell values are listed in **Table 2**.[19,29]

Jills are induced ovulators, and individuals that do not breed during estrus may exhibit prolonged estrus throughout the breeding season. After a month of prolonged estrus, high levels of estrogen in the bloodstream may cause bone marrow suppression with leucopenia, thrombocytopenia, and aplastic anemia. A decrease in PCV and total RBC numbers in jills is consistent with prolonged estrus. Jills with PCV values higher than 25% generally have a good prognosis, and ovariohysterectomy will quickly remove high circulating estrogen levels with a return to normal erythrocyte production in the bone marrow. Alternatively, hormone treatments such as proligestone, human chorionic gonadotrophin, or gonadotrophin-releasing hormone injections can be used to induce ovulation, resulting in decreased circulating estrogen levels. However, it might take up to 4 months for the anemia to fully resolve. PCV values between 15% and 25% in jills present a guarded prognosis, and supportive care, such as fluid replacement and blood transfusion, may be indicated before any surgery is attempted. As described previously, administration of hormone injections also can be considered. The prognosis for jills with a PCV lower than 15% is poor, and may require blood transfusions over several months.

A polychromatophil, an immature RBC that has lost its nucleus, appears bluer than a mature RBC (when Wright's stain is used), and it is usually larger than a mature RBC. Polychromatophilia is suggestive of an increased production of erythrocytes by the bone marrow (erythroid hyperplasia) in response to anemia. The presence of clinical signs of prolonged estrus with anemia can be confirmed with the presence of increased numbers of polychromatophils. A representative polychromatophil is shown in **Fig. 1**B.

Thrombocytes (Platelets)

The mean platelet diameter for male and female ferrets is reported to be 1.7 μm (range of 1.5–2.3 μm).[19,28] The mean number of circulating platelets reported in ferrets varies significantly between studies.[17,30] As noted previously, a jill with prolonged estrus may have a low platelet count. Referenced values for platelet counts in normal ferrets is provided in **Table 2**.

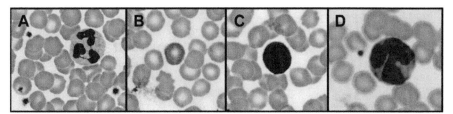

Fig. 1. Representative ferret blood cells. (*A*) Neutrophil, RBCs, and platelets. (*B*) Polychromatophil and RBCs. (*C*) Lymphocyte and RBCs. (*D*) Monocyte and RBCs. (Wright-Giemsa stain, original magnification 1000×).

Leukocytes (White Blood Cells)

Neutrophils are the predominant leukocyte observed in ferret blood, followed by lymphocytes, eosinophils and monocytes, and finally basophils. The ranges of total white blood cell (WBC) numbers and the WBC cell types observed in a standard differential count are provided in **Table 2**.

Neutrophils

The ferret neutrophil has a segmented nucleus, and its pale blue cytoplasm contains polychromatic granules. Comparative values of neutrophils observed in differential counts in normal ferrets, by age and sex, are provided in **Table 2**. A typical neutrophil is illustrated in **Fig. 1A**.

Lymphocytes

Ferret lymphocytes have a reported mean diameter of 7.7 μm (range of 6.2–9.2 μm) in males and 8.7 μm (range of 7.7–10.0 μm) in females.[19] Comparative values of lymphocytes observed in differential counts in normal ferrets, by age and sex, are provided in **Table 2**. A typical lymphocyte is illustrated in **Fig. 1C**.

Eosinophils

Eosinophils may have a 1-lobed or 2-lobed nucleus, and the cytoplasm is filled with numerous round red granules. Eosinophils have a mean diameter of 12.7 μm in males and 12.6 μm in females.[19,29] Comparative values of eosinophils observed in differential counts in normal ferrets, by age and sex, are provided in **Table 2**.

Basophils

Basophils have a segmented nucleus with a reported mean diameter of 13.5 μm in males and 13.8 μm in females.[19] Comparative values of basophils observed in differential counts in normal ferrets, by age and sex, are provided in **Table 2**.

Monocytes

Monocytes have a reported diameter between 12 and 18 μm. Comparative values of monocytes observed in differential counts in normal ferrets, by age and sex, are provided in **Table 2**. A typical lymphocyte is illustrated in **Fig. 1D**.

REFERENCES

1. American Veterinary Medical Association. 2012 U.S. pet ownership & demographic sourcebook. Schaumberg (IL): AVMA; 2012.
2. Joslin JO. Blood collection techniques in exotic small mammals. J EXOT PET MED 2009;18(2):117–39.
3. Hrapkiewicz K, Colby L, Denison P. Clinical laboratory animal medicine: an introduction. 4th edition. Ames (IA): Wiley Blackwell; 2013. p. 298–307.
4. Fox JG. Housing and management. In: Fox JG, editor. Biology and diseases of the ferret. 2nd edition. Baltimore (MD): Williams & Wilkins; 1998. p. 179–80.
5. Ballard B, Rockett J. Restraint and handling for veterinary technicians and assistants. Clifton Park (NY): Delmar; 2009. p. 70–2.
6. Drexel University. A compendium of drugs used for laboratory animal anesthesia, analgesia, tranquilization and restraint. Philadelphia: Drexel University IACUC; 2007.

7. Marini RP, Fox JG. Anesthesia, surgery, and biomethodology. In: Fox JG, editor. Biology and diseases of the ferret. 2nd edition. Baltimore: Williams & Wilkins; 1998. p. 464–72.

8. Ness RD. Clinical pathology and sample collection of exotic small mammals. Vet Clin North Am Exot Anim Pract 1999;2:591–620.

9. Marini RP. Effect of isoflurane on hematologic variables in ferrets. Am J Vet Res 1994;55:1479–83.

10. Marini R, Callahan R, Jackson L. Distribution of technetium 99m-labeled red blood cells during isoflurane anesthesia in ferrets. Am J Vet Res 1997;58:781–5.

11. Bleakley SP. Simple technique for bleeding ferrets (Mustela putorius furo). Lab Anim 1980;14:59–60.

12. Brown S. Clinical techniques in domestic ferrets. Seminar Avian Exotic Pet Med 1997;6:75–85.

13. Capello V. Application of the cranial vena cava venipuncture technique to small exotic mammals. Exot DVM 2006:8.3, Zoological Education Network.

14. Dyer SM, Cervasio EL. An overview of restraint and blood collection techniques in exotic pet practice. Vet Clin North Am Exot Anim Pract 2008;11:423–43.

15. Otto G, Rosenblad WD, Fox JG. Practical venipuncture techniques for the ferret. Lab Anim 1993;27:26–9.

16. Brown C. Blood collection from the cranial vena cava of the ferret. Lab Anim (NY) 2006;35(9):23–4.

17. Besch-Williford CL. Biology and medicine of the ferret. Vet Clin North Am Small Anim Pract 1987;17:1155–83.

18. Fox JG, Marini R. Diseases of the endocrine system. In: Fox JG, editor. Biology and diseases of the ferret. Baltimore (MD): Williams & Wilkins; 1998. p. 291–305.

19. Thornton PC. The ferret Mustela putorius furo, as a new species in toxicology. Lab Anim 1979;13:119–24.

20. Zimmerman KL, Moore MM, Smith SA. Hematology of the ferret. In: Weiss DJ, Wardrop KJ, editors. Schalm's veterinary hematology. Ames (IA): Wiley-Blackwell; 2010. p. 904–9.

21. Carpenter JW, Hill EF. Hematological values for the Siberian ferret. J Zoo Anim Med 1979;10:126–8.

22. Fox JG. Serum chemistry and hematology reference values in the ferret. Lab Anim Sci 1986;36:22–8.

23. Hoover JP, Baldwin CA. Changes in physiologic and clinicopathologic values in domestic ferrets from 12–47 weeks of age. Companion Anim Pract 1988;2: 40–4.

24. Lee EJ. Haematological and serum chemistry profiles of ferrets (Mustela putorius furo). Lab Anim 1982;16:133–7.

25. Ohwada K, Katahira K. Reference values for organ weight, hematology and serum chemistry in the female ferret (Mustela putorius furo). Jikken Dobutsu 1993;42:135–42.

26. Zeissler R. Hematological and clinical biochemical parameters in ferrets under various physiological and pathological conditions. 1. Comparative studies of changes in the hemograms of pregnant, lactating and non-pregnant females. Z Versuchstierkd 1981;23:244–54.

27. Marini R, Otto G, Erdman S. Biology and diseases of the ferret. In: Fox JG, Anderson L, Lowe F, editors. Laboratory animal medicine. London: Academic Press; 2002. p. 483–517.

28. Hillyer EV, Quesenberry KE. Ferrets rabbits, and rodents: clinical medicine and surgery. Philadelphia: WB Saunders; 1997. p. 432.

29. Siperstein LJ. Ferret hematology and related disorders. Vet Clin North Am Exot Anim Pract 2008;11:535–50.
30. Kawasaki TA. Normal parameters and laboratory interpretation of disease states in the domestic ferret. Semin Avian Exotic Pet Med 1994;3:40–7.

Hematological Assessment in Pet Rabbits

Blood Sample Collection and Blood Cell Identification

David M. Moore, MS, DVM, DACLAM[a],*,
Kurt Zimmerman, DVM, PhD, DACVP[b],
Stephen A. Smith, MS, DVM, PhD[b]

KEYWORDS

- Rabbit • Blood collection • Hematology • Hemogram
- White blood cell count morphology • Differential count

KEY POINT

- Part of the clinical care of pet rabbits is the assessment of overt and latent clinical conditions, and hematological assessments are an important part of the clinician's armamentarium.

The American Veterinary Medical Association (AVMA) has estimated that about 1.4 million households have pet rabbits, with a total of 3.2 million rabbits maintained as pets.[1] Because about two-thirds of pet owners consider their pets to be family members, it is important that Flopsy, Mopsy, and Cottontail receive the clinical care they need and deserve. Part of that clinical care is the assessment of overt and latent clinical conditions, and hematological assessments are an important part of the clinician's armamentarium. Because indoor-housed rabbits have a lifespan of 8 to 12 years (and outdoor-housed have a lifespan of about 4–8 years), visits to the veterinary clinic may add up over time. This article describes the methods for manual restraint, collection of blood, identification of blood cells, and interpretation of the hemogram in rabbits.

METHODOLOGY FOR BLOOD COLLECTION
Restraint

A rabbit presented for clinical evaluation may already be stressed from transport to the clinic, and from the sights, sounds, and smells in the clinic. Those stressors may

This article originally appeared in Veterinary Clinics of North America: Exotic Animal Practice, Volume 18, Issue 1, January 2015.
[a] Virginia Tech, 300 Turner Street Northwest, Suite 4120 (0497), Blacksburg, VA 24061, USA;
[b] Department of Biomedical Sciences and Pathobiology (0442), Virginia–Maryland Regional College of Veterinary Medicine, 245 Duck Pond Drive, Blacksburg, VA 24061, USA
* Corresponding author.
E-mail address: moored@vt.edu

engage the flight response in the rabbit, and attempts to flee from the examination table may have disastrous consequences. To avoid injury to its spine, be sure to support the rabbit's hindquarters when picking it up to move it from 1 location to another.

Although manual restraint may be used for auscultation and palpation of the rabbit, potentially stressful procedures, such as blood collection, are best accomplished with additional restraint devices, to reduce the risk of injury to the patient and to the technician or veterinarian. A rabbit can scratch and slash handlers with the claws on its forefeet and hind feet, and struggling and twisting by an inadequately restrained rabbit may result in spine and spinal cord injury in the animal, with either paresis or permanent paralysis as the outcome. Most clinics have cloth cat restraint bags in multiple sizes, and an appropriately sized bag can be used to restrain a rabbit. Alternatively, a bath towel can be used to wrap up the rabbit, leaving its head exposed. The slight pressure that both of those exert on the rabbit's body provides a calming effect, and the rabbit is unlikely to struggle and injure its spine. Chemical restraint may also be used to facilitate blood collection; however, anesthesia may be contraindicated in an already debilitated patient. Drugs that can be used in sedation, tranquilization, and anesthesia of rabbits have been described in the published literature.[2,3]

Blood Collection Sites—Location and Preparation, and Venipuncture Techniques

The 2 primary vessels used for blood collection from a rabbit are the marginal ear vein, yielding small-to-moderate quantities of blood (depending on the experience and expertise of the phlebotomist), and the central auricular artery, from which a larger volume of blood can be collected. Other veins/sites that may be used include the lateral saphenous vein of the hind leg, the cephalic vein on the foreleg, and the jugular vein. Restraint required for those alternate sites may be stressful to the animal. Thus the 2 preferred methods are emphasized in this article.

Table 1 provides a comparison of the advantages and disadvantages of the common blood collection sites in rabbits. **Fig. 1** illustrates the location of the 2 preferred vessels for blood collection in the rabbit.

The central auricular artery and the marginal ear vein(s) are approached on the outer, haired surface of the pinna of either ear. The fur should be plucked over the intended venipuncture site. This is not distressful to the rabbit, and the minor local irritation stimulates vasodilation. The venipuncture site should be cleansed with a suitable disinfectant solution or alcohol, recognizing that this may result in vasoconstriction. Induction of vasodilation, and thus facilitation of blood collection, can be accomplished by several procedures, and technicians and veterinarians may select among the methods listed to accomplish that aim:

- Fill an examination glove with water. Tie it off; microwave it until its temperature is warm to the touch, but not scalding, and apply that to the rabbit's era for about a minute.
- Swab the skin over the proposed venipuncture site with oil of wintergreen and then collect blood 1 to 2 minutes after its application, taking care to rinse any residual oil off the ear after the blood has been collected.
- Administer acepromazine subcutaneously (0.5–1.0 mg/kg) about 15 to 20 minutes before blood collection (the time involved is perhaps not practical in a busy practice).
- Gently stroke (milk) the vessel with the thumb and forefinger from the base of the ear toward the tip of the ear.

Recommended needle sizes range from 22 to 25 gauge, selecting the smallest gauge needle required to minimize discomfort and tissue trauma. Standard needles

Table 1
Comparison of blood collection sites in the rabbit

Collection Site	Advantages	Disadvantages
Marginal ear vein	• Easily visualized • Easily accessible • Vessel is not mobile • Does not require sedation/anesthesia • Good for collecting small volumes of blood	• The vein is small and easily collapsed with rapid aspiration • May be too small in smaller breeds or young rabbits • Cannot collect a large volume of blood • May result in thrombosis and sloughing of skin over site • Hematoma formation and bruising can occur
Central auricular artery	• Easily visualized • Easily accessible • Vessel is not mobile • Does not require sedation/anesthesia • Rapid collection of larger volume of blood	• May require topical application of a local anesthetic to prevent arteriospasm • If damage is done to the artery, blood supply to the pinna will be compromised • Hematoma formation and bruising can occur
Lateral saphenous vein	• Easily visualized • Easily accessible	• Vein is mobile, requires stabilization • Vein may collapse during aspiration • Sedation desirable to prevent injury to limb
Cephalic vein	• Good for collecting small-to-moderate volumes of blood	• May not be easily visualized • Vein is mobile, requires stabilization • Sedation desirable to prevent injury to limb and visual stress to rabbit • Skin may be contaminated with exudates from upper respiratory tract (URT) infection—foreleg used in grooming • Shorter length in smaller breeds, hard to access
Jugular vein	• Good for collecting larger volumes of blood	• Not easily visualized in obese rabbits or females with large dewlaps • Sedation/anesthesia recommended • Short nosed/dwarf breeds and rabbits with URT infections may become dypsneic when the neck is extended back during restraint

or butterfly catheters may be used. The vacuum associated with a vacutainer tube may collapse the vessel; thus use of a syringe is recommended to control the rate of aspiration.

The lateral, as opposed to the medial, marginal ear vein is the more accessible of the 2 veins. One individual, using a thumb and forefinger, should apply pressure to the vein near the base of the ear. The needle is inserted into the vein, directing it toward the base of the ear. The skin and vessel wall are thin enough to visualize the needle within the vessel. The phlebotomist should slowly aspirate the blood, pausing briefly if the flow has stopped, or slowly rotating the needle and syringe on its axis in case the bevel of the needle has been closed off by the vessel wall. When the needle is withdrawn, the assistant/technician should apply gentle pressure over the venipuncture site with a cotton swab or sterile gauze pad for about 1 to 2 minutes to prevent hematoma formation.

When collecting blood from the central auricular artery (**Fig. 2**), the phlebotomist should apply digital pressure to the artery near the tip of the era, and insert the needle in a distal direction, toward the base of the ear. Given the higher pressure in the artery,

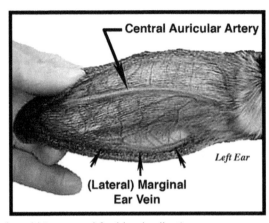

Fig. 1. Vessels of the rabbit ear used for blood collection.

gentle pressure should be applied over the venipuncture site for 2 to 4 minutes (or as needed) to prevent hematoma formation. A hematoma on the pinna may be irritating to the rabbit, causing head shaking and ear scratching, which can cause the hematoma to become even larger and more irritating.

Several publications are available that provide additional information on restraint and blood collection in rabbits.[4,5]

Volume Collected

Depending on the number and types of blood tests (eg, complete blood cell count [CBC], differential, and/or clinical chemistry) and the size and strain of rabbit, 0.5 to 10 mL of blood can be withdrawn using the methods described previously. The recommended maximum safe volume of blood that can be collected is 7.7 mL/kg of body weight.[6]

Handling of the Blood Sample

A drop of fresh blood, without anticoagulant, can be placed on a clean glass microscope slide for preparation of a peripheral blood smear for examination for the differential count of leukocytes, and for assessing erythrocyte abnormalities. Fresh blood can be drawn into heparinized microhematocrit tubes for determination of the packed cell volume (hematocrit).

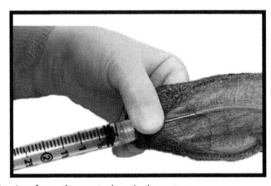

Fig. 2. Blood collection from the central auricular artery.

If additional tests are to be performed (eg, total/absolute white cell count or clinical chemistry testing), the blood should be placed in a vacutainer tube containing antico-agulant (a purple top tube containing Ethylenediaminetetraacetic acid [EDTA]). To minimize the risk of hemolysis of red blood cells, which would adversely affect test results, the following steps should be taken:

- Remove the rubber stopper from the vacutainer.
- Remove the needle from the syringe containing the blood.
- Slowly dispense the blood down an inside wall of the tube.
- Gently agitate the tube to mix the blood with the anticoagulant.

Samples may be stored at 4°C prior to testing, and timely processing (eg, within 1 hour after collection) is preferable. Overnight shipment to outside laboratories and testing within 48 to 72 hours should yield analytically acceptable results.[7]

MORPHOLOGY AND NUMBERS OF PERIPHERAL BLOOD CELLS
Erythrocytes

The rabbit erythrocyte is a biconcave disc with an average diameter of 6.7 to 6.9 μm,[8] and an average thickness of 2.15 to 2.4 μm.[9,10] The average lifespan of an erythrocyte ranges from 45 to 70 days.[6] There can be marked variability in the size of erythrocytes, referred to as anisocytosis, with some cells being one-fourth the diameter of normal cells.[11]

Polychromasia, a variation in staining of erythrocytes with Wright's stain, associated with the presence of young erythrocytes, those cells having a diffuse blue color, was observed in 1% to 2% of erythrocytes.[9] Young rabbits, 1 to 2 months of age, were found to have reticulocyte counts of 3% to 11%; adult males were found to have reticulocyte counts of 1.5% to 2.5%; and adult females were found to have reticulocyte counts of 2.5% to 3.5%.[10,11] Higher reticulocyte counts may be found after repeated blood collections, and are associated with regenerative anemia.[12,13]

Comparative values of erythrocyte parameters in rabbits are provided in **Tables 2** and **3**. Male rabbits have slightly higher numbers of erythrocytes and slightly higher hemoglobin concentrations compared with females.[6] Compared with adults, newborn rabbits have lower erythrocyte counts; however, their mean corpuscular volume (MCV) and mean corpuscular hemoglobin (MCH) values are higher than those in adults.

Thrombocytes (Platelets)

Comparative values of thrombocyte numbers are provided in **Table 2**. Thrombocytes may be observed singly or in groups in stained blood smears. They may be oblong, oval, or rounded, and they may be from 1 μm to 3 μm in diameter. When stained with Wright's stain, they appear to have a violet-hued center, with a pale blue to colorless periphery.[14] It was observed that in acute infectious processes, there is a decrease in thrombocyte counts and an increase in nucleated red blood cell (RBC) counts.[15]

Leukocytes (White Blood Cells)

The ranges of total white blood cell (WBC) numbers and the WBC types observed in a standard differential count are provided in **Tables 2** and **3**. The WBC count in rabbits may vary dramatically as a result of circadian rhythms (diurnal fluctuations and variation within a month), nutritional status and dietary differences, and differences in age, gender, and breed.[6] Total leukocyte counts are lowest in the late afternoon and evening.[16]

Table 2
Referenced ranges of normal hematological parameters in the New Zealand white rabbit
(*oryctolagus cuniculus*)

	Adult Male	Adult Female	Age 1 to 3 mo
RBC ($\times 10^6/\mu L$)	5.46–7.94	5.11–6.51	5.15–6.48
PCV (%)	33–50	31.0–48.6	38.1–44.1
Hgb (g/dL)	10.4–17.4	9.8–15.8	10.7–13.9
MCV (fL)	58.5–66.5	57.8–65.4	66.2–80.3
MCH (pg)	18.7–22.7	17.1–23.5	19.5–22.7
MCHC (%)	33–50	28.7–35.7	24.2–32.6
Platelets ($\times 10^3/\mu L$)	304–656	270–630	—
WBC ($\times 10^3/\mu L$)	5.5–12.5	5.2–10.6	4.1–9.79
Neutrophils (%)	38–54	36.4–50.4	18.8–46.4
Lymphocytes (%)	28–50	31.5–52.1	44.6–77.8
Eosinophils (%)	0.5–3.5	0.8–3.2	0–2.4
Basophils (%)	2.5–7.5	2.4–6.2	0.1–4.5
Monocytes (%)	4–12	6.6–13.4	0–13.1

Data from Refs.[6,8,11]

Neutrophils

The rabbit neutrophil, also referred to as a heterophil, is the second most common WBC seen in peripheral blood smears. The rabbit neutrophil contains small acidophilic granules and varying numbers of large red granules, leading some to call it a pseudoeosinophil.[11] The smaller pink granules outnumber the larger red granules by 80% to 90%.[17] The rabbit neutrophil is about 10 μm to 15 μm in diameter; its polymorphic nucleus stains light purple, and the nucleus is surrounded by a diffusely pink cytoplasm.[11] A typical rabbit neutrophil is illustrated in **Fig. 3**.

Table 3
Referenced ranges of normal hematological parameters in 3 additional rabbit species

	Dutch Belted (*Lepus europaeus*)	Eastern Cottontail (*Sylvilagus floridianus*)	Jackrabbit (*Lepus californicus*)
RBC ($\times 10^6/\mu L$)	4.8–6.3	4.2	6.59–8.56
PCV (%)	34.8–48.9	18–49	42–53
Hgb (g/dL)	12.2–16.3	—	13.7–17.5
MCV (fL)	62.7–88.1	—	57.6–70.0
MCH (pg)	22.0–29.4	—	18–23.1
MCHC (%)	28.5–38.1	—	28.8–36.8
Platelets ($\times 10^3/\mu L$)	126–490	—	170–798
WBC ($\times 10^3/\mu L$)	6–13	—	2.2–14.7
Neutrophils (%)	30–50	0.5–61.5	13.0–81.5
Lymphocytes (%)	28.5–52.5	22–93	25–83
Eosinophils (%)	0.5–5.0	0.0–9.5	0–8
Basophils (%)	2–8	0.0–6.5	0.0–1.5
Monocytes (%)	2–16	0–5	2–10

Data from Refs.[6,8,11,23–25]

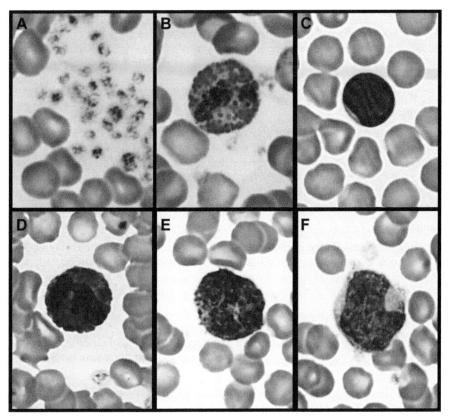

Fig. 3. Representative rabbit blood cells. (*A*) RBCs and platelets. (*B*) Heterophil, platelets, and RBCs. (*C*) Lymphocyte and RBCs. (*D*) Eosinophil and RBCs. (*E*) Basophil and RBCs. (*F*) Monocyte and RBCs. (Wright-Giemsa stain; 1000x).

The number of circulating neutrophils is lower in the early morning and highest in the late afternoon and evening.[16]

A rare homozygous genetic condition, the Pelger-Huet anomaly, has been observed in rabbits, and is characterized by severe skeletal deformities and higher mortality.[6] In this condition, neutrophils and monocytes are observed as having round-to-oval nuclei, without the typical segmentation. However, the presence of a few such cells in a blood smear from an otherwise normal rabbit are not indicative of the genetic condition.[14]

Lymphocytes

The lymphocyte is the most common WBC cell type observed in peripheral blood smears. The rabbit lymphocyte may be seen in both small and large forms, with the former about the size of an RBC, and the latter as large as a neutrophil.[14] The nucleus of the rabbit lymphocyte is condensed and round, and surrounded by a narrow band of blue-staining cytoplasm, which, in larger lymphocytes, may contain azurophilic granules.[18] The number of circulating lymphocytes is higher in the early morning, and lowest in the late afternoon and evening.[16] A typical rabbit lymphocyte is illustrated in **Fig. 3**.

Eosinophils

The rabbit eosinophil is slightly larger than a neutrophil (about 12–16 μm in diameter), and has a bilobed or horseshoe-shaped nucleus. Within the cytoplasm are numerous acidophilic granules that are about 3 to 4 times larger than those in neutrophils, which may occupy much of the space in the cytoplasm.[14,17] A low or absent eosinophil count is observed in healthy rabbits.[16] A typical rabbit eosinophil is illustrated in **Fig. 3**.

Basophils

Rabbits, in contrast to most other species, have small-to-moderate numbers of basophils in the peripheral circulation, in some instances constituting up to 30% of WBCs in differential counts in clinically normal animals.[17] The rabbit basophil is about the same size as the rabbit neutrophil. The basophil nucleus stains light purple, and the cytoplasm contains purple-to-black metachromic granules, which may sometimes obscure the nucleus.[14,17,18] A typical rabbit basophil is illustrated in **Fig. 3**.

Monocytes

The rabbit monocyte is the largest of the WBCs (around 15–18 μm in diameter). This cell has an amoeboid-shaped nucleus (lobulated, horseshoe, or bean-shaped), with diffuse, lightly stained nuclear chromatin.[11,18] The cytoplasm is blue in color, and it may occasionally contain vacuoles.[18] A typical rabbit lymphocyte is illustrated in **Fig. 3**.

INTERPRETATION OF THE HEMOGRAM

Differences in hematological values were assessed in 3 breeds of rabbits, and the results are provided; however, that same author reported that there was no significant difference between the breeds[19]:

Chinchilla—highest value for WBC, lymphocytes, monocytes, RBC, hemoglobon (Hb), packed cell volume (PCV) and MCV

New Zealand white—highest value for mean corpuscular hemoglobin concentration (MCHC) and MCH

Dutch—highest values in neutrophils, eosinophils, basophils, and platelets

Rabbits presenting with an infectious disease do not typically have a higher WBC count, but rather have a shift from lymphocyte-predominant to neutrophil-predominant differential counts. Sometimes rabbits with acute infections may have a normal differential count, but a decrease in total WBC count.[17] Leukemias are infrequently reported in rabbits, usually presented as lymphoblastic leukemia.[20] In cases of septicemia and in overwhelming bacterial infections, leucopenia with a degenerative left shift will be observed.

Rabbits transported at 28°C (82.4°F) for 1 to 3 hours were found to have elevated PCV, lymphocytopenia, and leukocytosis.[21] Cold stress has been shown to cause an increase in RBC numbers.[16] Clinicians should consider and note environmental temperatures associated with transport of rabbits to the clinic when conducting hematological examinations.

In an experimental study in rabbits of hepatic coccidiosis (caused by *Eimeria stiedai*), hematological findings 7 days after infection included anemia, leukocytosis, neutrophilia, and monocytosis.[22]

Erythrocytes

Low hematocrit/packed cell volume less than 30%
- Regenerative anemia (indicated by polychromasia, nucleated RBCs, and Howell-Jolly bodies [inclusions of nuclear chromatin remnants])[8]

- Varying degrees of anemia (present with chronic infectious conditions [eg, pasteurellosis], with associated abcessation of skin or internal organs such as testes, uterus, heart, lungs or lead toxicity)[15]
- Late pregnancy
- High doses of ivermectin

High hematocrit/packed cell volume greater than 50%
- Dehydration
  - Gastric stasis
  - Trichoezoar (hair ball)
  - Malocclusion
- Shock (associated with splenic contraction).

Reduced total RBCs with increased nucleated RBCs
- Acute infection

Regenerative anemia
- Acute blood loss
- Chronic blood loss
  - Uterine adenocarcinoma
  - Endometrial hyperplasia
  - Gastric hemorrhage
  - Urolithiasis

Nonregenerative anemia signs
- Acute blood loss (initial stages)
- Lymphoma or chronic renal disease
- Chronic diseases
  - Pasteurellosis (snuffles)
  - Tracheobronchitis
  - Pododermatitis
  - Mastitis
  - Endometritis
  - Osteomyelitis
- Dental disease

Thrombocytes

Thrombocytopenia
- Acute infection
- Hemorrhage
- Inadequate mixing of a sample with an anticoagulant, resulting in microclots
- Disseminated intravascular coagulation (DIC)

Leukocytes

Leukopenia
- Chronic stress
- Acute infection
- Chronic infection

Neutrophilia
- Acute infection (with associated lymphopenia)

  - ○ Pyogenic bacteria
  - ○ Tissue inflammation/necrosis
- Prolonged stress
- Hyperadrenocorticism

Neutropenia
- Overwhelming acute or chronic bacterial infections
- Viral infections
- Hypersplenism
- Endotoxic, septic, or anaphylactic shock
- Estrogen producing tumors (eg, Sertoli cell tumor)
- Toxemia (uremia)
- Neoplasia

Lymphopenia
- Acute infection
- Stress
- Chronic exogenous steroid administration

Lymphophilia
- Lymphoma
- Viral infection

Eosinophilia
- Chronic parasitism
- Chronic skin disease or atopy (with associated basophilia)

Eosinopenia
- Chronic stress

Monocytosis
- Chronic infection
- Inflammation

REFERENCES

1. American Veterinary Medical Association. U.S. pet ownership & demographic sourcebook. Schaumberg (IL): AVMA; 2012.
2. Carpenter JW, Mashima TY, Gentz EJ, et al. Caring for rabbits: an overview and formulary. Vet Med 1995;90(4):340–64.
3. Hawk CT, Leary S. Formulary for laboratory animals. 3rd edition. Ames (IA): Wiley-Blackwell; 2005.
4. Dyer SM, Cervasio EL. An overview of restraint and blood collection techniques in exotic pet practice. Vet Clin North Am Exot Anim Pract 2008;11(3):423–43.
5. Murray MJ. Rabbit and ferret sampling and artifact considerations. In: Fudge AM, editor. Laboratory medicine avian and exotic pets. Philadelphia: Saunders; 2000. p. 265–8.
6. Mitruka BJ, Rawnsley HM. Clinical biochemical and hematological reference values in normal experimental animals. New York: Masson Publishing; 1977.

7. Ameri M, Schnaars HA, Sibley JR, et al. Stability of hematologic analytes in monkey, rabbit, rat, and mouse blood stored at 4°C in EDTA using the ADVIA 120 hematology analyzer. Vet Clin Pathol 2011;40(2):188–94.
8. Jain NC. Normal values in blood of laboratory, furbearing and miscellaneous zoo, domestic and wild animals. In: Jain NC, editor. Schalm's veterinary hematology. Philadelphia: Lea & Febiger; 1986. p. 274–343.
9. Hawkey CM, Dennett TB. Color atlas of comparative veterinary hematology. Ames (IA): Iowa State University Press; 1989.
10. Schermer S. The blood morphology of laboratory animals. Philadelphia: Davis Company; 1967.
11. Zimmerman KL, Moore DM, Smith ST. Hematology of laboratory rabbits. In: Weiss DJ, Wardrop KJ, editors. Schalm's, Veterinary Hematology. Philadelphia: Lippincott Williams and Wilkins; 2010. p. 862.
12. Balin A, Koren G, Hasu M, et al. Evaluation of a new method for the prevention of neonatal anemia. Pediatr Res 1989;25:274.
13. Bartolotti A, Castelli D, Bonati M. Hematology and serum chemistry of adult, pregnant, and newborn New Zealand rabbits (Oryctolagus cuniculus). Lab Anim Sci 1989;39:437.
14. Kozma C, Macklin LM, Cummins R, et al. Anatomy, physiology, and biochemistry of the rabbit. In: Weisbroth SH, Flatt RE, Kraus AL, editors. The biology of the laboratory rabbit. Orlando (FL): Academic Press; 1974. p. 64.
15. McLaughlin RM, Fish RE. Clinical biochemistry and hematology. In: Manning PJ, Ringler DH, Newcomer CE, editors. The biology of the laboratory rabbit. 2nd edition. San Diego (CA): Academic Press; 1994. p. 119–24.
16. Washington IM, Van Hoosier GM. Clinical biochemistry and hematology. In: Suckow MA, Stevens KA, Wilson RP, editors. The laboratory rabbit, guinea pig, hamster, and other rodents. Academic Press; 2012. p. 97–100.
17. Benson KG, Paul-Murphy J. Clinical pathology of the domestic rabbit. Vet Clin North Am Exot Anim Pract 1999;2(3). 542.
18. Reagan WJ, Irizarry Rovira AR, DeNicola DB, et al. Normal white cell morphology. In: Reagan WJ, Rovira ARI, DeNicola DB, editors. Veterinary hematology: atlas of common domestic and non-domestic species. Ames (IA): Blackwell; 2008. p. 29–35.
19. Etim NN, Williams ME, Akpabio U, et al. Haematological parameters and factors affecting their values. Agricultural Science 2014;2(1):40.
20. Marshall KL. Rabbit hematology. Vet Clin North Am Exot Anim Pract 2008;11: 551–67.
21. Nakyinsige K, Sazili AQ, Aghwan ZA, et al. Changes in blood constituents of rabbits subjected to transportation under hot, humid tropical conditions. Asian-Australas J Anim Sci 2013;26(6):874–8.
22. Costa-Freitas FL, Yamamoto BL, Freitas WL, et al. Systemic inflammatory response indicators in rabbits experimentally infected with sporulate oocysts of *Eimeria stiedai*. Rev Bras Parasitol Vet 2011;20(2):121–6.
23. Jacobson HA, Kirkpatrick RL, Burkhart HE, et al. Hematologic comparisons of shot and live trapped cottontail rabbits. J Wildl Dis 1978;14:82–8.
24. Kramp WJ. Herpesvirus sylvilagus infects both B and T lymphocytes in vivo. J Virol 1985;56(1):60–5.
25. Lepitzki DA, Woolf A. Hematology and serum chemistry of cottontail rabbits of southern Illinois. J Wildl Dis 1978;27(4):82–8.

Hematologic Assessment in Pet Rats, Mice, Hamsters, and Gerbils

Blood Sample Collection and Blood Cell Identification

Nicole M. Lindstrom, MS, DVM[a], David M. Moore, MS, DVM, DACLAM[a],*, Kurt Zimmerman, DVM, PhD, DACVP[b], Stephen A. Smith, MS, DVM, PhD[b]

KEYWORDS

- Hamster • Mouse • Rat • Gerbil • Blood collection • Hematology • Hemogram

KEY POINTS

- Hamsters, gerbils, rats, and mice are presented to veterinary clinics and hospitals for prophylactic care and treatment of clinical signs of disease.
- Normal reference hematologic parameters are valuable for comparison with the results of clinical and diagnostic testing, and for development of treatment plans for small rodent patients.
- It is important to recognize that several variables affect hemogram results, including methods of sample collection, preparation of samples, equipment, reagents, methods of analysis, age, gender, circadian rhythm, breed, and environment of the animals being sampled.

Medical treatment of pocket pets has become an increasing component of veterinary clinical practice. According to the 2013 to 2014 American Pet Products Association National Pet Owners Survey, 68% of US households own a pet, which is approximately 82.5 million homes. Roughly 6.9 million of those homes (8.3% of the total) owned noncat/nondog small animal species.[1] About 1.3 million households have small rodent species (rat, mouse, hamster, gerbil) as pets.[2]

Normal reference hematologic parameters are valuable for comparison with the results of clinical and diagnostic testing, and for development of treatment plans for

This article originally appeared in Veterinary Clinics of North America: Exotic Animal Practice, Volume 18, Issue 1, January 2015.
[a] Virginia Tech, 300 Turner Street Northwest, Suite 4120 (0497), Blacksburg, VA 24061, USA;
[b] Department of Biomedical Sciences and Pathobiology (0442), Virginia-Maryland Regional College of Veterinary Medicine, 245 Duck Pond Drive, Blacksburg, VA 24061, USA
* Corresponding author.
E-mail address: moored@vt.edu

small rodent patients. It is important to recognize that several variables affect hemogram results, including methods of sample collection, preparation of samples, equipment, reagents, methods of analysis, age, gender, circadian rhythm, breed, and environment of the animals being sampled.[3,4] As a resource for veterinarians and their technicians, this article describes the methods for collection of blood, identification of blood cells, and interpretation of the hemogram in mice, rats, gerbils and hamsters.

BIOSAFETY AND OCCUPATIONAL HEALTH CONSIDERATIONS FOR CLINIC STAFF

Rodents from pet stores, from the wild, and pet rodents that may be exposed to wild rodents in the home, can carry several zoonotic diseases that can be easily transmitted to humans. A variety of publications are available that explain in detail the signs and symptoms of these diseases in both rodents and humans.[5–8] Zoonotic agents of concern are listed in **Table 1**, along with the modes of transmission, clinical signs in animals, and symptoms in humans.

Of equal importance for occupational safety in the clinic when handling small pet rodents is the recognition that these rodents produce allergens that can cause acute allergic reactions in handlers (dermatologic, such as wheal-and-flare reaction; eye and nasal passage irritation); in hypersensitized individuals there is a risk of anaphylactic shock. Allergens are secreted in the urine and saliva of rats, mice, and gerbils. It should be recognized that fur and dander may be contaminated with the allergens from grooming (saliva) or contact with urine in the cage environment.

Exposure risks for clinic staff can be mitigated by appropriate handling and restraint of the animals, wearing basic personal protective equipment (gloves, mask, long-sleeved coat or gown, eye protection), practicing good personal hygiene, sanitization of examination room surfaces the rodents came into contact with, and effective rodent pest control in the clinic.[5]

METHODOLOGY FOR BLOOD COLLECTION
Restraint

Proper restraint is an absolute necessity for venipuncture of small mammals. Most hamsters, gerbils, mice, and rats can undergo manual restraint alone for venipuncture. However, it is important to remember that the handling and restraint, transport to the veterinary hospital, and the hospital environment itself are stressful to these prey species. It is vital to approach these animals calmly and confidently and to minimize visual, olfactory, and auditory stimuli.[3,9,10] Anesthesia may be needed for adequate restraint to obtain samples from small mammals. However, anesthesia itself has been shown to produce changes in hematology parameters including decreased hematocrit, hemoglobin level, and red blood cell (RBC) count.[3] Handling and restraint, sedation, and anesthetic protocols for mice, rats, hamsters, and gerbils have been described in a variety of articles and books.[11–15]

Manual restraint
Mice Pet mice that are accustomed to being held can be lifted with both hands. To move single animals for short periods of time (2–3 seconds) from cage to examination table, grasp the animal gently at the base of the tail and lift. Do not lift mice by the tip of their tail, because that results in degloving injuries to the tail tip. The other hand can be placed under the mouse for additional support. Alternatively, mice can be picked up by the base of the tail or scruff of the neck using rubber-tipped forceps. Mice can also be coaxed, head first, into an appropriately sized disposable plastic syringe cover or large centrifuge tube, leaving the tail exposed for blood collection.

Table 1
Zoonotic disease agents in small rodents

Pathogen	Transmission	Animal Disease	Human Disease
Streptobacillus moniliformis, Spirillum minor (rat bite fever, Haverhill fever)	Animal bites, ingestion of contaminated food products	Usually a subclinical infection, but purulent lesions have been reported in some animals	Polyarthritis, myalgias, regional lymphadenopathy, fever
Salmonellosis (most rodents)	Fecal-oral, ingestion of contaminated products	Malaise, dehydration, bloody diarrhea	Dehydration, vomiting, abdominal pain, nausea
Leptospirosis (most rodents)	Direct contact with contaminated urine	Infertility, fever, anorexia, anemia	Headache, myalgia, conjunctivitis, nausea
Lymphocytic choriomeningitis	Exposure to saliva or urine from infected animals or to infected cell lines in the laboratory. Fomites may play a role	Viremia, viuria, and chronic wasting disease	Subclinical infection, mild flulike symptoms. Viral meningitis and encephalitis (rare)
Hantavirus (most rodents)	Exposure to aerosols, urine, and fecal material from infected animals. Fomites may play a role	Subclinical	Fever, myalgia, petechiation, abdominal pain, headache
Dermatophytosis (*Trichophyton mentagrophytes*)	Direct contact	Circular raised erythematous lesion with hyperkeratosis and hair loss	Circular raised erythematous lesions with hyperkeratosis and hair loss
Ornithonysisus bacoti (tropical rat mite)	Direct contact with cage materials	Asymptomatic to moderate pruritus	Severe pruritus
Sarcoptes scabei (guinea pigs and hamsters)	Direct contact with infected animal	Intense pruritus	Intense pruritus

Restraint for performing an examination, treatments, or procedures has been described in detail elsewhere.[16] Briefly, restraint can be performed by hand or using a commercially available restraint device. To restrain a mouse by hand, grasp the tail at its base with the nondominant hand and lift the mouse onto the cage lid or similar rough surface. If gentle traction is kept on the tail base, the animal moves forward and grasps onto the cage lid or other surface with its forepaws. The handler can tuck the base of the tail between the third and fourth finger, and then firmly grasp the mouse by the scruff with the same hand that is holding the tail. Gathering sufficient skin in the scruff-hold prevents the mouse from twisting or turning such that it can bite the handler. Recognize that drawing up loose skin in the scruff-hold can leave little room for respiratory movements of the ribs, which can result in asphyxiation of the mouse. The scruff-hold, therefore, should be used for only brief periods of time, and the handler should observe the pinna, nose, and paws for signs of cyanosis.

Rats Large pet rats should be restrained using an over- or under-the-shoulders grip with the thumb and fingers of one hand (thoracic encirclement), or using a commercially available restraint device or towel.[16] The over-the-shoulder grip can be performed by grasping the rat by the base of the tail and pulling gently backward with the dominant hand. Then place the nondominant hand over the back of the rat and grasp the rat around the thorax with the head of the rat between the index and middle fingers. It is important to not overcompress the rat's thorax and prevent respiratory movements of the ribs, resulting in anoxia. The body of the rat can then be stabilized by the handler's other hand, arm, or body. The under-the-shoulders grip is performed similarly, except the rat is grasped around the thorax, immediately under the shoulder blades. The forearms of the rat are gently pushed cranially with the thumb and index finger, and they cross under the chin, preventing the animal from biting the handler. Commercially available plastic restraint devices are very useful when performing blood draws on rats. Rats may be restrained in other ways, such as by wrapping in a small towel, or by simply cupping a hand over the animal.[16]

Gerbils Gerbils are usually docile animals and can simply be picked up and carefully restrained by the skin over the scruff of the neck. The gerbil can also be enclosed within one hand and held firmly in an upright position. Gerbils should not be picked up by the tip of the tail because of the risk of degloving injury.[12,17,18]

Hamsters Hamsters can be docile when handled frequently but care must be taken to avoid being bitten. To avoid startling a sleeping hamster before restraint, talk to the animal and gently touch its body one or two times to ensure that it is awake and aware of the handler's presence. Manual restraint of hamsters can be performed by gathering the loose skin over the scruff of the neck in one hand. Loose skin may be an understatement—there is generally enough skin that you could put in another two hamsters. In contrast to the scruff-hold in rats, mice, and gerbils, great care should be taken to gather enough of the hamster's loose skin into the scruff-hold such that the corners of the mouth are drawn back into a smile (a "smiling" hamster is one that cannot bite the handler). A hamster can also be placed in an appropriately sized plastic restraint tube for blood collection. These tubes should have air holes at the nose end, and be cleaned frequently to reduce the risk of cross-infection or stress from pheromones.[12,17,19]

Chemical restraint

Drugs that can be used for sedation, tranquilization, and anesthesia of mice, rats, hamsters, and gerbils have been described in published literature, and many online formularies for injectable anesthesia are available.[15,20] Inhalant anesthesia (isoflurane) is frequently used for rapid induction and anesthesia of small pet rodents.

Blood Collection Sites in Rats, Mice, Gerbils, and Hamsters: Location, Preparation, and Venipuncture Techniques

Several references are available that describe blood collection techniques in small pet rodents.[11–13] Recommended venipuncture sites for small pet rodents, used in clinical practice, are summarized in **Table 2**. A representative cross-section of a rodent's tail is provided in **Fig. 1**. Blood can be collected from the lateral tail veins and ventral caudal artery of mice, rats, and gerbils.

Collection from tail veins
The lateral tail veins run the length of the tail, and are more readily visualized in nonpigmented animals.[21] Vasodilation can be induced by placing the animal in an isolator at 104°F for a few minutes, or applying a warm water compress. "Milking" the vein, applying slight compression and stroking from base to tip, in an attempt to dilate the vessels, should not be done because this results in leukocytosis of the sample. After swabbing the venipuncture site with an appropriate disinfectant, a sterile hypodermic needle or a sterile lancet is used to prick the vein, and blood is collected in a microhematocrit tube or a microcentrifuge containing an appropriate volume of anticoagulant. Gentle pressure should be applied over the venipuncture site to stop the bleeding.

Collection from ventral caudal artery
This artery runs the length of the tail, but is not readily visualized. After the collection site has been disinfected, a 23- to 25-gauge needle (the smaller size for smaller species) is inserted in the ventral midline, about one-third the length of the tail from the body. The needle is inserted at a 30-degree angle, in a cranial direction, until it contacts the bone of the ventral surface of the caudal vertebra. The needle is then slightly withdrawn until blood begins to flow through the needle, and then is maintained in that position. Blood

Table 2 Recommended venipuncture sites in small pet rodent	
Species	**Vessel**
Mouse	Lateral saphenous vein Femoral vein Medial saphenous vein Jugular vein Lateral tail vein Ventral tail artery Facial vein (superficial temporal)
Rat	Saphenous vein Femoral vein Jugular vein Dorsal and lateral tail veins Ventral tail artery Cranial vena cava
Gerbil	Saphenous vein Metatarsal vein Lateral tail vein
Hamster	Lateral saphenous vein Cephalic vein Cranial vena cava

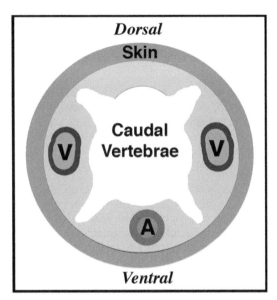

Fig. 1. Cross-section of rodent tail, showing vessels used for blood collection.

can be collected in a microhematocrit tube as it flows from the needle hub. In rats, a 1- or 3-mL syringe, with its plunger removed, can be affixed to the needle before arterial puncture is attempted, and blood is allowed to flow into the barrel of the syringe. After blood collection, gentle pressure should be applied to the arterial puncture site for several minutes to prevent continued blood flow.

Collection from hindlimb vessels
Blood can be collected from the lateral saphenous veins[22] and dorsal metatarsal veins of mice, rats, hamsters, and gerbils. The anatomic locations and procedures for blood collection from those vessels are provided in the article on guinea pig hematology elsewhere in this issue.

Blood can be collected from the facial vein after pricking it with a sterile lancet.[23] This technique has been used successfully in rats, mice, hamsters, and gerbils used in research. However, this method requires practice to accomplish successfully, and practice animals are generally not readily available in most veterinary practices. Thus the procedure has been referenced, but is not described herein.

Blood Volume Collected
Blood collection from small mammals is challenging because of limited blood volume available for sampling, and because the restraint or sedation necessary to obtain a sample may alter the results of some assays.[3,4,11,12,18] The maximum volume of blood that can be safely withdrawn in a single sample is approximately 7.5% to 10% of the circulating blood volume.[11] **Table 3** provides information to assist in determining the maximum safe blood sample volume in small pet rodents based on the animal's body weight. It is important to adhere to these recommended limits to prevent hypovolemic shock and anemia. The extracted volume is replaced within 24 hours in most healthy animals, although a return to normal levels of all blood constituents may take up to 2 weeks.[11] The volume and frequency of blood collection must also take into account the health status of the patient.

Table 3		
Determining maximum safe blood sample volumes in small rodents based on body weight		
Body Weight (g)	**Circulating Blood Volume (mL)**	**Draw No More than 7.5%–10% of Circulating Blood Volume (mL)**
20	1.10–1.40	0.082–0.14
25	1.37–1.75	0.10–0.18
30	1.65–2.10	0.12–0.21
35	1.93–2.45	0.14–0.25
40	2.20–2.80	0.16–0.28
125	6.88–8.75	0.52–0.88
150	8.25–10.50	0.62–1.0
200	11.00–14.00	0.82–1.4
250	13.75–17.50	1.0–1.8
300	16.50–21.00	1.2–2.1
350	19.25–24.50	1.4–2.5

Data from National Institutes of Health. NIH guidelines for survival bleeding of rats and mice. 2012.

MORPHOLOGY AND NUMBERS OF PERIPHERAL BLOOD CELLS

Referenced ranges of hematologic parameters in normal rats, mice, hamsters, and gerbils are provided in **Table 4**. Values listed for hamsters are for the Syrian (golden) hamster. Hematologic values for European and Djungarian hamsters have been described in the literature.[27–29] Reference values should be used as a tool for diagnosis and treatment, along with clinical signs and physical examination parameters, but not as the sole guide to determine if values are normal or abnormal.[3,4,11,12]

Erythrocytes

The approximate diameters of erythrocytes in small rodents are as follows: mouse, 5 to 7 μm; rat, 5.7 to 7 μm; and hamster, 5 to 7 μm.[3] Moderate anisocytosis is seen in mouse, rat, and hamster RBCs, with the diameter of some cells only one-third that of the standard RBC size. In rats and mice, Howell-Jolly bodies and nucleated RBCs are sometimes observed. RBCs of young rats and mice are morphologically variable, and young animals have more circulating reticulocytes than do older animals (10%–20% vs 2%–5%).[3] Neonatal gerbils have erythrocyte counts that are approximately one-half adult values, but increase to adult values by about 8 weeks of age.[9] Gerbils up to 20 weeks old have a large number of circulating reticulocytes and erythrocytes with basophilic stippling and polychromasia. These cells are also abundant in older gerbils and are probably associated with the short erythrocyte lifespan.[9] The lifespan of erythrocytes in small rodents is as follows: mouse, 41 to 52 days; rat, 56 to 69 days; hamster, 50 to 78 days; and gerbil, 10 days.[3] Hibernation (more correctly, pseudohibernation) in hamsters prolongs the life span of their erythrocytes. The end of hibernation in the hamster is associated with an increase in reticulocyte numbers.[3] Comparative values of erythrocyte numbers are provided in **Table 4**.

Thrombocytes (Platelets)

The mouse thrombocyte is round to oval to elongated in shape, and approximately 1 to 4 μm in diameter. Rat and mouse platelets have similar morphology. Round

Table 4
Referenced ranges of hematologic parameters in normal rats, mice, hamsters, and gerbils

	Rat		Mouse		Hamster		Gerbil	
	Male	Female	Male	Female	Male	Female	Male	Female
RBC ($\times 10^6$/µL)	8.15–9.75	6.76–9.2	6.9–11.7	6.86–11.3	4.7–10.3	3.96–9.96	7.1–8.6	8.0–9.4
PCV (%)	44.4–50.4	37.6–50.6	33.1–49.9	39.7–44.5	47.9–57.1	39.2–58.8	42–49	43–50
Hgb (g/dL)	13.4–15.8	11.5–16.1	11.1–11.5	10.7–11.1	14.4–19.2	13.1–18.9	12.1–13.8	13.1–16.9
MCV (fL)	49.8–57.8	50.9–65.5	47.5–50.5	47–52	64.8–77.6	64–76	46.6–60	46.64–60.04
MCH (pg)	14.3–18.3	15.6–19	11.7–12.7	11.1–12.7	19.9–24.9	20.2–25.8	16.1–19.4	16.3–19.4
MCHC (%)	26.2–35.4	26.5–36.1	23.2–31.2	22.3–29.5	27.5–36.5	27.8–37.4	30.6–33.3	30.6–33.3
Platelets ($\times 10^3$/µL)	150–450	160–460	157–412	170–410	367–573	300–490	432–710	540–632
WBC ($\times 10^3$/µL)	8.0–11.8	6.6–12.6	12.5–15.9	12.1–13.7	5.02–10.2	6.48–10.6	4.3–12.3	5.6–12.8
Neutrophils (%)	6.2–42.6	4.4–49.2	13.2–21.6	15.7–18.5	17.1–27.1	22.8–35.2	9.3–23.6	10.7–25.8
Lymphocytes (%)	57.6–83.2	50.2–84.5	62.4–82.8	65.9–77.9	54.7–92.3	50.9–84.9	68–76.8	58.9–78.1
Eosinophils (%)	0.1–0.63	0–1.96	1.37–2.81	2.05–2.77	0.26–1.54	0.22–1.18	0–1.6	0–2.3
Basophils (%)	0–0.6	0–0.4	0.22–0.82	0.13–0.85	0–5	0–2.1	0–1.6	0–0.8
Monocytes (%)	0–0.65	0–1.81	2.22–2.47	0.98–1.11	0.9–4.1	0.4–4.4	0–6.5	1.7–6.2

Abbreviations: Hgb, hemoglobin; MCH, mean corpuscular hemoglobin; MCHC, mean corpuscular hemoglobin concentration; MCV, mean corpuscular volume; PCV, packed cell volume.
Data from Refs.[9,24–26]

platelets the size of RBCs and platelet clumps may be frequently observed.[3] The margins of platelets appear indistinct in Wright-Giemsa–stained blood smears.[3] The cytoplasm of mouse and rat thrombocytes has a faint pink to gray color, and toward the center of the cell, blue angular granules may be observed, and occasionally red granules may be present.[3] In hamsters, platelets appear to be amorphous veils of a gray-blue ground substance with violet-stained granules.[9,30] Comparative values of thrombocyte numbers are provided in **Table 4**.

Leukocytes (White Blood Cells)

Leukocyte concentrations in these small pet rodents demonstrate diurnal variation,[3] and thus laboratory results are affected by the time of day when the sample is collected.

Acute stress in rats results in elevated serum corticosterone but with a normal neutrophil/lymphocyte ratio, whereas chronic stress (distress) yields the opposite— normal serum corticosterone concentrations with an elevated neutrophil/lymphocyte ratio.[31] Although neutrophilia and lymphopenia were seen in chronically stressed rats, the values for each were with normal referenced ranges.[31] A similar picture is seen in aging mice and rats, when the proportion of lymphocytes decreases and the proportion of neutrophils increases.[3]

The ranges of total WBC numbers and the white blood cell (WBC) types observed in a standard differential count are provided in **Table 4**. Typical WBCs for each of the small pet rodents are provided in the following figures: mouse WBCs (**Fig. 2**), rat WBCs (**Fig. 3**), hamster WBCs (**Fig. 4**), and gerbil WBCs (**Fig. 5**).

Neutrophils

The nucleus of the neutrophil in rodents has several indentations, giving it a hyperseg-mented appearance. Band forms may be seen in normal animals, but this is usually seen in association with inflammation.[3] Ring forms may be seen, but are usually asso-ciated with accelerated ganulopoiesis.[3] The cytoplasm of neutrophils is pale with faint pink granules. In hamsters, neutrophils (heterophils) resemble eosinophils, with a lobular nucleus and dense pink cytoplasmic granules. Comparative values of neutro-phils observed in differential counts in normal mice, rats, hamsters, and gerbils are provided in **Table 4**.

Lymphocytes

In mice, rats, hamsters, and gerbils, lymphocytes comprise approximately 75% of the leukocytes in the peripheral blood. Lymphocytes in rats and mice may be small or large with variable amounts of cytoplasm, varying from deep to pale blue, and sometimes containing large, dark-staining, azurophilic granules. In hamsters, lympho-cytes are small round cells with a dark blue nucleus that fills most of the cell and is

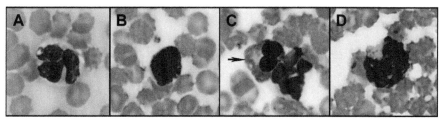

Fig. 2. Representative mouse blood cells. (*A*) Neutrophil and RBCs. (*B*) Lymphocyte and RBCs. (*C*) Eosinophil and RBCs. (*D*) Monocyte and RBCs. The *arrow* is pointing out the eosin-ophil. (Wright-Giemsa stain; 1000x).

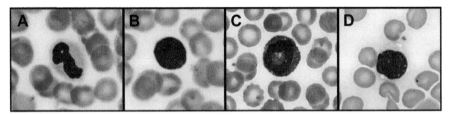

Fig. 3. Representative rat blood cells. (*A*) Neutrophil and RBCs. (*B*) Lymphocyte and RBCs. (*C*) Eosinophil and RBCs. (*D*) Monocyte, platelet, and RBCs. (Wright-Giemsa stain; 1000x).

surrounded by a rim of lighter blue cytoplasm. Comparative values of lymphocytes observed in differential counts in normal mice, rats, hamsters, and gerbils are provided in **Table 4**.

Eosinophils
In mice, eosinophils have a band-shaped and occasionally ring-shaped nucleus that is partially obscured by the presence of ruddy orange to red granules. The granules are large, round, and fairly uniform in size, but have indistinct borders.[3] In rats, eosinophils have nuclei that are usually less segmented than neutrophils and contain small, round, reddish granules that fill the cytoplasm. In hamsters, the nucleus is annual-shaped, sometimes twisted, that fills the periphery of the call as a wide band. The nucleus is surrounded by a narrow zone of cytoplasm, which is tightly packed with rod-shaped azurophilic granules.[3] Comparative values of eosinophils observed in differential counts in normal mice, rats, hamsters, and gerbils are provided in **Table 4**.

Basophils
In rats, mice, and hamsters, basophils are rarely observed on peripheral blood smears. They lack tertiary granules but have larger and less numerous mature granules. Basophil nuclei are lobulated, and the cytoplasm contains large, round purple granules that may be few in number or so numerous that they obscure the nucleus. Comparative values of basophils observed in differential counts in normal mice, rats, hamsters, and gerbils are provided in **Table 4**.

Monocytes
Monocytes are the largest-sized WBC in these small rodents. Monocyte morphology is similar to that seen in other species with pleomorphic nuclei that may be round, indented, or lobular, an extensive cytoplasm that stains pale gray blue, and often

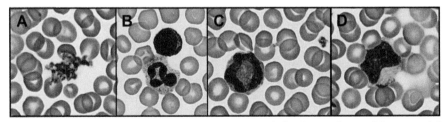

Fig. 4. Representative hamster blood cells. (*A*) Clumped platelets and RBCs. (*B*) Neutrophil, lymphocyte, and RBCs. (*C*) Eosinophil, platelet, and RBCs. (*D*) Monocyte and RBCs. (Wright-Giemsa stain; 1000x).

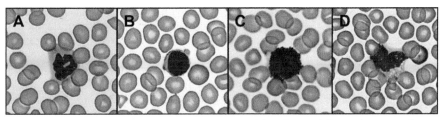

Fig. 5. Representative gerbil blood cells. (*A*) Neutrophil and RBCs. (*B*) Lymphocyte and RBCs. (*C*) Basophil and RBCs. (*D*) Monocyte and RBCs. (Wright-Giemsa stain; 1000x).

contains vacuoles.[3] Comparative values of monocytes observed in differential counts in normal mice, rats, hamsters, and gerbils are provided in **Table 4**.

REFERENCES

1. American Pet Products Association. 2013–2014 National Pet Owners Survey. Greenwich (CT): American Pet Products Manufacturers Association; 2014.
2. American Veterinary Medical Association. 2012 U.S. pet ownership & demographic sourcebook. Schaumberg (IL): AVMA; 2012.
3. Provencher Bollinger A, Everds NE, Zimmerman KL. Hematology of laboratory animals. In: Weiss DJ, Wardrop KJ, editors. Schalm's veterinary hematology. Philadelphia: Lippincott Williams and Wilkins; 2010. p. 852–62.
4. Washington IM, Van Hoosier G. Clinical biochemistry and hematology. In: Suckow MA, Stevens KA, Wilson RP, editors. The laboratory rabbit, guinea pig, hamster, and other rodents. 1st edition. London: Academic Press; 2012. p. 57–116.
5. Hill WA, Brown JP. Zoonoses of rabbits and rodents. Vet Clin North Am Exot Anim Pract 2011;14(3):519–31, vii.
6. Chomel BB. Zoonoses of house pets other than dogs, cats and birds. Pediatr Infect Dis J 1992;11:479–87.
7. American Biological Safety Association. Zoonotic diseases fact sheet. Mundelein (IL): ABSA; 2012.
8. Committee on Occupational Health and Safety in Research Animals Facilities, Institute of Laboratory Animal Resources, Commission of Life Sciences, National Research Council. Occupational health and safety in the care and use of research animals. Washington, DC: National Academic Press; 1997.
9. Zimmerman KL, Moore DM, Smith SA. Hematology of the Mongolian gerbil. In: Weiss DJ, Wardrop KJ, editors. Schalm's veterinary hematology. Philadelphia: Lippincott Williams and Wilkins; 2010. p. 899–903.
10. Smith SA, Zimmerman KL, Moore DM. Hematology of the Syrian (golden) hamster. In: Weiss DJ, Wardrop KJ, editors. Schalm's veterinary hematology. Philadelphia: Lippincott Williams and Wilkins; 2010. p. 904–9.
11. Ott Joslin J. Blood collection techniques in small mammals. J Exotic Pet Medicine 2009;18:117–39.
12. Hrapkiewicz K, Colby L, Denison P. Clinical laboratory animal medicine: an introduction. 4th edition. Ames (IA): Wiley Blackwell; 2013.
13. Dyer SM, Cervasio EL. An overview of restraint and blood collection techniques in exotic pet practice. Vet Clin North Am Exot Anim Pract 2008;11(3):423–43.
14. Fowler ME. Restraint and handling of wild and domestic animals. 3rd edition. Ames (IA): Wiley-Blackwell; 2008.

15. Longley LA. Anesthesia of exotic pets. Philadelphia: Saunders Elsevier; 2008.
16. Machholz E, Mulder G, Ruiz C, et al. Manual restraint and common compound administration routes in mice and rats. J Vis Exp 2012;(67):e2771. http://dx.doi.org/10.3791/2771.
17. Harkness JE, Wagner JE. The biology and medicine of rabbits and rodents. 4th edition. Baltimore (MD): Williams and Wilkins; 1995.
18. Batchelder M, Keller LS, Sauer MB, et al. Gerbils. In: Suckow MA, Stevens KA, Wilson RP, editors. The laboratory rabbit, guinea pig, hamster, and other rodents. 1st edition. London: Academic Press; 2012. p. 1131–55.
19. Fenyk-Melody J. The European hamster. In: Suckow MA, Stevens KA, Wilson RP, editors. The laboratory rabbit, guinea pig, hamster, and other rodents. 1st edition. London: Academic Press; 2012. p. 923–33.
20. Hawk CT, Leary S. Formulary for laboratory animals. 3rd edition. Ames (IA): Wiley-Blackwell; 2005.
21. Brown C. Blood collection from the tail of a rat. Lab Anim (NY) 2006;35(8):24–5.
22. Hem A, Smith AJ, Solberg P. Saphenous vein puncture for blood sampling of the mouse, rat, hamster, gerbil, guinea pig, ferret and mink. Lab Anim 1998;32(4):364–8.
23. Golde WT, Gollobin P, Rodriguez LL. A rapid, simple, and humane method for submandibular bleeding of mice using a lancet. Lab Anim (NY) 2005;34:39–43.
24. Mitruka BJ, Rawnsley HM. Clinical biochemical and hematological reference values in normal experimental animals. New York: Masson Publishing; 1977. p. 82–3.
25. Mays A Jr. Baseline hematological and blood biochemical parameters of the Mongolian gerbil (*Meriones unguiculatus*). Lab Anim Care 1969;19:838–42.
26. Ruhren R. Normal values for hemoglobin concentration and cellular elements in the blood of Mongolian gerbils. Lab Anim Care 1965;15:313–20.
27. Mitchell MA, Tully TN. Manual of exotic pet practice. St Louis (MO): Saunders Elsevier; 2009. p. 414.
28. Moore DM. Hematology of the Syrian (golden) hamster (*Mesocricetus auratus*). In: Feldman BF, Zinkl JG, Jain NC, editors. Schalm's veterinary hematology. 5th edition. Philadelphia: Lippincott Williams & Wilkins; 2000. p. 1115–9.
29. Moore DM. Hematology of the Mongolian gerbil (*Meriones unguiculatus*). In: Feldman BF, Zinkl JG, Jain NC, editors. Schalm's veterinary hematology. 5th edition. Philadelphia: Lippincott Williams & Wilkins; 2000. p. 1111–4.
30. Schermer S. The blood morphology of laboratory animals. 3rd edition. Philadelphia: FA Davis; 1967.
31. Swan MP, Hickman DL. Evaluation of the neutrophil-lymphocyte ratio as a measure of distress in rats. Lab Anim (NY) 2014;43(8):276–82.

Hematological Assessment in Pet Guinea Pigs (*Cavia porcellus*)

Blood Sample Collection and Blood Cell Identification

Kurt Zimmerman, DVM, PhD, DACVP[a],*, David M. Moore, MS, DVM, DACLAM[b],
Stephen A. Smith, MS, DVM, PhD[a]

KEYWORDS

- Guinea pig • Guinea pig blood collection • Guinea pig hematology
- Guinea pig hemogram • Guinea pig WBC morphology • Guinea pig differential count

KEY POINTS

- Pet guinea pigs are presented to veterinary clinics for routine care and treatment of clinical diseases.
- In addition to obtaining clinical history and physical exam findings, diagnostic testing may be required, including hematological assessments.
- Guinea pigs are subject to dental problems (malocclusion), nutritional problems (vitamin C deficiency), bacterial infections (cervical lymphadenitis, pneumonia), reproductive/metabolic problems (dystocia, pregnancy toxemia), internal and external parasites, and musculoskeletal problems (fracture of the spine), some of which may require hematological assessment by veterinary clinicians.

Approximately 1.3 million guinea pigs are maintained as pets in about 0.84 million homes in the United States.[1] They have a long lifespan (5–7 years)[2,3] compared with other, smaller rodents, and are more likely to be presented for clinical care than other rodent species. Guinea pigs are subject to dental problems (malocclusion), nutritional problems (vitamin C deficiency), bacterial infections (cervical lymphadenitis, pneumonia), reproductive/metabolic problems (dystocia, pregnancy toxemia), internal

This article originally appeared in Veterinary Clinics of North America: Exotic Animal Practice, Volume 18, Issue 1, January 2015.

[a] Department of Biomedical Sciences and Pathobiology (0442), Virginia-Maryland Regional College of Veterinary Medicine, Duck Pond Drive, Blacksburg, VA 24061, USA; [b] Department of Biomedical Sciences and Pathobiology, Virginia Tech, 300 Turner Street Northwest, Suite 4120 (0497), Blacksburg, VA 24061, USA
* Corresponding author.
E-mail address: kzimmerm@vt.edu

and external parasites, and musculoskeletal problems (fracture of the spine), some of which may require hematological assessment by veterinary clinicians. As a resource for veterinarians and their technicians, this article describes the methods for manual restraint, collection of blood, and identification of blood cells in guinea pigs.

METHODOLOGY FOR BLOOD COLLECTION
Restraint

Although guinea pigs may be naturally curious, they dislike change (eg, changes in diet, environment, handlers, unfamiliar noise), and may make an attempt to flee to avoid restraint. Some people refer to them as whistle pigs, because they make high-pitched vocalizations when excited or frightened; this sound should not be interpreted as pain when standard, nonpainful procedures, including manual restraint, are used. Some handlers abandon efforts to restrain a vocalizing animal for fear of causing harm, even though the restraint is needed for proper clinical diagnosis and treatment of the animal.

The handler should not attempt to restrain or pick up the animal by grasping the skin over the scruff of the neck; that is distressing to the animal, and should not be attempted. When picking up the guinea pig for examination or to move it from one area to another, the handler should place one hand over the dorsum, behind the shoulders, and grasp the animal gently but securely with the thumb and fingers around the rib cage, taking care not to restrict respiratory movements of the ribs. When lifting the animal, the other hand should be placed under the hindquarters for support. If the hindquarters are not supported, the animal may struggle and twist, causing injury to the spine, with resultant paresis or paralysis of the hind limbs.

Guinea pigs may become distressed if restrained in lateral or dorsal recumbency.[4] Guinea pigs may be wrapped securely in a towel, which seems to calm or comfort them. However, swaddling a guinea pig tends to make most vessels used for venipuncture inaccessible. Thus, additional care should be taken when wrapping the animal to allow access to the intended venipuncture site.

Compared with other pet rodent species and rabbits, the guinea pig is unlikely to bite the handler.

Drugs that can be used in sedation, tranquilization, and anesthesia of guinea pigs have been described in published literature.[5–7] However, professional judgment should be used to assess whether it is safe, based on the animal's clinical status, to anesthetize the animal.

Blood Collection Sites: Location and Preparation, and Venipuncture Techniques

Several veins are used as common venipuncture sites in guinea pigs, including the lateral saphenous and metatarsal veins of the hind limbs, and the cephalic veins of the forelegs.[8–10] Additional methods include the jugular vein, cranial vena cava, femoral vein, pricking a tiny vein in the pinna, or close clipping of a nail. **Table 1** provides a comparison of the advantages and disadvantages of the various blood collection sites in guinea pigs.

Given the small diameters of the commonly used veins, the phlebotomist should select an appropriately sized needle (eg, 22–30 gauge).

To induce vasodilation and facilitate blood collection, the animal can be placed in an incubator with an internal temperature of $40^\circ C$ ($104^\circ F$) for several minutes. As an alternative, an examination glove can be filled with water, tied off, microwaved until its temperature is warm but not scalding to the touch, and applied to the venipuncture site for about a minute.

Table 1
Comparison of blood collection sites in the guinea pig

Collection Site	Advantages	Disadvantages
Lateral saphenous vein	• Easily visualized • Easily accessible • Does not require sedation/anesthesia • Good for collecting small to moderate volumes of blood	• The vein is small and easily collapsed with rapid aspiration • Restraint may injure leg
Lateral metatarsal vein	• Easily visualized • Easily accessible • Does not require sedation/anesthesia • Good for collecting small volumes of blood	• The vein is small and easily collapsed with rapid aspiration • Restraint may injure leg • Free-flow sample is not sterile
Cephalic vein	• Good for collecting small volumes of blood	• Vein is mobile, requires stabilization • Vein may collapse during aspiration • Forelimb is short, making access difficult
Cranial vena cava	• Good for collecting moderate volumes of blood	• Cannot be visualized or palpated; rely on landmarks • Sedation/anesthesia required • Risk of internal bleeding
Jugular vein	• Good for collecting moderate volumes of blood	• Cannot be visualized or palpated; rely on landmarks • Sedation/anesthesia recommended • May become dyspneic when the neck is extended back during restraint
Ear veins	• Easily visualized • Easily accessible • Does not require sedation/anesthesia • Collecting small volumes of blood	• Could be irritating/painful • Free-flow sample is not sterile
Toenail clip	• Easily visualized • Easily accessible • Does not require sedation/anesthesia • Collecting small volumes of blood	• Could be irritating/painful • Free-flow sample is not sterile

Fig. 1 shows the location of the primary venipuncture sites on the hind limb. The fur over the selected site should be removed with electric clippers, and the site swabbed with an appropriate disinfectant solution.

The lateral saphenous vein runs dorsoventrally and then laterally over the tarsal joint. The foot should be grasped and traction applied to extend the leg. An assistant should apply digital pressure, gently squeezing the leg between the thumb and forefinger, proximal to the venipuncture site. Blood collection may be accomplished using a needle and syringe, or the vessel may be pricked/punctured using a sterile needle or

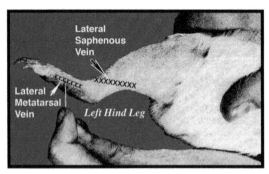

Fig. 1. Location of the lateral saphenous and lateral metatarsal veins in the guinea pig.

sterile lancet.[11] With the needle-and-syringe method, a needle of 23 to 25 gauge on a 1.0-mL syringe is inserted in the vein in a distal to proximal direction and, with slow aspiration to avoid collapse of the vessel, about 0.5 to 1.0 mL of blood can be collected.[4] For the free-flow method, pressure is applied (as described earlier) to dilate the vein, then a sterile needle of 20 to 23 gauge or a sterile lancet can be used to prick the vessel, with from 0.1 to 3 mL of blood collected in a microhematocrit tube, Pasteur pipette, or a snap-cap microcentrifuge tube that contains an appropriate volume of anticoagulant solution. Following either collection method, gentle pressure should be applied to the venipuncture site to stop the flow of blood and to prevent hematoma formation.

The lateral metatarsal vein is located on the lateral aspect of the foot. Preparation of the venipuncture site is the same as described earlier. Free-flow collection of blood from this vein and prevention of hematoma formation is also as described earlier. From 0.1 to 3 mL of blood may be collected by this method.[4,12] The dorsal metatarsal vein (not shown) may also be used for blood collection, using the techniques described earlier.

The procedure for cephalic venipuncture is similar to that in dogs and cats, but is more difficult because of the short length of the guinea pig forearm.

A small free-flow sample of blood may be collected by pricking/puncturing one of the small veins in the pinna, using appropriate presampling and postsampling procedures as described earlier.

Clipping a toenail to the quick yields some blood, but the procedure is painful and may lead to a secondary infection in the nail.

Volume Collected

In general, up to 50 μL of blood can collected in a microhematocrit tube from the saphenous vein, metatarsal vein, ear veins, or clipped toenail in adult guinea pigs.[13] Larger volumes of blood may be collected, within a range of 0.5 to 0.7 mL/100 g of body weight.[4,8,14] That range is based on the consensus that 7% to 10% of blood volume can safely be collected at any 1 time, with an average adult blood volume of 69 to 75 mL/kg of body weight.[4,15,16]

MORPHOLOGY AND NUMBERS OF PERIPHERAL BLOOD CELLS
Erythrocytes

Guinea pig erythrocytes appear as biconcave disks when stained with modified Wright stain (**Fig. 2**). Females have slightly fewer erythrocytes than males. Guinea pig erythrocytes, with a mean cell volume of 84 fL, are larger than erythrocytes in other common laboratory animal species.[17] Anisocytosis is moderate, with width ranging

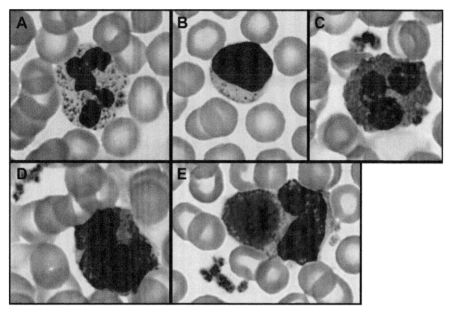

Fig. 2. Representative guinea pig blood cells. (A) Heterophil and red blood cells (RBCs). (B) Lymphocyte and RBCs. (C) Eosinophil, platelets, and RBCs. (D) Monocyte, platelets, and RBCs. (E) Kurloff cell, platelets, and RBCs. (Wright-Giemsa stain, original magnification 1000x).

between 6.6 and 7.9 μm. An increase in the relative numbers of polychromatophils in the blood smear indicates a regenerative response to anemia. In normal nonanemic cavies, polychromatic erythrocytes may total 25% of circulating erythrocytes in neonates, 4.5% in juveniles, and 1.5% in adults.[17–20] Comparative values of erythrocyte numbers are provided in **Table 2**.

Table 2
Reference ranges of normal hematological parameters in the guinea pig (*Cavia porcellus*)

	Adult Male	Adult Female	Age 2–90 d
RBC ($\times 10^6$/μL)	4.36–6.84	3.35–6.15	4.06–6.02
PCV (%)	37–47	40.9–49.9	33.8–48.8
Hgb (g/dL)	11.6–17.2	11.4–17.0	10.13–15.1
MCV (fL)	71–83	86.1–95.9	77.5–88.7
MCH (pg)	24.2–27.2	23.1–26.3	—
MCHC (%)	29.7–38.9	28.2–34.4	28.3–32.4
Platelets ($\times 10^3$/μL)	260–740	266–634	—
WBC ($\times 10^3$/μL)	5.5–17.5	5.2–16.4	2.66–10.1
Neutrophils (%)	28–56	20.3–41.9	14.8–42.6
Lymphocytes (%)	40.0–62.5	46.4–80.4	52.6–83.2
Eosinophils (%)	1–7	0–7	0.1–3.6
Basophils (%)	0–1.7	0–0.8	0–0.58
Monocytes (%)	3.3–5.3	1.0–2.6	0–3.7

Abbreviations: Hgb, Hemoglobin; MCH, Mean corpuscular hemoglobin; MCHC, Mean corpuscular hemoglobin concentration; MCV, Mean cell volume; PCV, Packed cell volume; RBC, Red blood cell; WBC, white blood cell.
Data from Refs.[13,25,32]

Thrombocytes (Platelets)

In blood smears, guinea pig platelets appear as irregular oval cytoplasmic fragments 2 to 3 μm in diameter with concentric dark inner and lighter outer staining regions (see **Fig. 2**). Reported normal platelet numbers range from 120 to 850/mm³.[2–4,8,13,16,19,21–26] Comparative values of thrombocyte numbers are provided in **Table 2**.

Leukocytes (White Blood Cells)

A variety of factors can influence white blood cell (WBC) total count and differential counts: circadian rhythm (time of day the sample is collected), time of last feeding, breed, and gender.[25] The ranges of total WBC numbers and the WBC cell types observed in a standard differential count are provided in **Table 2**.

Neutrophils (Heterophils)

Guinea pigs heterophils or pseudoeosinophils are the functional counterparts of neutrophils seen in other species and are the next most commonly noted white cell type (see **Fig. 2A**).[8,19] These cells measure 10 to 12 μm in width, with dense nuclei with 5 or more segments. Cytoplasm of heterophils contains multiple pale round eosinophilic inclusions versus the more elongated inclusions seen in eosinophils. Toxicity (accelerated marrow production and shortened maturation time) manifests, as seen in other small animal species, by the presence of increased small basophilic Dohle bodies, cytoplasmic basophilia, and occasionally increased cytoplasmic vacuolation.[27] Reduced nuclear segmentation (bands, left shift) typically accompanies these toxic changes and in most cases can be viewed as markers for the presence of inflammation. Comparative values of neutrophils observed in differential counts in normal guinea pigs are provided in **Table 2**.

Lymphocytes

Lymphocytes are the predominant WBC type in guinea pig blood.[3,4,8,13,16,21,27] Both small and large forms of lymphoid cells are seen, but most are small cells (see **Fig. 2B**).[2,8,13,19] The larger forms can be double the size of the small cells (about the same size as erythrocytes), and may contain a few azurophilic cytoplasmic granules. Comparative values of lymphocytes observed in differential counts in normal guinea pigs are provided in **Table 2**.

Eosinophils

The granules in eosinophils are more pointed than those in heterophils, and they stain more prominently. Eosinophils are larger (10–15 μm wide) with less nuclear segmentation (see **Fig. 2C**).[8,13,17,19] Comparative values of eosinophils observed in differential counts in normal guinea pigs are provided in **Table 2**.

Basophils

Basophils are slightly larger than heterophils with lobulated nuclei and many round variably sized reddish purple to black cytoplasm granules. Comparative values of basophils observed in differential counts in normal guinea pigs are provided in **Table 2**.

Monocytes

Guinea pig monocytes are morphologically similar to those seen in common domestic species, being larger and having darker grey-blue cytoplasm compared with the previously mentioned large lymphocytes (see **Fig. 2D**). Their nuclei tend to be oval to ameboid with a loose lacy chromatin pattern. Comparative values of monocytes observed in differential counts in normal guinea pigs are provided in **Table 2**.

Kurloff Cells

Kurloff cells are a leukocyte type observed in guinea pigs and capybaras (a close relative). The cell is considered a normal incidental feature, appearing as larger mononuclear cells, possibly of lymphoid origin, containing a single reticulated eosinophilic cytoplasmic inclusion 1 to 8 μm wide and present in 3% to 4% of the lymphoid cells or 1% to 2% of the total leukocytes (see **Fig. 2**E).[2] These inclusions consist of a mucopolysaccharide that is toluidine blue, periodic acid-Schiff, and Lendrum stain positive.[2,17] The exact origin and function of these cells is unknown, although it has been speculated that they may function as natural killer cells in the general circulation or as protectors of fetal antigen in the placenta because their numbers can increase under the influence of increased estrogens.[8,13,17,19,28-31]

REFERENCES

1. American Veterinary Medical Association. 2012 U.S. pet ownership & demographic sourcebook. Schaumburg (IL): Membership & Field Services, American Veterinary Medical Association; 2012.
2. Percy DH, Barthold SW. Pathology of laboratory rodents and rabbits. 3rd edition. Ames (IA): Blackwell Pub; 2007. p. 325.
3. Vanderlip SL. The guinea pig handbook. Hauppauge (NY): Barron's; 2003.
4. Harkness JE, Turner PV, VandeWoude S, et al. Harkness and Wagner's biology and medicine of rabbits and rodents. 5th edition. Ames (IA): Wiley-Blackwell; 2010. p. 111.
5. Hawk CT, Leary S. Formulary for laboratory animals. 3rd edition. St Louis (MO): Wiley-Blackwell; 2005.
6. Mitchell MA, Tully TN. Manual of exotic pet practice. St Louis (MO): Saunders Elsevier; 2009. p. 470.
7. Gaertner DJ, Hallman TM, Hankenson FC, et al. Anesthesia and analgesia for laboratory rodents. In: Fish RE, Brown MJ, Danneman PJ, et al, editors. Anesthesia and analgesia in laboratory animals. 2nd edition. San Diego (CA): Academic Press; 2008. p. 279–80.
8. Marshall KL. Clinical hematology of rodent species. Vet Clin North Am Exot Anim Pract 2008;11:523–33.
9. Ott Joslin J. Blood collection techniques in exotic small mammals. J Exot Pet Med 2009;18:117–39.
10. Reuter RE. Venipuncture in the guinea pig. Lab Anim Sci 1987;37:245–6.
11. Hem A, Smith AJ, Solberg P. Saphenous vein puncture for blood sampling of the mouse, rat, hamster, gerbil, guinea pig, ferret and mink. Lab Anim 1998;32:364–8.
12. Dolence D, Jones HE. Pericutaneous phlebotomy and intravenous injection in the guinea pig. Lab Anim Sci 1975;25(1):106–7.
13. Zimmerman LK, Moore MD, Smith SA. Hematology of the guinea pig. In: Weiss DJ, Wardrop KJ, Schalm OW, editors. Schalm's veterinary hematology. 6th edition. Ames (IA): Wiley-Blackwell; 2010. p. 893–8.
14. Hillyer EV, Quesenberry KE. Biology, husbandry, and clinical techniques (of guinea pigs and chinchillas). In: Ferrets, rabbits, and rodents: clinical medicine and surgery. Philadelphia: WB Saunders; 1997. p. 432.
15. Osmond DG, Everett NB. Bone marrow blood volume and total red cell mass of the guinea-pig as determined by 59-Fe-erythrocyte dilution and liquid nitrogen freezing. Q J Exp Physiol Cogn Med Sci 1965;50:1–14.
16. Quesenberry KE, Carpenter JW. Ferrets, rabbits, and rodents: clinical medicine and surgery. 3rd edition. St Louis (MO): Elsevier/Saunders; 2012.

17. Thrall MA. Veterinary hematology and clinical chemistry. 2nd edition. Ames (IA): Wiley-Blackwell; 2012.

18. Albritton EC, American Institute of Biological Sciences, Committee on the Handbook of Biological Data. Standard values in blood, being the first part of a handbook of biological data. Dayton (OH): Air Force, Wright Air Development Center; 1951.

19. Campbell TW, Ellis C. Avian and exotic animal hematology and cytology. 3rd edition. Ames (IA): Blackwell Pub; 2007.

20. Schermer S. The blood morphology of laboratory animals. 3rd edition. Philadelphia: FA Davis; 1967.

21. Suckow MA, Stevens KA, Wilson RP. The laboratory rabbit, guinea pig, hamster, and other rodents. 1st edition. London; Waltham (MA): Academic Press/Elsevier; 2012.

22. Johnson-Delaney CA. Exotic companion medicine handbook for veterinarians. Lake Worth (FL): Wingers Pub; 1995.

23. Kaspareit J, Messow C, Edel J. Blood coagulation studies in guinea pigs (*Cavia porcellus*). Lab Anim 1988;22:206–11.

24. Jones TC, Garner FM, Benirschke K, et al. Pathology of laboratory animals. New York: Springer-Verlag; 1978.

25. Mitruka BM, Rawnsley HM. Clinical biochemical and hematological reference values in normal experimental animals. New York: Masson Pub. USA; 1977.

26. Valenciano CA, Decker SL, Cowell LR. Interpretation of feline leukocyte responses. In: Weiss DJ, Wardrop KJ, Schalm OW, editors. Schalm's veterinary hematology. 6th edition. Ames (IA): Wiley-Blackwell; 2010. p. 335–43.

27. Banks RE. Guinea pig. Exotic small mammal care and husbandry. Ames (IA): Wiley-Blackwell; 2010. p. 115–24.

28. Izard J, Barrellier MT, Quillec M. The Kurloff cell. Its differentiation in the blood and lymphatic system. Cell Tissue Res 1976;173:237–59.

29. Eremin O, Wilson AB, Coombs RR, et al. Antibody-dependent cellular cytotoxicity in the guinea pig: the role of the Kurloff cell. Cell Immunol 1980;55:312–27.

30. Debout C, Quillec M, Izard J. New data on the cytolytic effects of natural killer cells (Kurloff cells) on a leukemic cell line (guinea pig L2C). Leuk Res 1999;23: 137–47.

31. Marshall AH, Swettenham KV, Vernon-Roberts B, et al. Studies on the function of the Kurloff cell. Int Arch Allergy Appl Immunol 1971;40:137–52.

32. Jain NC. Normal values in blood of laboratory, furbearing and miscellaneous zoo, domestic and wild animals. In: Jain NC, editor. Schalm's veterinary hematology. Philadelphia: Lea & Febiger; 1986. p. 274–343.

Avian Hematology

Michael P. Jones, DVM, DABVP (Avian)

KEYWORDS

- Avian hematology • Erythrocyte • Leukocyte • Anemia • Leukocytosis • Leukopenia

KEY POINTS

- Hematology is an invaluable part of the clinical management of avian patients.
- The half-life of avian erythrocytes is shorter than mammalian erythrocytes.
- Acute blood loss is the most common cause of regenerative anemia in birds.
- Nonregenerative anemia is the most common type of anemia described in birds.
- The heterophil is the most common granulocyte found in the peripheral blood of birds.
- Lymphocytes are second to heterophils in frequency in most avian species except Amazon parrots and canaries, in which the lymphocytes may be the predominate leukocytes and may account for up to 70% of circulating leukocytes.

AVIAN HEMATOLOGY

Hematology is an invaluable part of the clinical management of avian patients. To evaluate the health of their patients, the clinical progression of disease, and response to therapy, avian veterinarians should be well versed in sample collection, cellular identification, and interpretation of results of the hemogram. Avian erythrocytes and leukocytes may be evaluated with automated or manual techniques. Packed cell volume (PCV), total erythrocyte count, hemoglobin concentration, Wintrobe indices, reticulocyte count, erythrocyte morphology, total white blood cell (WBC) count, and leukocyte differentials are all used to evaluate the avian hemogram. It should be noted that although hematologic reference intervals and ranges have been established for many avian species, determined values may vary by age, sex, season/environment, and hormonal influences.[1–4] In one study, PCV and total erythrocyte count tended to be higher in male birds compared with female birds, and also increased with age. In another study,[5] only the erythrocyte count tended to increase significantly with age in bald eagles.

 The reader should know that although an understanding of avian hematologic techniques is essential, methods of sample collection, processing, and analysis of blood samples are elaborated in detail elsewhere.[1,6–8]

This article originally appeared in Veterinary Clinics of North America: Exotic Animal Practice, Volume 18, Issue 1, January 2015.
The author has nothing to disclose.
Department of Small Animal Clinical Sciences, College of Veterinary Medicine, University of Tennessee, 2407 River Drive, Room C247, Knoxville, TN 37996, USA
E-mail address: mpjones@utk.edu

Clin Lab Med 35 (2015) 649–659
http://dx.doi.org/10.1016/j.cll.2015.05.013
0272-2712/15/$ – see front matter © 2015 Elsevier Inc. All rights reserved.
labmed.theclinics.com

AVIAN ERYTHROCYTE MORPHOLOGY

Avian erythrocytes are oval or elliptical in shape with a central, oval nucleus and are mostly uniform in appearance among avian species (**Fig. 1**). Comparatively, they are larger than mammalian erythrocytes. When stained with Wright or Romanowsky stains, healthy, mature erythrocytes have an orange-pink–colored cytoplasm. The nucleus, which is uniformly clumped in appearance, stains a dark purple color and becomes more condensed with age.[1,3]

Polychromatophilic Erythrocytes and Reticulocytes

The half-life of avian erythrocytes is relatively short (28–45 days), which results in the regular appearance of polychromatophilic erythrocytes (approximately 1%–5% of the total erythrocyte count) in the circulating blood pool.[9] These polychromatic erythrocytes are more rounded in appearance, their cytoplasm stains more basophilic, and their nuclei are more rounded with less densely packed chromatin when compared with mature erythrocytes. They, along with reticulocytes, are indicative of bone marrow activity and erythrocyte regenerative capacity in avian species.[1,3] Polychromatophilic erythrocytes appear as reticulocytes when stained with Wright or new methylene blue stains. However, a significant number of avian erythrocytes contain basophilic granular material when supravitally stained; therefore, reticulocytes are defined as having a distinct ring of reticular material (characteristic clumps of residual cytoplasmic RNA) partially or completely encircling the nucleus.[3,9,10] Although the percentages of polychromatophils parallel the percentage of reticulocytes, the reticulocyte percentage is a more precise measurement of erythrocyte regeneration.[11] Immature erythrocytes with basophilic staining cytoplasm and a smaller, more rounded appearance than mature red blood cells are most commonly rubricytes.[1,3] They are an indication of a marked regenerative response in avian patients.

Anisocytosis

Variation in size and of avian erythrocytes is occasionally seen in peripheral blood smears.[1] Slight anisocytosis is considered an insignificant finding in birds.[3] Automated methods of performing erythrocyte counts can calculate the degree of anisocytosis using the red cell distribution width (RDW%), which measures variation in red blood cell size, or mean corpuscular volume.[7] RDW% may vary depending on the patient's age or even between laboratories. Normal psittacine RDW% is 10% to 11%. Percentages above those indicate an increase in anisocytosis.[7]

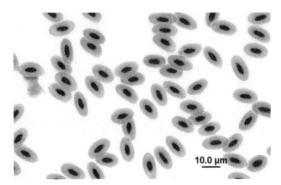

Fig. 1. Erythrocytes in the blood film of a hawk (*Buteo jamaicensis*) (Wright-Giemsa stain).

Poikilocytes

Erythrocytes that exhibit variations in shape are termed poikilocytes. These cells are more susceptible to damage, and as a result, have a shorter half-life than other erythrocytes. These may appear round, elongated, or irregular. The erythrocyte nucleus also may vary in appearance, location, and number, or on rare occasions may be absent.[7,12] Erythrocytes that are anucleated are termed erythroplastids.[8] Erythrocytes, which appear round with oval nuclei, are indicative of asynchronous maturation associated with accelerated erythropoiesis.[1,9] Binucleate erythrocytes, which indicate abnormal erythropoiesis, are often associated with severe, chronic inflammatory or neoplastic processes.[12]

Anemia

Most birds have a PCV between 35% and 55%; however, reference ranges and reference intervals for individual species should be considered. Anemias are usually the result of increased loss or destruction of erythrocytes or decreased production and are demonstrated by a decrease in the total erythrocyte count and PCV. Anemias due to decreased production appear to be mild anemias in contrast to more severe anemias caused by disease processes that affect the peripheral blood or bone marrow. Anemias are classified as regenerative, nonregenerative, hemolytic, or hemorrhagic.

Regenerative anemia
Regenerative anemias are characterized by the presence of polychromasia, reticulocytosis, macrocytosis, increased RDW%, and anisocytosis. Acute blood loss is the most common cause of a regenerative anemia in birds.

Nonregenerative anemia
Nonregenerative anemias seem to be the most common type of anemia described in birds, and indicate a lack of appropriate bone marrow response.[7] Etiologies include chronic inflammatory conditions, chronic infectious diseases (tuberculosis, colibacillosis, salmonellosis, aspergillosis), some viral diseases (West Nile virus), acute or chronic chlamydophilosis, and toxicosis (lead or aflatoxicosis), iron deficiency, endocrinopathies (hypothyroidism), and leukemia.[1-3]

Hemolytic anemia
Hemolytic anemias are often regenerative in nature and indicated by increased polychromasia, macrocytosis, anisocytosis, and reticulocytosis. Disorders that may cause a hemolytic anemia include erythrocyte destruction by parasites (*Plasmodium* spp and *Aegyptianella* sp), bacterial septicemia, acute toxicosis (oil ingestion, lead, zinc, petroleum products, and aflatoxicosis) and immune-mediated conditions.[1] However, the latter has not been well documented in birds.[13]

Hemorrhagic anemia
Hemorrhagic anemias result from blood loss due to trauma, gastrointestinal parasitism, coagulation disorders (as in conure bleeding syndrome, rodenticide toxicosis, and aflatoxicosis), organ rupture or ulceration, aneurysms, and some viral diseases. Following acute hemorrhage there is often a rapid increase (in hours) during which erythropoiesis increases dramatically.[1,14]

Polycythemia

Polycythemia is defined as an elevated PCV and erythrocyte count and is considered uncommon in birds.[1,3,7] Polycythemia may be categorized as absolute or relative polycythemia. Relative polycythemia is due to either redistribution of erythrocytes or the result of hemoconcentration or loss of plasma volume as a result of dehydration.[2,8] Birds do not store reserve erythrocytes in their spleen so relative polycythemia due to redistribution of erythrocytes is not seen in birds. Absolute polycythemia is further divided into primary polycythemia (polycythemia vera) or secondary polycythemia. Polycythemia vera is rare in birds[1,3] and is caused by a myeloproliferative disease that results in an increased production of erythrocytes.[3,8] Secondary polycythemia is a response to hypoxia, which results in an increased production of erythropoietin. Disease conditions that lead to secondary polycythemia include chronic pulmonary diseases, cardiac disease, iron storage disease, rickets, renal disease or renal neoplasia, or a physiologic response to high altitude.[3,8] Polycythemia is often a diagnosis of exclusion of possible etiologies. Treatment of polycythemia involves alleviation of the underlying cause and phlebotomy.[3]

Hemoparasites

Hemoparasites are seen in many species of captive and free-ranging birds. The most commonly identified hemoparasites include *Hemoproteus* spp, *Plasmodium* spp, and *Leukocytozoon* spp. Many avian species are susceptible to infection with hemoparasites, although clinical disease seems to be more significant in some species than others. *Hemoproteus* and *Leukocytozoon* may be found in large numbers within the bloodstream with no apparent clinical signs. Both *Hemoproteus* (**Fig. 2**) and *Leukocytozoon* (**Fig. 3**) are generally considered to be of low pathogenicity unless there is concurrent disease. However, once the underlying disease process is treated or alleviated, the presence of these hemoparasites in the blood seems to dissipate. *Hemoproteus* spp are sometimes confused with *Plasmodium* spp when evaluating a blood smear, except that *Hemoproteus* gametocytes tend to encircle more than half of the erythrocyte nucleus without displacing it from its central position and are not found in any other blood cells.[3]

   Plasmodium spp, the causative agent of avian malaria, can be pathogenic in a number of avian species, especially passerines (canaries), waterfowl, birds of prey, penguins, and poultry.[3] Intraerythrocytic gametocytes appear round or elongated and commonly displace the erythrocyte nucleus.[1,3,8] In addition, schizonts (containing merozoites) may be found in erythrocytes, and gametocytes and schizonts can be identified in other blood cells.[3,8] Clinical signs of *Plasmodium* infections include lethargy and depression, anorexia, weight loss, increased respiratory effort, biliverdinuria,

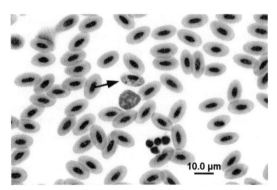

Fig. 2. *Hemoproteus* gametocyte (*arrow*) within an erythrocyte in the blood film of a hawk (*Buteo jamaicensis*) (Wright-Giemsa stain).

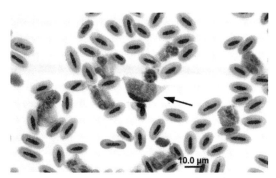

Fig. 3. *Leukocytozoon* gametocyte (*arrow*) in the blood film of a hawk (*Buteo jamaicensis*) (Wright-Giemsa stain).

and acute death. Laboratory diagnostics test results also may reveal hemolytic anemia, leukocytosis, and lymphocytosis.[1,3,8]

AVIAN LEUKOCYTE MORPHOLOGY

Avian leukocytes include granulocytes (heterophils, eosinophils, and basophils), mononuclear cells (lymphocytes and monocytes), and thrombocytes. Total WBC count, estimated WBC count, and leukocyte differential performed by automated or manual techniques are all used to evaluate leukocytes in the avian hemogram. Specific methods of sample collection, processing, and analysis of blood samples are elaborated in detail elsewehere.[1,2,8]

Leukocytosis refers to an elevation of the total WBC count and is most often associated with inflammatory diseases (gout, egg-yolk coelomitis, degenerative joint disease, or allergy), infectious diseases (bacteria, fungi, or parasites), or stress, or may actually be a normal finding in young birds.[2,6–8] When a marked leukocytosis (total WBC >30,000 $10^3/\mu$L) is noted, infectious diseases, such as chlamydophila, aspergillosis, mycobacteriosis, pneumonia, coelomitis, salpingitis, coelomitis, toxicosis (lead), neoplasia, and some and viral infections should be strongly considered. Stress leukograms have been reported in macaws, African gray parrots, cockatoos, and ratites, as well as other avian species, and may occur following travel, capture and restraint for physical examination, exercise, and trauma.[6,7,14,15] Although considered rare, excessively high leukocyte counts may indicate leukemia.

Leukopenia is often associated with chronic infectious or inflammatory diseases, severe, overwhelming bacterial or viral infections (circovirus infections in young birds, herpes virus, or polyomavirus), toxicosis, chemotherapeutic agents, or septicemia.[2,6,7] Improper sample handling may cause an artifactual decrease in WBC count due to blood clotting.[2]

Heterophil

The heterophil is the most common granulocyte found in peripheral blood and is usually the most predominant WBC. Avian heterophils contain eosinophilic, oval or spindle shaped granules which tend to cover most of the heterophil's nucleus (**Fig. 4**).[14] The nucleus contains coarsely clumped chromatin and usually has two to three lobes.[1,14]

Heterophilia may be associated with acute or chronic inflammatory and infectious diseases, stress, or may be normal in young birds.[2] In many instances, the severity of the leukocytosis associated with a heterophilia may correlate with the severity of

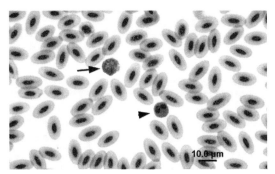

Fig. 4. Heterophil (*arrow*) and eosinophil (*arrowhead*) in the blood film of a hawk (*Buteo jamaicensis*) (Wright-Giemsa stain).

the disease.[10] The differential diagnoses for heterophilia mirror those for leukocytosis. Chlamydophila, aspergillosis, and mycobacteriosis, pneumonia, coelomitis, salpingitis, coelomitis, toxicoses (lead and zinc), neoplasia, and viral infections are all likely causes of a heterophilic inflammatory response.[1,6,7]

True heteropenia is rare in avian patients, but is usually associated with a leukopenia.[15] Overwhelming infectious diseases, bacterial septicemia, and some viral diseases, especially circovirus infections in African gray parrots (*Psittacus erithacus erithacus*), may cause a heteropenia.[1,3,6,7] In some instances, heteropenia occurs when significant numbers of ruptured leukocytes (smudge cells), likely heterophils, are present in a blood smear.[15] In some species, such as canaries and Amazon parrots, lymphocytes may be the predominate leukocyte in the hemogram.

Immature (band) heterophils are rarely seen in peripheral blood smears; however, when present, they may indicate severe, acute inflammation in which the demand for heterophils exceeds their release from the bone marrow.[3] Band heterophils are seen in peripheral blood smears within the first 12 to 24 hours after the onset of inflammatory disease, and are released in response to cytokines and other inflammatory mediators.[1,3,8] A degenerative left shift occurs when the increase in immature heterophils is greater than the number of mature heterophils and is associated with a persistent leukopenia. Left shifts may result from acute chlamydophila infections or other overwhelming diseases (such as mycobacteriosis, systemic fungal disease, septicemia).[1,2,7,15] A degenerative left shift indicates a poor to guarded prognosis. Band heterophils are characterized by an indistinctly lobulated or even horseshoe-shaped nucleus, cytoplasm that stains basophilic, and fewer granules that are round and stain deeply basophilic.[2] Care must be taken not to confuse them with basophils.

Toxic heterophils are a significant finding on an avian blood smear and are seen with severe diseases that affect production and release from the bone marrow.[7] Toxic heterophils have increased cytoplasmic basophilia, vacuolization of the cytoplasm, hypersegmentation and degeneration of the nucleus, degranulation or abnormal granules, and basophilic cytoplasmic inclusions (**Fig. 5**).[1,2,7,14,16]

Eosinophil

The avian eosinophil is a round cell with a pale blue cytoplasm in contrast to the colorless cytoplasm of the heterophil (see **Fig. 4**).[1,7] Typically, avian eosinophil granules are round in shape, although size, shape, and color may vary among species. Eosinophil granules are brighter in color when compared with the heterophil granules. This difference is due to a higher concentration of arginine in the eosinophil granules.[1,7,14]

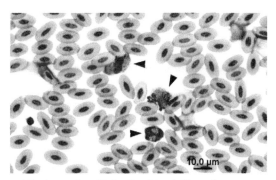

Fig. 5. Toxic heterophils (*arrowheads*) in the blood film of a cormorant (*Phalacrocorax auritus*) (Wright-Giemsa stain).

Eosinophil granules also lack the refractile central body of the heterophil granule.[1,6,7] Eosinophilia is often relative in that there may be an increased percentage of eosinophils but not a change in the absolute value of circulating eosinophils.[7] Etiologies for eosinophilia in birds often can be a mystery. Eosinophilia is rare in many avian species but common in others. When an eosinophilia is present, it may be due to marked tissue damage, parasitic diseases, such as giardiasis, ascaridiasis, and cestodiasis, or allergic conditions, but this is not always the case.[1,3,6,7,12] Eosinopenia is rarely reported in birds.[7]

Basophil

Basophils are also uncommon in peripheral blood smears of avian species; however, when seen, they should not be confused with toxic heterophils (**Fig. 6**). Avian basophils are slightly smaller than heterophils, with clear cytoplasm, a lightly blue stained nucleus that is nonlobed, and round basophilic granules that often obscure the nucleus.[2,3] Very little is known about the avian basophils; they appear to participate in early inflammatory responses and possibly allergic (hypersensitivity) reactions. Basophilia may be observed in birds with respiratory disease or tissue damage, and may be common in active chlamydial infections (particularly in budgerigars and Amazon parrots).[1,3,6,7,16] In Amazon parrots, such as the green-cheeked Amazon parrot (*Amazona viridigenalis*), the basophil granules appear to be larger and more prominent than in other psittacine species.[17] It is common for normal hemograms to not show any basophils.

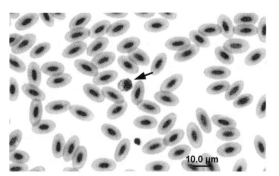

Fig. 6. Basophil (*arrow*) in the blood film of a hawk (*Buteo jamaicensis*) (Wright-Giemsa stain).

Lymphocyte

Lymphocytes are second only to the heterophil in frequency in most species except in Amazon parrots and some passerines (canaries). These species are often called "lymphocytic" because lymphocytes appear to be the predominate WBC and may account for up to 70% of circulating leukocytes.[3,7] Lymphocytes are typically round cells with a large nucleus-to-cytoplasmic ratio, but they may be somewhat irregular in shape due to molding around adjacent cells.[1] Lymphocytes have a round, centrally located, or slightly eccentric nuclei with densely clumped or reticulate nuclear chromatin and high nuclear-to-cytoplasmic (N/C) ratio (**Fig. 7**).[1,3] Their cytoplasm is clear or slightly basophilic and homogeneous, with no vacuolization.[2,3] Lymphocytes are usually characterized as small, medium, or large. Small or medium lymphocytes are the most common of the 3 in the peripheral blood. Small lymphocytes may be difficult to distinguish from avian thrombocytes, which have a clear, lightly blue or pale gray-colored cytoplasm, vacuolization, a larger more rounded darkly basophilic nucleus, and 2 small basophilic inclusions at the poles.[1–3] Reactive lymphocytes are medium to large in size with densely clumped chromatin, a deeply basophilic cytoplasm, a distinct pale Golgi zone, and cytoplasmic vacuoles.[1–3,6,7] Reactive lymphocytes may be present in small number in the peripheral blood smear and indicate antigenic stimulation often due to infectious diseases such as viral diseases (herpes virus or circovirus), chlamydophila infections, aspergillosis, tuberculosis, and salmonellosis.[2,6,7] Large lymphocytes with smooth disperse chromatin, nucleoli, abundant blue cytoplasm, and a prominent Golgi zone can be neoplastic and an indication of lymphoid leukemia or a leukemic phase of lymphoma.[3]

Lymphocytosis is not a common occurrence in birds, although an apparent increase may be seen in the previously mentioned "lymphocytic" species.[7] Lymphocytosis may result from antigenic stimulation of the immune system associated with infectious or inflammatory conditions or lymphocytic leukemia.[3,15,18]

Lymphopenia may occur relative to a marked increase in heterophils.[6,7,15] More commonly, lymphopenia may result from excessive endogenous or exogenous corticosteroids, and viral infections and diseases that cause bursal damage or bone marrow suppression (pancytopenia).[1,3]

Monocyte

Monocytes are the largest of the mononuclear leukocytes, but are rarely seen in peripheral blood smears.[7] They are most often confused with large lymphocytes.

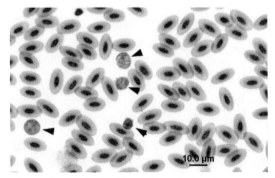

Fig. 7. Lymphocytes (*arrowheads*) in the blood film of a hawk (*Buteo jamaicensis*) (Wright-Giemsa stain).

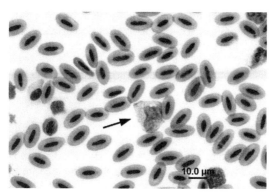

Fig. 8. Monocyte (*arrow*) in the blood film of a hawk (*Buteo jamaicensis*) (Wright-Giemsa stain).

Monocytes are round or amorphously shaped, with eccentric nuclei that are round, elongated, or indented, and the cytoplasm typically stains a blue-gray color with occasional vacuoles and fine eosinophilic granules (**Fig. 8**).[1–3,7] Monocytes are phagocytic, and once they enter into tissues they are transformed into macrophages.[3] Chlamydophila infections, and other chronic infectious diseases, such as tuberculosis, mycoses, and bacterial granulomatous diseases, are often but not always characterized by a monocytosis.[1,7,15] Monocytosis and basophilia have been described as the only hematological abnormalities seen in budgerigars with chlamydial infections. Because monocytes are not common in the peripheral blood, low or zero counts are not uncommon.[1,7]

Thrombocyte

Thrombocytes are small, oval or round cells, with dense nuclear chromatin, clear, faintly blue or pale gray cytoplasm, and one or more distinct granules at the poles (**Fig. 9**).[2,3,6,7] Thrombocytes are smaller than erythrocytes; however, they have a high N/C ratio and the nucleus is more rounded than that of erythrocytes. Avian thrombocytes arise from a stem cell, in contrast to mammalian platelets, which arise from megakaryocytes.[1,3,7] Thrombocyte counts are not commonly done, but instead, thrombocytes are reported as either adequate, increased, or decreased. The function of avian thrombocytes is not completely clear; however, they function in hemostasis

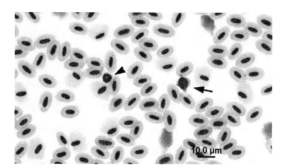

Fig. 9. Lymphocyte (*arrow*) and thrombocyte (*arrowhead*) in the blood film of a parrot (*Poicephalus senegalus*) (Wright-Giemsa stain).

and also are considered to be phagocytic, assisting in the removal of foreign material within the blood.[3,19] Thrombocytosis, although not well documented, may arise as an appropriated response to thrombocytopenia or chronic inflammatory disease in birds. Thrombocytopenia may occur due to increased destruction or excessive demand, as in septicemia or disseminated intravascular coagulation, bone marrow suppression (pancytopenia), and in some viral diseases (circovirus, reovirus, or polyomavirus).[1,7]

SUMMARY

Avian veterinarians often rely heavily on the results of various diagnostic tests, including hematology results. As such, cellular identification and evaluation of the cellular response are invaluable tools that help veterinarians understand the health or condition of their patient, as well as to monitor severity and clinical progression of disease and response to treatment. Therefore, it is important to thoroughly understand how to identify and evaluate changes in the avian erythron and leukon, as well as to interpret normal and abnormal results.

REFERENCES

1. Campbell TW, Ellis CK. Hematology of birds. In: Campbell TW, Ellis CK, editors. Avian and exotic animal hematology and cytology. 3rd edition. Ames (IA): Blackwell Publishing Professional; 2007. p. 3–50.
2. Doneley B. Interpreting diagnostic tests. In: Avian medicine and surgery in practice: companion and aviary birds. London: Manson Publishing Ltd; 2011. p. 69–91.
3. Mitchell EB, Johns J. Avian hematology and related disorders. Vet Clin North Am Exot Anim Pract 2008;11:501–22.
4. Herbert R, Nanney J, Spano JS, et al. Erythrocyte distribution in ducks. Am J Vet Res 1989;50:958–60.
5. Jones MP, Arheart KL, Cray C. Reference intervals, longitudinal analyses, and index of individuality of commonly measured laboratory variables in captive bald eagles (Haliaeetus leucocephalus). J Avian Med Surg 2014;28:118–26.
6. Fudge AM. Avian complete blood count. In: Fudge AM, editor. Laboratory medicine: avian and exotic pets. Philadelphia: WB Saunders Co; 2000. p. 9–18.
7. Fudge AM. Avian clinical pathology—hematology and chemistry. In: Altman RB, Clubb SL, Dorrestein GM, et al, editors. Avian medicine and surgery. Philadelphia: WB Saunders Co; 1997. p. 142–57.
8. Clark P, Boardman WSJ, Raidal SR. General hematological characteristics of birds. In: Atlas of clinical avian hematology. Ames (IA): Wiley-Blackwell; 2009. p. 33–53.
9. Campbell TW. Hematology of psittacines. In: Weiss DJ, Wardrop KJ, editors. Schalm's veterinary hematology. 6th edition. Hoboken (NJ): Wiley-Blackwell; 2010. p. 968–76.
10. Campbell TW. Avian hematology. In: Avian hematology and cytology. 2nd edition. Ames (IA): Iowa State University Press; 1995. p. 3–19.
11. Johns JL, Shooshtari MP, Christopher MM. Development of a technique for quantification of avian reticulocytes. Am J Vet Res 2008;69:1067–72.
12. Capitelli R, Crosta L. Overview of psittacine blood analysis and comparative retrospective study of clinical diagnosis, hematology and blood chemistry in selected psittacine species. Vet Clin North Am Exot Anim Pract 2013;16:71–120.
13. Johnston MS, Son TT, Rosenthal KL. Immune-mediated hemolytic anemia in an eclectus parrot. J Am Vet Med Assoc 2007;230:1028–31.

14. Campbel1 TW. Hematology. In: Ritchie BW, Harrison GJ, Harrison LR, editors. Avian medicine: principles and applications. Lake Worth (FL): Wingers Publishing; 1994. p. 176–98.

15. Fudge AM, Joseph V. Disorders of avian leukocytes. In: Fudge AM, editor. Laboratory medicine: avian and exotic pets. Philadelphia: WB Saunders Co; 2000. p. 19–25.

16. Scope A, Filip T, Gabler C, et al. The influence of stress from transport and handling on hematologic and clinical chemistry blood parameters of racing pigeons (*Columbia livia domestica*). Avian Dis 2002;46:I224–9.

17. Woerpel RW, Rosskopf WJ. Clinical experience with avian laboratory diagnostics. Vet Clin North Am Small Anim Pract 1984;14(2):249–80.

18. Schoemaker NJ, Dorrestein GM, Latimer KS, et al. Severe leukopenia and liver necrosis in young African grey parrots (*Psittacus erithacus erithacus*) infected with psittacine circovirus. Avian Dis 2000;44(2):470–8.

19. Grecchi R, Saliba AM, Mariano M. Morphological changes, surface receptors and phagocytic potential of fowl mono-nuclear phagocytes and thrombocytes in vivo and in vitro. J Pathol 1980;130:23–31.

Reptile Hematology

John M. Sykes IV, DVM, DACZM[a],*,
Eric Klaphake, DVM, DACZM, DABVP (Avian), DABVP (Reptile/Amphibian)[b]

KEYWORDS

- Reptile • Hematology • Leukogram • Phlebotomy • Snake • Chelonian • Lizard
- Crocodilian

KEY POINTS

- Sample collection and processing: Most reptile species have accessible sites for blood sample collection. The anticoagulant of choice is heparin, although slides made from fresh nonanticoagulated blood are best if possible. Syringes and needles can be coated with heparin before collection to prevent clotting in small patients. A Romanowsky-type stain is preferred for cytology (eg, Giemsa). Rapid stains can be used to produce acceptable hemogram results but may understain some cell types.
- Lymph contamination: In most reptiles, the lymphatic drainage system is closely paired with the venous system such that lymph contamination of blood samples is a common occurrence. Grossly contaminated samples should not be used for hematology. In addition, samples with low packed cell volume, no evidence of regeneration (polychromasia), and a high percentage of small lymphocytes are likely to be significantly lymph contaminated, and the hemogram results should be interpreted with caution.
- Variation: The normal hemogram of reptiles varies by many factors including species, age, gender, season, environmental parameters, geographic location, and sample collection method. Because of this variation, values should be compared with reference intervals most closely matching the species and situation for each individual reptile. As these values are often not available, interpretation of the hemogram may rely heavily on cell morphology and on changes over the progression of a disease rather than on absolute values at a single point in time.

INTRODUCTION

The basic principles of hematology used in mammalian medicine can be applied to reptiles. This article outlines techniques for sample collection, processing, and analysis that are unique to reptiles, and provides a review of factors influencing interpretation of the results.

This article originally appeared in Veterinary Clinics of North America: Exotic Animal Practice, Volume 18, Issue 1, January 2015.
[a] Zoological Health Program, Wildlife Conservation Society, Bronx Zoo, 2300 Southern Boulevard, Bronx, NY 10460, USA; [b] Cheyenne Mountain Zoo, 4250 Cheyenne Mountain Zoo Road, Colorado Springs, CO 80906, USA
* Corresponding author.
E-mail address: jsykes@wcs.org

RESTRAINT AND BLOOD COLLECTION TECHNIQUES
General Comments

Before collecting a blood sample, the maximum safe volume that can be collected should be determined. Reptiles have a lower total blood volume than a similarly sized mammal, 5% to 8% of their body weight,[1,2] and 10% of this volume may be safely collected from healthy reptiles (eg, 0.5–0.8 mL in a 100-g animal). Smaller samples should be collected from compromised individuals.

Lithium heparin is generally the anticoagulant of choice in reptiles, as ethylenediaminetetraacetic acid (EDTA) has been reported to cause hemolysis, particularly in chelonians.[3,4] However, other studies of multiple reptilian species that suggest EDTA produces blood smears of comparable or better quality to those using heparin.[5–8] Ideally, hematology slides should be prepared from samples immediately after collection to avoid complications related to the anticoagulant. However, when drawing a sample from small individuals, it can be helpful to heparinize the needle and syringe before collection to prevent clot formation in the syringe. A study of slide preparation using blood obtained from green iguanas (*Iguana iguana*)[9] found that both the coverslip-slide method and bevel-edge slide techniques produced adequate quality smears, whereas the slide-slide method produced lower quality smears (higher numbers of ruptured cells). Slides are stained with a Romanowsky-type stain for morphologic analysis (eg, Giemsa, Wright, or Wright-Giemsa).[10,11] Rapid stains, such as Diff-Quik, may result in understaining or damage to some cell types, but can be used to produce adequate hemogram results.[11] For all venipuncture attempts, cleaning the skin with a dilute chlorhexidine solution before phlebotomy is prudent.

Snakes

There are 2 common venipuncture sites in snakes: the caudal tail vein (**Fig. 1**) and the heart (**Fig. 2**).[12,13] For either site, proper restraint of the snake's head is critical for handler safety. The caudal tail vein is accessed by holding the snake in dorsal recumbency and stabilizing the tail caudal to the cloaca. Holding the tail ventral to the body, such as over the end of a table, aids in successful collection. The needle is inserted on the midline between one-third and one-half the distance from the cloaca to the tip of the tail (usually 6–12 scutes caudal to the cloaca) at a 45° angle directed cranially. Avoid puncture of the hemipenes and scent glands that lie on either side of the midline. The needle is advanced with slight negative pressure. If vertebrae are encountered,

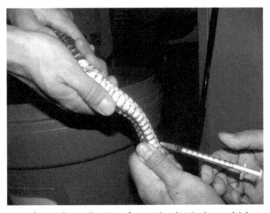

Fig. 1. Blood collection from the tail vein of a snake (*Naja kaouthia*).

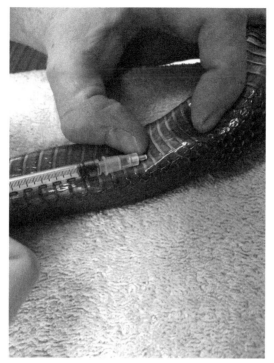

Fig. 2. Blood collection from the heart of a snake (unknown species).

the needle should be backed out and redirected. Restraint for this site is easy, but it can be difficult to collect a large volume from the tail, and risks include lymphatic contamination and trauma or infection to the hemipenes or scent glands. This site is useful for larger snakes and rattlesnakes, but is often more difficult to access in some colubrids and smaller boids.

For direct cardiac puncture, the snake is restrained in dorsal recumbency. The heart is usually located one-fourth to one-third the distance from the head to the tail.[12,14] It is found by visual inspection, palpation, or occasionally an ultrasound probe, particularly in larger snakes. Stabilize the heart with a finger cranial and the thumb caudal to the heart, taking care not to apply too much pressure, which may occlude blood flow in and out of the heart. The needle is inserted at a 45° angle into the ventricle of the heart. The syringe will fill slowly with each heart beat using only minimal negative pressure. Moderate digital pressure for up to 1 minute after the needle is withdrawn can decrease hematoma formation.[12] This technique can be performed safely in nonsedated snakes with adequate restraint provided the needle is minimally moved when in the body, although cardiac tamponade can occur if significant amounts of blood fill the pericardial space after puncture. If redirection is required, the needle should be withdrawn to the skin, redirected, and then advanced again.

Venipuncture of the palatine vein of snakes[15] is not recommended because of difficulties in restraint, minimal blood flow, and significant hematoma formation.

Lizards

Blood collection in lizards is usually from the tail vein with the lizard restrained in ventral or dorsal recumbency. Species that perform tail autotomy may need to be anesthetized (eg, with intramuscular ketamine)[16] before using this technique. One may also use the vagal technique (for calming lizards) by applying pressure over both eyes either digitally or by taping cotton balls over closed eyes. The tail vein can be accessed either ventrally or laterally. The ventral approach is performed as described for snakes. For the lateral approach, the needle is inserted at a 90° angle to the tail, just ventral to the lateral processes of the vertebrae, and directed medially. This site is identified by the longitudinal groove where the dorsal and ventral musculatures meet, although the groove can be difficult to locate on obese individuals.

The ventral abdominal vein lies within the coelomic cavity just dorsal to the ventral midline between the umbilicus and sternum. The lizard must be well restrained or anesthetized in dorsal recumbency, and the needle inserted along the ventral midline at a shallow angle and directed cranially. There is a risk of lacerating the vessel without the ability to apply pressure postprocedure, and puncture of other visceral structures is possible.[12,17]

Chelonians

Many venipuncture sites for chelonians have been described, including the heart; jugular, subcarapacial (**Fig. 3**), femoral, brachial (**Fig. 4**), and coccygeal veins (**Fig. 5**) and the occipital sinus.[12,18,19] The optimal site varies with the size and species, sedation level, medical condition, and experience of the phlebotomist. Samples collected from the jugular vein may be least likely to result in hemodilution because the vein can be visualized.[20] Regardless of site, pressure should be applied after collection for hemostasis.

The subcarapacial site is useful and easy to access in many species, particularly if access to the neck or limbs is difficult.[18,21] The head and neck can be either in extension or withdrawn into the shell. The needle is inserted on the midline where the skin of the neck meets the carapace. The exact angle of the needle to the body varies with the shape of the carapace, but is advanced along the ventral aspect of the carapace using mild negative pressure.[21] For larger animals, a spinal needle may be needed to reach the site. This site is the preferred alternative to toenail clipping for nonmedical personnel.[22]

Although the jugular vein may be preferred, its use is accompanied by difficult restraint. To access the site, the chelonian is positioned in ventral recumbency with the head held in a slightly more "head-down" position and with pressure applied to

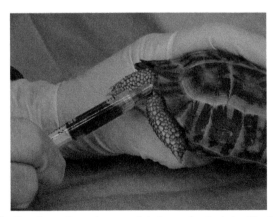

Fig. 3. Blood collection from the subcarapacial sinus of a tortoise (*Pyxis* sp). (*Courtesy of* Dr Bonnie L. Raphael, Bronx, NY.)

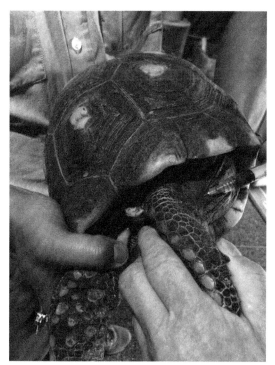

Fig. 4. Blood collection from the brachial plexus of a tortoise (*Chelonoidis carbonaria*). (*Courtesy of* Dr Bonnie L. Raphael, Bronx, NY.)

the back legs. The head is grasped using a ventral approach to avoid the normal defensive retraction response to dorsal threats. Grasping an extended foreleg prevents hinged tortoises from "boxing-up." Do not forcibly extract the head using instruments. Doing so can cause significant trauma to the beak. Once the head is restrained and extended, the vein is raised and visualized by applying pressure laterally at the thoracic inlet, either digitally or using a cotton-tipped applicator in smaller individuals.

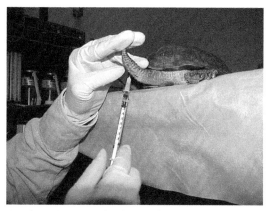

Fig. 5. Blood collection from the ventral tail vein of a turtle (unknown species). (*Courtesy of* Dr Bonnie L. Raphael, Bronx, NY.)

The presence and location of coccygeal veins in chelonians vary by species and may be dorsal, lateral, and/or ventral.[12] The dorsal vein can be accessed by flexing the tail ventrally and inserting the needle in a cranioventral direction as far cranially as possible on the dorsal midline. Lateral and ventral veins may be accessed with a technique similar to that already described for lizards.

The brachial vein (also called brachial plexus or ulnar plexus)[18] is located near the tendon of the triceps at the radiohumeral joint (elbow).[19] The foreleg is grasped and extended. The triceps tendon is palpated near the caudal aspect of the elbow joint, and the needle is inserted ventral to the tendon with the syringe held parallel to the forearm (see **Fig. 3**). Aldabra tortoises (Geochelone gigantean) have been trained for voluntary blood collection at this site.[23]

Cardiocentesis may be performed if other sites are not available, but in the clinical situation it is generally reserved for administration of euthanasia solution.[18,19] A needle is placed directly through the plastron on the midline near the junction of the pectoral and abdominal scutes.[12,19] Access via the thoracic inlet is difficult because of the inability to stabilize the heart and the required needle length.[19]

Two different approaches to the occipital sinus have been described.[19,24] In sternal recumbency, extend the head, aim the nose ventrally, then direct the needle caudally on the dorsal midline of the neck, just caudal to occiput.[19] Alternatively, position the chelonian vertically, extending and then flexing the head to make a 90° angle with the shell, and cranially direct the needle into the sinus at the dorsal midline of the neck.[24] With either method, a 25- or 23-gauge needle is used, and adequate manual or chemical restraint is critical.

The dorsal cervical sinuses (lateral occipital sinuses) are unique to sea turtles.[18] The turtle is restrained in sternal recumbency with the head flexed ventrally. The sinuses are dorsal and lateral to the cervical vertebrae. The needle is directed at up to a 90° angle into the sinus. These sinuses cannot be palpated and may be fairly deep (up to 3 cm).[13] Neck-restraining boxes and/or use of an ultrasound machine may help locate the proper site in larger sea turtles.

Sampling from cut toenails is not recommended. The sample size from this location will be small and contaminated with lymph, as the lymphatics of the area will be cut along with the blood vessels. This procedure is also considered to be painful, and may carry a greater risk of infection in comparison with collection from other sites.[13]

Crocodilians

The tail vein (**Fig. 6**) and the supravertebral sinus are the most commonly used sites in crocodilians. The tail vein is accessed as for lizards, either from a ventral or lateral approach. Collection from larger crocodilians can be facilitated by operant conditioning. The supravertebral sinus is accessed by restraining the animal in ventral recumbency with the head controlled. The needle (22- or 23-gauge) is placed on the ventral dorsal midline just caudal to the occiput and directed ventrally at a 90° angle. Negative pressure should be applied as the needle is advanced, and care should be taken, as spinal cord trauma (ie, pithing) can occur if needle is advanced too deeply.[12]

SAMPLE ANALYSIS
Erythrocytes

The packed cell volume (PCV), total erythrocyte count (RBC), and erythrocyte morphology should always be evaluated.[11,13] The PCV can be measured using hematocrit tubes as for mammals. The total RBC can be obtained using automated

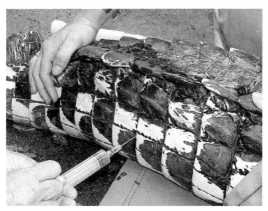

Fig. 6. Blood collection from the lateral approach to the tail vein on a crocodile (*Crocodylus rhombifer*). (*Courtesy of* Dr Bonnie L. Raphael, Bronx, NY.)

cell counters or manually.[25] Manual methods involve a hemocytometer and some type of staining/dilution system. The erythrocyte Unopette (Becton-Dickinson, Rutherford, NJ, USA) is one such system; an alternative system uses Natt and Herrick solution and a diluting pipette. Use of the Natt and Herrick solution allows determination of the RBC and total leukocyte count using the same sample in the hemocytometer.[10]

Mature reptilian erythrocytes are oval with an irregularly margined nucleus (**Figs. 7–15**).[10,11,26] New erythrocytes are created from the bone marrow, extramedullary sites such as the liver and spleen, or mature circulating cells dividing to form daughter cells.[10] Thus mitotic figures in circulating reptile erythrocytes may be normal. Compared with mature erythrocytes, immature cells appear smaller, rounder, have a basophilic cytoplasm, and have less dense chromatin in the nucleus (see **Fig. 7**).[11] Reticulocytes can be observed using a new methylene blue stain, and are 2.5% or less of the normal total RBC.[11] Hemoglobin, mean cell volume, and mean cell hemoglobin concentration are calculated as for mammals.

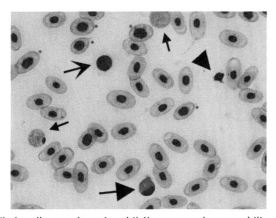

Fig. 7. Heterophils (*small arrows*), eosinophil (*large arrow*), azurophilic monocyte (*curved arrow*), lymphocyte (*arrowhead*), and immature erythrocytes (*asterisks*) in a bog turtle (*Glyptemys muhlenbergii*) (Diff-Quik stain, original magnification ×1000).

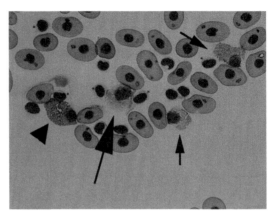

Fig. 8. Heterophils (*small arrows*), eosinophil (*arrowhead*), monocyte (*large arrow*), and thrombocytes (*asterisks*) in a tortoise (*Astrochelys radiata*) (Diff-Quik stain, original magnification ×1000).

Leukocytes

Complete leukocyte analysis includes a total leukocyte count (WBC), differential, and morphologic assessment.[11,13] Owing to the nucleated nature of reptile erythrocytes, automated methods of obtaining a WBC and differentials are not accurate. Manual methods for obtaining a WBC include estimated counts from blood smears, the semidirect method with phloxine B solution (eg, Unopette system), and the direct method (eg, using Natt and Herrick solution). Each method has advantages and disadvantages, and the accuracy of results depends on the cytologist's experience.

The estimated count method is performed by counting the total number of leukocytes in at least 10 fields of a stained blood smear using the high-dry (40× or 45×) objective. The average number of leukocytes per field is multiplied by 1500, resulting in the estimated leukocytes per microliter. This method is rapid and simple, but is prone to error if cells are clumped or not evenly distributed on the slide.[27]

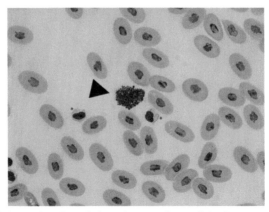

Fig. 9. Eosinophil (*arrowhead*) and thrombocytes (*asterisks*) of a pit viper (*Cryptelytrops macrops*) (Diff-Quik stain, original magnification ×1000).

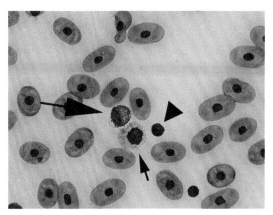

Fig. 10. Eosinophil (*large arrow*), basophil (*small arrow*), and a small lymphocyte (*arrowhead*) in a snapping turtle (*Chelydra serpentine*) (Diff-Quik stain, original magnification ×1000). Note that the basophil is understained using this staining technique.

The semidirect method is performed by staining acidophilic granulocytes with phloxine B solution. These stained granulocytes are counted in a hemocytometer, and a differential cell count is performed on a stained slide. The total WBC is then calculated using the number of heterophils and eosinophils counted in the hemocytometer and the percentage of such cells on the differential: Total WBC/μL = number of cells stained in hemocytometer chamber × 1.1 × 16 × 100/percentage of heterophils and eosinophils on differential.[25,28] This method requires an accurate differential for calculation of the WBC. If the heterophil count is low (due to true heteropenia or lysis of heterophils during creation of the blood smear), the total WBC can be artificially elevated.

The direct method is performed by staining all leukocytes with a solution such as Natt and Herrick, which are counted using a hemocytometer, and the total WBC is calculated. This method relies on distinguishing small lymphocytes from thrombocytes in the hemocytometer.[11,29] Inaccurately counting thrombocytes as lymphocytes will artificially elevate the result.

Heterophils (see **Figs. 7** and **8**) are the most common granulocyte in reptile blood and are analogous to the neutrophil.[10,13] Heterophils are round, may have

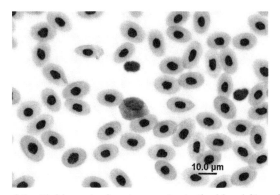

Fig. 11. An eosinophil with blue cytoplasmic granules in the blood film of a lizard (*Iguana iguana*) (Wright-Giemsa stain). (*Courtesy of* Dr Terry Campbell, Fort Collins, CO.)

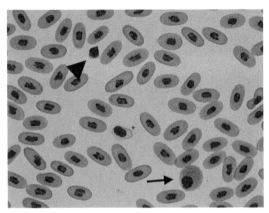

Fig. 12. Azurophil (*arrow*), lymphocyte (*arrowhead*), and thrombocyte (*asterisk*) in a python (*Morelia viridis*) (Diff-Quik stain, original magnification ×1000).

pseudopodia, and have clear cytoplasm.[10,13] The nucleus is round, eccentric, and may be bilobed.[13,29] The granules are eosinophilic, elongated, or spindle-shaped, and may be very numerous.[11,29] The morphology of heterophils may vary within an individual, particularly in the staining qualities of the granules. This variation has been hypothesized to be due to different stages of maturation of the heterophil, as this cell may mature while in circulation.[30–32] Toxic changes may be represented by the presence of a basophilic cytoplasm, abnormal granules, and vacuoles.[29,33] Degranulation may also be an indication of toxicity, although it may also be an artifact. A left shift may be indicated by the presence of myelocytes and metamyelocytes in circulation.[13] The presence of intracellular bacteria within leukocytes may indicate infection (see **Fig. 14**).

Eosinophils (see **Figs. 7–11**) are of similar size and shape to heterophils, and an eccentric nucleus is present. The distinguishing morphologic feature is that the eosinophilic granules of eosinophils are usually spherical, rather than the oval or elongated granules of heterophils.[10,11,29] Eosinophils of green iguanas (*I iguana*) are unusual because of their bluish-green spherical granules, the function of which is unknown

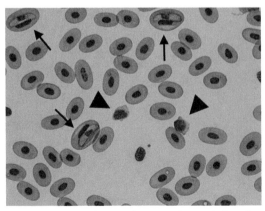

Fig. 13. Hemogregarine parasites within erythrocytes (*arrows*), lymphocytes (*arrowheads*), and a thrombocyte (*asterisk*) in a rattlesnake (*Crotalus horridus*) (Diff-Quik stain, original magnification ×1000).

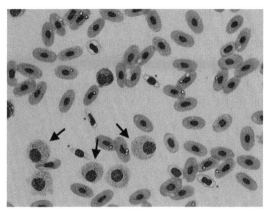

Fig. 14. Intracellular bacteria within azurophils (*arrows*), and thrombocytes (*asterisks*) in a python (*Python bivittatus*) (Diff-Quik stain, original magnification ×1000).

(see **Fig. 11**).[34] Eosinophils are not present in all species, particularly snakes[13]; they have been found in king cobras (*Ophiophagus hannah*),[32] but not in diamondback rattlesnakes (*Crotalus adamanteus*)[30] or yellow rat snakes (*Elaphae obsoleta quadrivitatta*).[8] Some investigators contend that eosinophils in snakes are actually variations of heterophils.[30] Variation of eosinophils within individuals, as described for heterophils, has been observed in green turtles (*Chelonia mydas*).[35]

Basophils (see **Fig. 10**) are small granulocytes with darkly basophilic granules that obscure the centrally located, nonlobed nucleus.[10,11] Care should be taken to distinguish between a normal basophil and a toxic heterophil where granules are basophilic and round.[29]

Lymphocytes (see **Figs. 7, 10, 12,** and **13**) of reptiles are morphologically similar to those of mammals. Lymphocytes lack granules, may be small or large, have a high nucleus to cytoplasm ratio, and have basophilic cytoplasm.[11,26] These cells may have phagocytosed particles or erythrocytes,[10,29] and typically contour to the shape of adjacent cells.[8,29] Reactive lymphocytes may indicate antigenic stimulation and are typically larger, with more basophilic cytoplasm that may contain discrete punctuate vacuoles.[13]

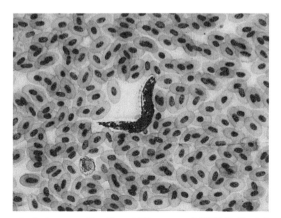

Fig. 15. Filarid nematode in a monitor lizard (*Varanus* sp) (Diff-Quik stain, original magnification ×1000).

Monocytes (see **Figs. 7** and **8**) are also similar to those of mammals. Monocytes are often the largest leukocyte (species dependent), with variably shaped contour and nucleus.[11,13] Monocytes of many nonsquamate reptiles contain azurophilc granules. These cells may be reported as "azurophils" or "azurophilic monocytes" but are a variation of the normal monocyte rather than a distinct cell type.[11,34] By contrast, azurophils of snakes (see **Figs. 12** and **14**) are a distinct cell type whose function is similar to that of the neutrophil.[30] The azurophils of snakes have finer granules and round nuclei in comparison with the azurophilic monocytes of other reptiles that have coarser granules and a lobulated nucleus.[36] Reactive monocytes may contain cytoplasmic vacuoles.[37]

Thrombocytes (see **Figs. 8, 9, 12, 13,** and **14**) are small, oval basophilic cells with a central basophilic nucleus and pale-blue or colorless cytoplasm.[10,11] It is important to distinguish between small lymphocytes and thrombocytes when performing differential counts or using the direct method of obtaining the total WBC (see **Fig. 13**). Small lymphocytes are more round, with darker cytoplasm and more clumped chromatin in their nuclei in comparison with thrombocytes.[13,29]

FACTORS AFFECTING THE NORMAL HEMOGRAM

Species, slide staining and evaluation technique, health status, nutritional status, age, reproductive status, stress levels, gender, venipuncture site, season, hibernation status, captivity status, and environmental factors can affect the values and the presentation of blood cells. It is important to compare results from an individual with reference intervals that most closely match that individual. The following examples from recent articles highlight the range in variation within species, and demonstrate that these changes are not consistent across species or different situations.

Demographics

In a study of yellow-headed temple turtles (*Hieremys annandalii*), males were found to have higher WBC in comparison with females.[38] By contrast, a study of free-ranging cobras (*Naja naja*) found that females had higher WBC than did males.[39] The relative numbers of leukocytes may be different across genders, as demonstrated in yellow-marginated box turtles (*Cuora flavomarginata*) where males had higher eosinophil counts and females had higher monocyte counts.[40] Age may also play a role in altering parameters. For a population of loggerhead sea turtles (*Caretta caretta*), PCV and WBC were both lower in younger animals than in older juveniles. The differential counts were also different across ages, with younger animals having lower lymphocytes and higher granulocytes compared with older animals, and monocytes were lower in older animals.[41]

Biological Activity

In one study, nesting female leatherback turtles (*Dermochelys coriacea*) had lower eosinophil percentages than green (*C mydas*) and loggerhead turtles (*C caretta*). This finding was attributed to lower helminth parasite loads in leatherbacks resulting from their diet of jellyfish.[42] Another study comparing foraging, nesting, and stranded loggerhead sea turtles found significant differences between the groups for PCV and lymphocyte, monocyte, and total WBC counts.[43]

Season and Environmental Conditions

Environmental parameters affect the hemogram, but unfortunately changes are not always predictable. For example, PCV increases in desert tortoises (*Gopherus agassizii*) during dry periods,[44] similar to findings in yellow-marginated box turtles (*C flavomarginata*) whereby PCV was highest in summer months. These turtles also had lower monocyte counts in the summer.[40] By contrast, a study of Asian yellow pond turtles (*Ocadia sinensis*) found that all hematology parameters except monocytes varied with the season.[45] Differences can be found across a geographic range even for the same species and season. The numbers of heterophils, basophils, and azurophils varied across different locations for free-ranging giant garter snakes (*Thamnophis gigas*).[46] Captive reptiles may have values different from those of free-ranging individuals of the same species. For example, in Mediterranean pond turtles (*Mauremys leprosa*), the percentage of lymphocytes was 4.2% to 7.7% in free-ranging animals but 64.9% to 57.8% in captive animals, compared with 4.2% to 7.7% in free-ranging turtles.[47]

Restraint

Another factor to consider is immobilization or restraint of the reptile. Stress was induced in captive estuarine crocodiles (*Crocodylus porosus*) by 2 different handling methods: manual restraint (noosing with ropes) and immobilization by electrostunning. The investigators found that both groups showed a significant increase in PCV and hemoglobin concentration; however, the magnitude of change was significantly reduced and recovery was faster in stunned animals.[48] Another study found higher basophil counts in anesthetized free-ranging carpet pythons (*Morelia spilota imbricata*) when compared with those manually restrained.[49]

DISORDERS OF HEMATOLOGY

Much of the literature regarding the interpretation of reptilian hematologic results and their etiology is anecdotal and based on mammalian assumptions. Association of etiology with diagnostic results and correct treatment are often lacking in the peer-reviewed literature. What follows are personal anecdotal observations combined with reports from the literature when applicable.

Erythrocytic Disorders

Anemia

Because lymphatic vessels/sinuses usually run in tandem with veins, lymphodilution can occur with any sample. Even cardiocentesis can have contamination/dilution with pericardial fluid. Removal of some of the lymph in a particular venipuncture site before withdrawal of the needle may result in a "cleaner" sample on the next venipuncture attempt from the same site. Grossly contaminated samples are easily recognized and should be discarded. However, in other situations the degree of lymph contamination may be difficult to determine. In general, if the PCV is decreased (especially <15%), there is no evidence of regeneration (no polychromasia), and there are increased small lymphocytes in the sample, the degree of contamination is high and hematology results are likely invalid.

Because of this high frequency of hemodilution when collecting reptilian samples, the diagnosis of anemia may be difficult to make. If artifactual causes have been ruled out, true anemia may be due to blood loss, destruction, or decreased production. In many cases, a thorough history will suggest whether acute blood loss has occurred, such as from trauma. The presence of regeneration may be determined based on the degree of polychromasia, but reptile RBC are long-lived (up to 600–800 days)[50] and so the regenerative response is muted in comparison with mammals or birds. Anemia attributable to decreased production from chronic disease is the most common cause seen by the authors, as reptiles are often debilitated for an extended time before clinical signs are seen and veterinary care is sought. Causes for chronic anemia are many and may include infection, chronic exposure to improper environment and diet, chronic organ failure, toxin exposure, or neoplasia.

Polycythemia
Polycythemia has been suggested when the PCV exceeds 40%.[11] The most common cause is dehydration. One of the authors has encountered several cases of reptiles with PCV of this level and higher, many with concurrent elevations of total proteins or solids. Tentative diagnosis of dehydration has been made in these individuals, often subclinical, but polycythemia has also been noted in healthy reproductively active female iguanas (Klaphake, personal observation).

Inclusions
Erythrocyte inclusion bodies may be due to artifact from staining, viral particles, or the presence of hemoparasites (see **Fig. 13**). Iridovirus-related inclusion bodies have been observed incidentally and as causes of anemia in reptiles. In a fer-de-lance (*Bothrops moojeni*) evaluated for renal carcinoma, erythrocytes contained 2 types of inclusions, 1 viral and 1 crystalline. The snake was markedly anemic and exhibited a strong regenerative response. Ultrastructural analysis identified the virus to be an iridovirus consistent with snake erythrocyte virus, and the crystalline structures to be of a different nature to hemoglobin.[51] Inclusions of viral particles consistent with iridovirus have also been found in the erythrocytes and erythroblasts of free-ranging northern water snakes (*Nerodia sipedon sipedon*) from Canada[52] and free-ranging flap-necked chameleons (*Chamaeleo dilepis*) from Tanzania.[53]

The presence of hemoparasites has often been noted in nonclinical captive animals, leading to questions of their significance in captive reptiles.[54] Several free-ranging snakes in Florida inhabit the same environment with distinctive *Hepatozoon* species characteristic of each host species, none of which had apparent clinical signs.[55] There are, however, reports of disorder caused by hemoparasites. For example, blood cell composition (percent of immature erythrocytes) and blood hemoglobin were altered by infection with *Plasmodium* spp (severity varied depending on species of parasite) in eastern Caribbean island anoles (*Anolis sabanus*). Substantial data on 2 other lizard-malaria systems, *Sceloporus occidentalis* infected with *Plasmodium mexicanum* in northern California and *Agama agama* infected with *Plasmodium giganteum* and *Plasmodium agamae* in Sierra Leone, showed malaria was virulent in those 2 species as well.[56] In addition, hemogregarine parasites were thought to increase the monocyte count in a study of free-ranging lizards (*Ameiva ameiva*).[57] Fortunately, as many hemoparasites require an invertebrate as part of its life cycle, captive-raised reptiles, unless housed outdoors, seem to be at low risk for infection by these parasites.

Leukocytic Disorders
Infection is a challenging diagnosis to make in reptiles based on a single leukogram. Leukopenia, leukocytosis, and even a normal leukogram can all be present during infection. For example, in a study of siadenovirus in Sulawesi tortoises (*Indotestudo forsteni*), changes in affected animals included anemia, leukopenia or leukocytosis, heteropenia or heterophilia, lymphopenia or lymphocytosis, eosinophilia, and azurophilic monocytosis.[58] In another study of free-living spiny-tailed lizards (*Uromastyx* spp), one animal with a compound fracture of the humerus and associated abscess and osteolysis had an elevated RBC, leukocytosis, and heterophilia, whereas another

individual with osteomyelitis of the stifle had a low RBC and leukopenia.[59] As with anemia, many illnesses in reptiles are due to chronic disease, whereby the WBC would be expected change over time and may regress back into a normal or leukopenic range through the weeks or months before presentation. This observation may explain the variation in leukocyte counts in the aforementioned examples.

Leukocytosis

As already mentioned, leukocytosis in reptiles is often associated anecdotally with infection. Elevated total WBC may reflect inflammation/immune response, infection, and/or stress. Following the WBC in an individual over time may be of more value than a single point sample. For example, in a study of cold-stunned Kemp's ridley turtle (*Lepidochelys kempii*), total WBC in convalescent animals were lower than those of cold-stunned animals, suggesting that as animals improved their WBC decreased.[60]

Often the more important parameters to interpret in the WBC are the differential and leukocyte morphology, rather than total WBC. For example, in a study of captive green turtles (*C mydas*) with or without ulcerative dermatitis, there was no difference seen in total WBC, but the heterophil/lymphocyte ratio was significantly increased in affected turtles. Along with a reduced delayed-type hypersensitivity reaction, it was postulated that the affected turtles were immunosuppressed.[61] Changes in the hemogram over time may also be important to monitor. In a study of the pathology associated with implanting radiotransmitters in eastern massasauga rattlesnakes (*Sistrurus catenatus catenatus*), all implanted animals had elevated heterophil and basophil counts 1 month after surgery. In one implanted group, this pattern had changed to higher lymphocyte counts many months later.[62] Reptilian monocytosis often is observed in immune responses to bacterial infections and parasitic infestations that result in tissue granuloma formation,[63] and eosinophilia may occasionally be caused by parasite infestation.[64]

Documented cases of leukocytosis have also been reported to be due to neoplastic leukemias. Hematopoietic malignancies are most commonly reported in lizards[65] and snakes,[66] occurring sporadically in other reptiles. These neoplasias may present as multiple discrete masses, such as with lymphosarcoma, as circulating neoplasms (leukemia), or as a combination of both forms.[63,67–69] Typically they occur as sporadic cases, but outbreaks or clusters of lymphoid neoplasms have been reported.[70]

Leukopenia

Leukopenia caused by toxicosis associated with fenbendazole was noted in a 125-day study of Hermann's tortoises (*Testudo hermanni*). Serial blood samples found that although the tortoises remained healthy, an extended heteropenia occurred. It was suggested that the risk of mortality of an individual from nematode infection should be assessed relative to the potential for metabolic alteration and secondary septicemia following damage to hematopoietic and gastrointestinal systems by fenbendazole.[71]

Inclusions/hemoparasites

As with erythrocytic inclusions, the differentials of artifact, virus, and hemoparasite should be considered. A free-ranging adult female eastern box turtle (*Terrapene carolina*) had intracytoplasmic inclusions consistent with iridovirus within heterophils and large mononuclear leukocytes on routine blood smear examination.[72] In a report of blood films examined from 170 specimens of 15 *Chamaeleo* spp in Tanzania, 3 *C dilepis* had an intracytoplasmic inclusion within monocytes. One of the lizards was maintained in captivity and, at 46 days, a second type of inclusion was occasionally seen within monocytes. Transmission electron microscopic examination of monocytes revealed the presence of a chlamydia-like organism and pox-like virus.[73]

ACKNOWLEDGMENTS

The authors thank Karen Ingerman, LVT, for her help with image acquisition and assistance with this article. This article was adapted from a previous version written by the authors: Reptile hematology. In: Hematology and related disorders. Vet Clin Exp Anim Pract 2008; 11.

REFERENCES

1. Lillywhite HB, Smits AW. Lability of blood volume in snakes and its relation to activity and temperature. J Exp Biol 1984;110:267–74.
2. Smits AW, Kozubowski MM. Partitioning of body fluids and cardiovascular responses to circulatory hypovolemia in the turtle *Pseudemys scripta elegans*. J Exp Biol 1985;116:237–50.
3. Jacobson ER. Blood collection techniques in reptiles. In: Fowler ME, editor. Zoo and wild animal medicine, current therapy 3. Philadelphia: WB Saunders Co; 1993. p. 144–52.
4. Muro J, Cuenca R, Pastor J, et al. Effects of lithium heparin and tripotassium EDTA on hematologic values of Hermann's tortoises (*Testudo hermanni*). J Zoo Wildl Med 1998;29(1):40–4.
5. Harr KE, Raskin RE, Heard DJ. Temporal effects of 3 commonly used anticoagulants on hematologic and biochemical variables in blood samples from macaws and Burmese pythons. Vet Clin Pathol 2005;34(4):383–8.
6. Hanley CS, Hernandez-Divers SJ, Bush S, et al. Comparison of the effect of dipotassium ethylenediaminetetraacetic acid and lithium heparin on hematologic values in the green iguana (*Iguana iguana*). J Zoo Wildl Med 2004;35(3):328–32.
7. Martinez-Jimenez D, Hernandez-Divers SJ, Floyd TM, et al. Comparison of the effects of dipotassium ethylenediaminetetraacetic acid and lithium heparin on hematologic values in yellow-blotched map turtles, *Braptemys flavimaculata*. J Herp Med Surg 2007;17(2):36–41.
8. Dotson TK, Ramsay ER, Bounous DI. A color atlas of blood cells of the yellow rat snake. Compend Contin Educ Pract Vet 1995;17:1013–6.
9. Perpinan D, Hernandez-Divers SM, McBride M, et al. Comparison of three different techniques to produce blood smears from green iguanas, *Iguana iguana*. J Herp Med Surg 2006;16(3):99–101.
10. Frye FL. Hematology as applies to clinical reptile medicine. In: Biomedical and surgical aspects of captive reptile husbandry. 2nd edition. Malabar (FL): Krieger Publishing Co; 1991. p. 209–79.
11. Campbell TW. Clinical pathology of reptiles. In: Mader DR, editor. Reptile medicine and surgery. 2nd edition. St Louis (MO): Saunders; 2006. p. 453–70.
12. Hernandez-Divers SJ. Diagnostic techniques. In: Mader DR, editor. Reptile medicine and surgery. 2nd edition. St Louis (MO): Saunders; 2006. p. 490–532.
13. Strik NI, Alleman AR, Harr KE. Circulating inflammatory cells. In: Jacobson ER, editor. Infectious diseases and pathology of reptiles color atlas and text. Boca Raton (FL): CRC Press; 2007. p. 167–218.
14. Jacobson ER. Overview of reptile biology, anatomy, and histology. In: Jacobson ER, editor. Infectious diseases and pathology of reptiles color atlas and text. Boca Raton (FL): CRC Press; 2007. p. 1–130.

15. Olson GA, Hessler JR, Faith RE. Techniques for blood collection and intravascular infusions of reptiles. Lab Anim Sci 1975;25:783–6.
16. Schumacher J, Yelen T. Anesthesia and analgesia. In: Mader DR, editor. Reptile medicine and surgery. 2nd edition. St Louis (MO): Saunders; 2006. p. 442–52.
17. Redrobe S, MacDonald J. Sample collection and clinical pathology of reptiles. Vet Clin North Am Exot Anim Pract 1999;2(3):709–30.
18. Barrows MS, McAurthur S, Wilkinson R. Diagnostics. In: McArthur S, Wilkinson R, Meyer J, editors. Medicine and surgery of tortoises and turtles. Oxford (United Kingdom): Blackwell Publishing Ltd; 2004. p. 109–40.
19. Lloyd M, Morris P. Chelonian venipuncture techniques. Bull Assoc Reptilian Amphibian Vet 1999;9(1):26–8.
20. Gottdenker NL, Jacobson ER. Effect of venipuncture sites on hematologic and clinical biochemical values in desert tortoises (Gopherus agassizzi). Am J Vet Res 1995;56:19–21.
21. Hernandez-Divers SM, Hernandaz-Divers SJ, Wyneken J. Angiographic, anatomic and clinical technique descriptions of a subcarapacial venipuncture site for chelonians. J Herp Med Surg 2002;21(2):32–7.
22. Johnson JD. Nail trimming for blood collection from desert tortoises, Gopherus agassizii: panel summary. J Herp Med Surg 2006;16(2):61–2.
23. Weiss W, Willson S. The use of classical and operant conditioning in training Aldabra tortoises (Geochelone gigantean) for venipuncture and other husbandry issues. J Appl Anim Welf Sci 2003;6(1):33–8.
24. Martinez-Silvestre A, Perpinan D, Marco I, et al. Venipuncture technique of the occipital venous sinus in freshwater aquatic turtles. J Herp Med Surg 2002; 12(4):31–2.
25. Pierson FW. Laboratory techniques for avian hematology. In: Feldman BF, Zinkl JG, Jain NC, editors. Schalm's veterinary hematology. 5th edition. Philadelphia: Lippincott Williams and Wilkins; 2000. p. 1145–7.
26. Saint Girons MC. Morphology of the circulating blood cell. In: Gans C, Parsons TC, editors. Biology of the reptilia, vol. 3. New York: Academic Press; 1970. p. 73–91.
27. Latimer KS, Bienzle D. Determination and interpretation of the avian leukogram. In: Feldman BF, Zinkl JG, Jain NC, editors. Schalm's veterinary hematology. 5th edition. Philadelphia: Lippincott Williams and Wilkins; 2000. p. 417–32.
28. Campbell TW. Avian hematology. In: Avian hematology and cytology. Ames (IA): Iowa State University Press; 1988. p. 3–17.
29. Wilkinson R. Clinical pathology. In: McArthur S, Wilkinson R, Meyer J, editors. Medicine and surgery of tortoises and turtles. Oxford: Blackwell Publishing Ltd; 2004. p. 141–86.
30. Alleman AR, Jacobson ER, Raskin RE. Morphological, cytochemical staining, and ultrastructural characteristics of blood cells from eastern diamondback rattlesnakes (Crotalus adamaneus). Am J Vet Res 1999;60:507–14.
31. Bounous DI, Dotson TK, Brooks RL, et al. Cytochemical staining and ultrastructural characteristics of peripheral blood leucocytes from the yellow rat snake (Elaphe obsolete quadrivitatta). Comp Haematol Int 1996;6:86–91.
32. Salakiji C, Salakij J, Apibal S, et al. Hematology, morphology, cytochemical staining, and ultrastructural characteristics of blood cells in king cobras (Ophiophagus hannah). Vet Clin Pathol 2002;31(3):116–26.
33. LeBlanc CJ, Heatley JJ, Mack EB. A review of the morphology of lizard leukocytes with a discussion of the clinical differentiation of bearded dragon, Pogona vitticeps, leukocytes. J Herp Med Surg 2000;19(2):27–30.

34. Harr KE, Alleman AR, Dennis PM, et al. Morphologic and cytochemical character-istics of blood cells and hematologic and plasma biochemical reference ranges in green iguanas. J Am Vet Med Assoc 2001;218(6):915–21.

35. Work TM, Raskin RE, Balazs GH, et al. Morphological and cytochemical charac-teristics of blood cells from Hawaiian green turtles. Am J Vet Res 1998;59:1252–7.

36. Alleman AR, Jacobson ER, Raskin RE. Morphologic and cytochemical character-istics of blood cells from the desert tortoise (*Gopherus agassizii*). Am J Vet Res 1992;53:1645–51.

37. Stacy NI, Alleman AR, Sayler KA. Diagnostic hematology of reptiles. Clin Lab Med 2011;31:87–108.

38. Chansue N, Sailasuta A, Tangtrongpiros J, et al. Hematology and clinical chem-istry of adult yellow-headed temple turtles (*Hieremys annandalii*) in Thailand. Vet Clin Pathol 2011;40:174–84.

39. Parida SP, Dutta SK, Pal A. Hematology and plasma biochemistry of wild-caught Indian cobra *Naja naja* (Linnaeus, 1758). J Venom Anim Toxins Incl Trop Dis 2014; 20:14.

40. Yang PY, Yu PH, Wu SH, et al. Seasonal hematology and plasma biochemistry refer-ence range values of the yellow-marginated box turtle (*Cuora flavomarginata*). J Zoo Wildl Med 2014;45:278–86.

41. Rousselet E, Stacy NI, LaVictoire K, et al. Hematology and plasma biochemistry analytes in five age groups of immature, captive-reared loggerhead sea turtles (*Caretta caretta*). J Zoo Wildl Med 2013;44:859–74.

42. Deem SL, Dierenfeld ES, Sounguet GP, et al. Blood values in free-ranging nesting leatherback sea turtles (*Dermochelys coriacea*) on the coast of the Republic of Gabon. J Zoo Wildl Med 2006;37(4):464–71.

43. Deem SL, Norton TM, Mitchell M, et al. Comparison of blood values in foraging, nesting, and stranded loggerhead turtles (*Caretta caretta*) along the coast of Georgia, USA. J Wildl Dis 2009;45:41–56.

44. Dickinson VM, Jarchow JL, Trueblood MH. Hematology and plasma biochemistry reference range values for free-ranging desert tortoises in Arizona. J Wildl Dis 2002;38:143–53.

45. Chung CS, Cheng CH, Chin SC, et al. Morphologic and cytochemical charac-teristics of Asian yellow pond turtle (*Ocadia sinensis*) blood cells and their hematologic and plasma biochemical reference values. J Zoo Wildl Med 2009;40:76–85.

46. Wack RF, Hansen E, Small M, et al. Hematology and plasma biochemistry values for the giant garter snake (*Thamnophis gigas*) and valley garter snake (*Thamnophis sirtalis fitchi*) in the Central Valley of California. J Wildl Dis 2012; 48:307–13.

47. Hidalgo-Vila J, Diaz-Paniagua C, Perez-Santigosa N, et al. Hematologic and biochemical reference intervals of free-living Mediterranean pond turtles (*Mauremys leprosa*). J Wildl Dis 2007;43(4):798–801.

48. Franklin CE, Davis BM, Peucker SK, et al. Comparison of stress induced by manual restraint and immobilisation in the estuarine crocodile, *Crocodylus porosus*. J Exp Zool A Comp Exp Biol 2003;298(2):86–92.

49. Bryant GL, Fleming PA, Twomey L, et al. Factors affecting hematology and plasma biochemistry in the southwest carpet python (*Morelia spilota imbricata*). J Wildl Dis 2012;48:282–94.

50. Frye FL. Hematology as applied to clinical reptile medicine. In: Frye FL, editor. Biomedical and surgical aspects of captive reptile husbandry, vol. 1, 2nd edition. Melbourne (Australia): Krieger Publishing Cp; 1991. p. 209–77.

51. Johnsrude JD, Raskin RE, Hoge AY, et al. Intraerythrocytic inclusions associated with iridoviral infection in a fer de lance (*Bothrops moojeni*) snake. Vet Pathol 1997;34(3):235–8.

52. Smith TG, Desser SS, Hong H. Morphology, ultrastructure and taxonomic status of *Toddia* sp. in northern water snakes (*Nerodia sipedon sipedon*) from Ontario, Canada. J Wildl Dis 1994;30(2):169–75.

53. Telford SR, Jacobson ER. Lizard erythrocytic virus in East-African chameleons. J Wildl Dis 1993;29(1):57–63.

54. Campbell TW. Hemoparasites. In: Mader DR, editor. Reptile medicine and surgery. 2nd edition. St Louis (MO): Elsevier; 2006. p. 801–5.

55. Telford SR, Wozniak EJ, Butler JF. Haemogregarine specificity in two communities of Florida snakes, with descriptions of six new species of Hepatozoon (Apicomplexa: Hepatozoidae) and a possible species of *Haemogregarina* (Apicomplexa: Haemogregarinidae). J Parasitol 2001;87(4):890–905.

56. Schall JJ, Staats CM. Virulence of lizard malaria: three species of plasmodium infecting *Anolis sabanus*, the endemic anole of Saba, Netherlands Antilles. Copeia 2002;(1):39–43.

57. Bonadiman SF, Miranda FJ, Ribeiro ML, et al. Hematological parameters of *Ameiva ameiva* (Reptilia: Teiidae) naturally infected with hemogregarine: confirmation of monocytosis. Vet Parasitol 2010;171:146–50.

58. Rivera S, Wellehan JF, McManamon R, et al. Systemic adenovirus infection in Sulawesi tortoises (*Indotestudo forsteni*) caused by a novel siadenovirus. J Vet Diagn Invest 2009;21:415–26.

59. Naldo JL, Libanan NL, Samour JH. Health assessment of a spiny-tailed lizard (*Uromastyx* spp.) population in Abu Dhabi, United Arab Emirates. J Zoo Wildl Med 2009;40:445–52.

60. Innis CJ, Ravich JB, Tlusty MF, et al. Hematologic and plasma biochemical findings in cold-stunned Kemp's ridley turtles: 176 cases (2001-2005). J Am Vet Med Assoc 2009;235:426–32.

61. Muñoz FA, Estrada-Parra S, Romero-Rojas A, et al. Immunological evaluation of captive green sea turtle (*Chelonia mydas*) with ulcerative dermatitis. J Zoo Wildl Med 2013;44:837–44.

62. Lentini AM, Crawshaw GJ, Licht LE, et al. Pathologic and hematologic responses to surgically implanted transmitters in eastern massasauga rattlesnakes (*Sistrurus catenatus catenatus*). J Wildl Dis 2011;47:107–25.

63. Gregory CR, Latimer KS, Fontenot DK, et al. Chronic monocytic leukemia in an Inland Bearded Dragon, *Pogona vitticeps*. J Herp Med Surg 2004;14(2):12–6.

64. Hidalgo-Vila J, Martínez-Silvestre A, Ribas A, et al. Pancreatitis associated with the helminth *Serpinema microcephalus* (Nematoda: Camallanidae) in exotic red-eared slider turtles (*Trachemys scripta elegans*). J Wildl Dis 2011;47:201–5.

65. Hernandez-Divers SM, Orcutt CJ, Stahl SJ, et al. Lymphoma in lizards—three case reports. J Herp Med Surg 2003;13(1):14–21.

66. Garner MM, Hernandez-Divers SM, Raymond JT. Reptile neplasia: a retrospective study of case submissions to a specialty diagnostic service. Vet Clin North Am Exot Anim Pract 2004;7(3):653–71.

67. Tocidlowski ME, McNamara PL, Wojcieszyn JW. Myelogenous leukemia in a bearded dragon (*Acanthodraco vitticeps*). J Zoo Wildl Med 2001;32(1):90–5.

68. Schultze AE, Mason GL, Clyde VL. Lymphosarcoma with leukemic blood profile in a Savannah monitor lizard (*Varanus exanthematicus*). J Zoo Wildl Med 1999;30(1):158–64.

69. Schilliger L, Selleri P, Frye FL. Lymphoblastic lymphoma and leukemic blood profile in a red-tail boa (*Boa constrictor constrictor*) with concurrent inclusion body disease. J Vet Diagn Invest 2011;23:159–62.

70. Gyimesi ZS, Garner MM, Burns RB, et al. High incidence of lymphoid neoplasia in a colony of Egyptian spiny-tailed lizards (*Uromastyx aegyptius*). J Zoo Wildl Med 2005;36(1):103–10.

71. Neiffer DL, Lydick D, Burks K, et al. Hematologic and plasma biochemical changes associated with fenbendazole administration in Hermann's tortoises (*Testudo hermanni*). J Zoo Wildl Med 2005;36(4):661–72.

72. Allender MC, Fry MM, Irizarry AR, et al. Intracytoplasmic inclusions in circulating leukocytes from an eastern box turtle (*Terrapene carolina carolina*) with iridoviral infection. J Wildl Dis 2006;42(3):677–84.

73. Jacobson ER, Telford SR. Chlamydial and poxvirus infections of circulating monocytes of a flap-necked chameleon (*Chamaeleo dilepis*). J Wildl Dis 1990; 26:572–7.

Fish Hematology and Associated Disorders

Krystan R. Grant, DVM

KEYWORDS

- Fish • Teleost • Elasmobranch • Hematology • Erythrocytes • Leukocytes
- Thrombocytes • Blood cells

KEY POINTS

- This article reviews blood-collecting techniques including restraint, venipuncture sites, and sample handing.
- The section on hematologic evaluation includes the steps necessary to perform manual counts for total red and white blood cells, and cell descriptions for identification.
- Tables are included summarizing the reported etiology of changes in cell counts, packed cell volume, and red blood cell indices.

INTRODUCTION

There are scientific descriptions of approximately 27,300 different species of fish, which exceeds that of all other vertebrates combined.[1,2] With this many different types of known fish, the intrigue of their diversity is understandable. Ownership of captive pet fish shows an upward trend with approximately 148 million fish, or more than 41% of owned pets in the United States, in more than 69 million households.[3] In addition to pet fish, captivity also encompasses those in public aquaria, other educational facilities, and aquaculture. With the growing number and value of freshwater and marine fishes in captivity, the demand for their medical care increases. Fish handling, diagnostics, medicine, and surgery are often more challenging than in terrestrial and arboreal animals simply because of their aquatic nature.

One diagnostic tool that may assist the veterinary staff with detecting disease or identifying change is hematologic evaluation. As with other animals, normal variation from intrinsic or extrinsic factors or diseases affecting blood cells and counts may be evaluated by clinical hematology. Obtaining even a small blood sample may reveal information helpful in guiding treatment options.

This article originally appeared in Veterinary Clinics of North America: Exotic Animal Practice, Volume 18, Issue 1, January 2015.
The author has nothing to disclose.
Colorado State University, Department of Clinical Sciences, 300 West Drake Road, Fort Collins, CO 80523, USA
E-mail address: Krystan.grant@colostate.edu

The volume of information pertaining to reference intervals and interpretation of blood test results is relatively limited, which is expected given the number of different fish. Other challenges involved with hematologic evaluation in fish include the differences between publications regarding the nomenclature and function of blood cells. Research is ongoing, and the purpose of this article is to summarize the value, technique, and general interpretation of fish hematology.

BLOOD COLLECTION
Restraint Techniques

Blood collection from fish may be accomplished with either physical or chemical restraint. Physical restraint is the method used if the patient is cooperative or severely debilitated, and when the clinician is comfortable doing so without causing a great amount of stress to the animal. The integument of fish provides many functions, and should be approached and handled with caution for protection of the fish and the handler. Appropriate gloves should be worn to protect the handler from zoonotic disease and from physical and chemical defense mechanisms of the fish, and to protect the mucous layer of the fish.[4] Most small fish can be approached by using one hand to grasp near the base of the tail while supporting the body with the other hand.[5,6] The use of ancillary equipment, such as nets or stretchers, may be required depending on the size of the animal (**Fig. 1**). Some elasmobranchs may enter a hypnotic state referred to as tonic immobility when placed in dorsal recumbency (**Fig. 2**).[7–10] Tonic immobility has been noted in several species, and offers a short duration of decreased activity allowing for minor procedures such as physical or ultrasonographic examination, venipuncture, or administration of medications.

When physical restraint cannot be accomplished and the animal can withstand anesthesia, chemical assistance typically is used. There are many agents used for fish anesthesia but one of the most commonly used Food and Drug Administration–approved agents is tricaine methanesulfonate (Tricaine-S, previously Finquel). Tricaine methanesulfonate is also commonly referred to as tricaine, TMS, MS-222, or triple-2. Tricaine requires buffering with 2 parts sodium bicarbonate and is used to create induction and anesthetic baths. Many factors, such as physical characteristics of the fish, environmental conditions, and the procedure, will contribute to the optimum dose and therefore should be considered before use. Suggested initial doses

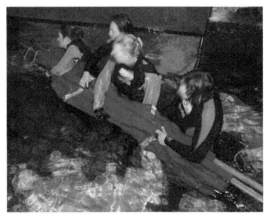

Fig. 1. Four aquarists restraining a sandbar shark (*Carcharhinus plumbeus*) in the red stretcher in preparation for examination.

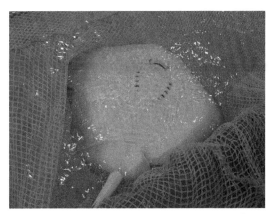

Fig. 2. Tonic immobility of a southern stingray (*Dasyatis americana*).

have been published (ranging from 50 to 400 mg/L), with a typical induction range for most fish at 50 to 150 mg/L, but it is recommended to begin conservatively.[10–15] A summary of the stages of anesthetic depths is provided in **Table 1**. Once the procedure is completed or nearly completed, the fish is gently ram-ventilated in appropriate untreated recovery water. Induction, anesthetic, and recovery baths should all be properly aerated.

Venipuncture Sites

A blood sample is often collected from the caudal vein by approaching it via the lateral or ventral tail. The lateral approach in teleosts (bony fish) begins with the fish in lateral recumbency and identification of the lateral line. An appropriately sized needle and syringe should be used. The needle is inserted into the skin between the scales, if applicable, just ventral to the lateral line. As the needle penetrates through the skin, mild negative pressure can be applied to the syringe as the needle is advanced deeper into the tissue until blood enters the syringe (**Fig. 3**). If bone is detected with the needle, the needle should be repositioned ventrally (below the spine). The ventral approach begins with the fish in dorsal recumbency. The needle is inserted on midline

Table 1
Summary of stages of anesthetic depth when using MS-222 in fish

Stage	Response	Reaction to External Stimuli	Opercular Rate
1	Light sedation	Slight loss	Slight decrease
2	Deep sedation	Total loss (except with strong pressure)	Slight decrease
3	Partial loss of equilibrium and muscle tone, hyperactive behavior	Total loss (except with strong pressure)	Increase
4	Total loss of equilibrium and muscle tone	Loss of spinal reflexes	Slow and regular
5	Loss of reflex activity	Total loss	Slow and irregular
6	None	None	Asphyxia, ceased

Data from Carter KM, Woodley CM, Brown RS. A review of tricaine methanesulfonate for anesthesia of fish. Rev Fish Biol Fisheries 2011;21(1):51–9.

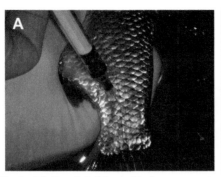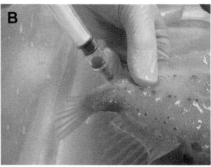

Fig. 3. (A) The tinfoil barb (*Barbonymus schwanenfeldii*) is in right lateral recumbency for collection of a blood sample from the caudal vein using the lateral approach. (B) The lumpfish (*Cyclopterus lumpus*) is in right lateral recumbency for collection of a blood sample from the caudal vein using the lateral approach.

of the ventral tail. Slight aspiration of the plunger is applied once the needle has penetrated the skin, and advanced deeper into the tissue until blood enters the syringe. Again, if bone is detected then the needle should be slightly retracted or repositioned left or right, depending on the position of the bone with respect to the needle.

Elasmobranch (cartilaginous fish) blood samples may also be collected from the caudal vein, and in larger sharks the dorsal venous sinus may be used. A ventral approach is often used with the animal in dorsal recumbency, the needle being inserted into the ventral midline of the tail. Once the needle has penetrated the skin, negative pressure is applied to the plunger. The needle is carefully advanced deeper into the tissue and possibly through a thin layer of cartilage to reach the vein (**Fig. 4**). Blood collection in larger sharks can be done at the dorsal venous sinus near the dorsal fin. With the shark in ventral recumbency, the caudal flap of the dorsal fin is lifted to expose the denticle-free skin. The needle is inserted in the center of the flesh pocket with negative pressure applied to the syringe. The needle may need to be repositioned or advanced to find the sinus (**Fig. 5**).

Cardiocentesis is another option for obtaining a blood sample, although this method may put the fish at a greater risk of injury or death.[16,17]

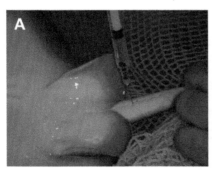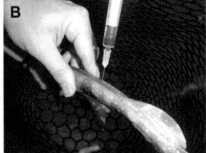

Fig. 4. (A) The southern stingray (*Dasyatis americana*) is in dorsal recumbency for collection of a blood sample from the caudal vein using the ventral approach. (B) The white-spotted bamboo shark (*Chiloscyllium plagiosum*) is in dorsal recumbency for collection of a blood sample from the caudal vein using the ventral approach.

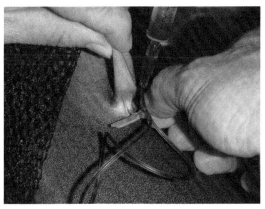

Fig. 5. The blacktip reef shark (*Carcharhinus melanopterus*) is in ventral recumbency for collection of a blood sample from the dorsal venous sinus.

Sample Handling

The amount of blood that can be safely obtained from a healthy fish has been reported at 30% to 50% of total blood volume.[18] Typically sample collection is approximately 1% of the body weight.[17,18] Once blood is retrieved it should be placed in a microtainer containing an anticoagulant, such as lithium heparin or ethylenediaminetetraacetic acid (EDTA). For hematologic evaluation the preferred anticoagulant is species specific, although heparin seems to be most commonly used.[19,20] For elasmobranch blood, although heparin can be used, a combination of heparin and EDTA or use of another modified anticoagulant solution is ideal to match the osmolarity of the blood.[21] Preferably fresh blood smears should be made at the time of blood collection, although they may also be made from the collected sample in anticoagulant.

HEMATOLOGIC EVALUATION
Erythrocyte Structure and Function

Most fish have nucleated erythrocytes, the exceptions being the silvery lightfish (*Maurolicus muelleri*) and other members of the Gonostomidae family (*Valenciennellus tripunctatus* and *Vinciguerria* sp), which have anucleated erythrocytes.[2,22,23] The structure of erythrocytes in fish is generally oval to elliptical with a centrally positioned, basophilic nucleus and pale, slightly eosinophilic cytoplasm.[2,24,25] The number and size of erythrocytes vary among species, but elasmobranch red blood cells (RBCs) are generally larger and more rounded in comparison with bony fish.[2,25,26] It has been reported that erythrocyte size is proportional to its genome size (or nucleus size determined by the amount of deoxyribonucleic acid)[27] and inversely related to the standard metabolic rate.[28] The primary function of RBCs is oxygen transport, the extent of which depends on the amount of hemoglobin concentration within the cell and the gas-exchange mechanism.[22]

Approximately 1% of the peripheral RBC population may be immature erythrocytes, likely derived from circulatory erythropoiesis.[16] Immature erythrocytes will contribute to polychromasia and anisocytosis because of their smaller, round shape and dark-staining nucleus and cytoplasm in comparison with their mature counterparts. The nucleus to cytoplasm ratio is much greater in young RBCs and decreases as the cells mature, allowing the hemoglobin content to increase. Because the presence of immature erythrocytes in peripheral blood may be normal, noting it in cases of anemic fish does not necessarily translate into a regenerative process. Although erythropoiesis occurs in peripheral blood, the primary site of hematopoiesis in general is the kidney in teleosts and the Leydig organ, epigonal organ, thymus, and spleen in the elasmobranch.[21,22]

Packed Cell Volume

The most common diagnostic tool used to evaluate the amount of RBCs is the packed cell volume (PCV). The PCV, or hematocrit, is the concentration of RBCs per volume of blood and is expressed as a percentage. The 2 terms are used interchangeably, but the hematocrit usually represents a calculated result whereas the PCV is a direct measurement from centrifuged blood. The normal range in teleosts is approximately 20% to 45%.[19,22] The normal range in sharks is more difficult because of the significant difference in results based on venipuncture site. The PCV tends to be lower in samples collected from the venous sinus near the dorsal fin than from those collected from the caudal vein of the tail.[29,30] Other factors that may contribute to PCV variation in healthy animals include stress (handling, anesthesia, water intake), physical characteristics (size, species), sex, environmental factors (water temperature, dissolved oxygen, population density, photoperiod), activity level (thermodynamics), reproductive status, life stage, and diet. Anemia is classified as hematocrit less than 20%, and may be due to blood loss (hemorrhagic anemia), cell destruction (hemolytic anemia), or decreased production (hypoplastic anemia).[25] Polycythemia is classified as hematocrit greater than 45% and may due to dehydration, sexually mature males, hypoxia, stress, splenic contraction, or erythrocyte swelling.[25] Some of the causes for a change in the PCV are summarized in **Table 4**. There is also a summary available regarding anemia in another report.[25]

Red Blood Cell Indices

In addition to hematocrit, other measures involving the RBCs include the total count, hemoglobin, and the indices mean cell volume (MCV), mean corpuscular hemoglobin concentration (MCHC), and mean cell hemoglobin (MCH). The preferred method of determining the total RBC count is manually, as automatic blood analyzers are not able to differentiate between RBCs and white blood cells (WBCs), thereby accruing a small margin of error. Determination of both types of cell counts is done manually using two different methods (one for erythrocytes and one for leukocytes) with a hemacytometer. For both types of cell counts, the Natt-Herricks solution kit (Natt-Pette) is used for fish, as they tend to be more lymphocytic. The kit contains prefilled Natt-Herricks stain reservoirs, a pipette calibrated for 5 μL (to make the 1:200 dilution), and tips for the pipette. The following steps are taken to establish the total RBC count:

1. Draw 5 μL of blood using the pipette and tip, and wipe the tip of any excess blood with a lint free cloth or tissue.
2. Add blood to the Natt-Herricks stain reservoir and gently flush sample from the tip with the plunger of the pipette.
3. Apply a rocking motion to the reservoir to mix the sample and allow to set for at least 5 minutes.
4. Set up the hemacytometer with a specifically designed coverslip, fill each chamber with the solution using capillary action, and allow to set for 5 to 10 minutes (**Fig. 6**).
5. Using the 10× objective on the microscope, note the grid of 9 large squares. Center the large center square and adjust to the 40× objective (**Fig. 7**).

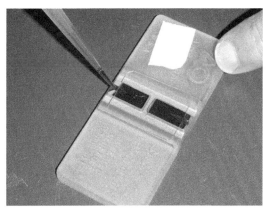

Fig. 6. The hemacytometer is loaded with a blood sample mixed with Natt-Herricks solution.

6. Count all the RBCs in the center square and 4 corner squares within the large center square. The RBCs will be elliptical cells with a centralized nucleus. The cytoplasm intensity may vary within a single sample depending on stain uptake for that particular cell (see **Fig. 7**).
7. Multiply the count for the 5 squares by 10,000 to calculate the total number of RBCs/mm^3 (or μL).

The hemoglobin concentration is typically measured using the cyanomethemoglobin method. The combination of the reagent and blood mixture should be centrifuged before measuring to remove the free nuclei.[16,19] Most teleost hemoglobin concentrations range from 5 to 10 g/dL.[19]

The MCV, MCHC, and MCH are collectively known as the RBC indices. The standard method for calculating the indices for other vertebrates can be used for fish. The equations and typical reference intervals for teleosts are shown in **Table 2**. The intervals shown are merely an estimate, as many factors may contribute to slight variation. For example, active fish will have a higher demand for oxygen and, therefore, a smaller RBC count and a lower MCV.[19,28] Elasmobranchs, in general, have larger and fewer erythrocytes that contain more hemoglobin in comparison with bony fish, which translates into increased MCV, MCHC, and MCH but decreased PCV, hemoglobin

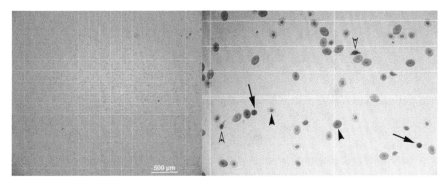

Fig. 7. (*Left*) The 9-square grid of the hemacytometer chamber. (*Right*) The hemacytometer chamber at 40× magnification for cell evaluation. The solid arrowheads indicate red blood cells. The open arrowheads indicate thrombocytes. The solid arrows indicate leukocytes. ([*Left*] *Courtesy of* Eric Carlson, BS, Denver, CO.)

Table 2 Red blood cell indices and their corresponding reference interval for teleost fish	
Red Blood Cell Indices	**Reference Interval for Teleosts[19]**
MCV (fL) = [PCV (%) × 10]/Total RBC	150–350 fL
MCH (pg) = [Hb (g/dL) × 10]/Total RBC	30–100 pg
MCHC (g/dL) = [Hb (g/dL) × 100]/PCV (%)	18%–30% (or g/dL)

Abbreviations: Hb, hemoglobin; MCH, mean cell hemoglobin; MCHC, mean corpuscular hemoglobin concentration; MCV, mean cell volume; PCV, packed cell volume; RBC, red blood cells.

concentration, and total RBCs.[31] Similar to PCV, other factors that may contribute to changes in these values are cell maturity (the more mature, the larger the cell, thereby increasing values), species, season, and diet.

Leukocyte Structure and Function

Similar to other vertebrates, fish have granulocytes and agranulocytes, with the agranulocytes being lymphocytes and monocytes. There is warranted confusion regarding the nomenclature of fish granulocytes, owing to their apparent diversity. Some fish granulocytes have an appearance similar to that of avian (heterophil) or mammalian (neutrophil) cells, hence the adoption of those terms in some cases. Analyzing the cellular ultrastructure with the use of an electron microscope and cytochemical staining can be done to help standardize the classification of teleost granulocytes. One study showed that koi, *Cyprinus carpio*, possessed neutrophils, eosinophils, and basophils, and confirmed the presence of lymphocytes and monocytes by using electron microscopy and cytochemical staining.[32] The same study suggested that cell identification might be more effectively accomplished by using more than 1 evaluation method. An example supporting this claim is with channel catfish, *Ictalurus punctatus*. One study[33] identified these fish as having neutrophils, basophils, lymphocytes, and monocytes using both electron microscopy and cytochemical staining while another[34] declared heterophils as the primary granulocyte, using electron microscopy only. In most cases of bony fish, the predominant leukocyte will have a similar appearance to the Romanowsky-stained avian or reptile heterophil, but may have the cytochemical properties of a mammalian neutrophil. From here on the primary teleost leukocyte is referred to as a neutrophil. Neutrophils are generally round with an eccentric nucleus. The basophilic nucleus can vary in shape: round, elongated, kidney-shaped, or segmented. The cytoplasm may be clear, light blue, or gray, and filled with colorless

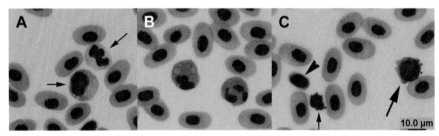

Fig. 8. Various blood cells from a white sturgeon (*Acipenser transmontanus*). All images show an abundance of red blood cells (not labeled). (*A*) Arrow on the left indicates a monocyte and arrow on the right indicates a neutrophil. (*B*) Two eosinophils. (*C*) Arrowhead indicates a thrombocyte, small arrow indicates a small lymphocyte, and large arrow indicates a large lymphocyte. Wright-Giemsa stain, 100×. (*Courtesy of* Terry Campbell, DVM, PhD, Fort Collins, CO.)

to slightly stained granules (**Fig. 8**A). Neutrophils play a primary role in the inflammatory process. In most species, neutrophils are involved with phagocytosis, but the time at which it occurs with respect to the initial insult and the duration varies among species.[35]

Eosinophils in bony fish are rare, but when seen are of similar size to slightly larger than the neutrophil, round with a round or lobed basophilic nucleus, and eosinophilic granules (see **Fig. 8**B). The cytoplasm is often a pale blue color. Eosinophils can be involved the defense against parasite infestation; however, fish that do not possess eosinophils rely on other cells to facilitate in this role.[35]

Basophils are also rare in teleosts but have been reported in some species.[18,35] Basophils are small, round cells with basophilic granules and nucleus. Many times the granules are so densely packed in the cytoplasm that the nucleus is difficult to see.

In elasmobranchs, the same apparent leukocytes exist; however, the discrepancy is not necessarily between whether a particular cell is a heterophil or neutrophil, but rather the term associated with that cell. Moreover, a single species may contain both types. The leukocytes of elasmobranchs have been determined to be G_1 (also referred to as type I, heterophil, and fine eosinophilic granulocyte or FEG), G_2 (also referred to as type II and neutrophil), and G_3 (also referred to as type III, eosinophil, and coarse eosinophilic granulocyte or CEG). It is likely species dependent, but these 3 cell types are similar in size.[30,36] The G_1 cell is usually round with an eccentric and round, indented, or segmented nucleus with fine eosinophilic granules (**Fig. 9**A). When evaluating the blood film of elasmobranchs, leukocytes that may have segmented or nonsegmented nuclei may contain both types, and should be recognized as the same cell. The G_2 cell is often round with an eccentric and round, indented, or segmented nucleus and indistinct granules. The granules and margin or the cell are often difficult to view and can be easily overlooked (see **Fig. 9**C). The G_3 cell is also typically round with a round nucleus and relatively large, round eosinophilic granules (see **Fig. 9**). This cell is often referred to as an eosinophil, but compared with bony fish is more commonly seen in elasmobranchs. Basophils may occasionally be found in the

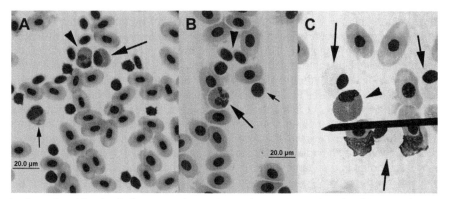

Fig. 9. Various blood cells from a southern stingray (*Dasyatis americana*). All images show an abundance of red blood cells in addition to several lymphocytes and thrombocytes (not labeled). (*A*) Large arrow indicates a G_1 (heterophil) cell, arrowhead indicates a G_3 (eosinophil) cell, and small arrow indicates a monocyte. (*B*) Large arrow indicates a segmented G_1 (heterophil) cell, small arrow indicates a lymphocyte, and arrowhead indicates 2 thrombocytes. (*C*) Large arrows indicate G_2 (neutrophils) cells; arrowhead indicates a G_1 (heterophil) cell. Wright-Giemsa stain, 100×.

peripheral blood of elasmobranchs, appearing as round cells with dark purple-stained granules. The amount of granules varies from sparse to obliterating the nucleus.

The lymphocytes and monocytes of teleosts and elasmobranchs are the most abundant cell type,[19,21,24] and have an appearance similar to that of lymphocytes of other vertebrates. Lymphocytes are occasionally described by size (small, medium, large), with the smaller cells being more mature and allowing the nucleus to occupy more cytoplasmic "real estate."[21] Combinations of different sizes may appear in one sample. Small lymphocytes are the most commonly seen in the peripheral blood of fish, being usually round with a high nucleus to cytoplasm ratio (see **Figs. 8C** and **9B**). The nucleus is round and contains dark basophilic chromatin. The cytoplasm is dark blue, occupying the occasional smooth but often irregular margins of the cell. This cell may also conform to the shape of the cells surrounding it.

Monocytes, as with other animals, are the largest leukocyte found in the peripheral blood of fish. Their shape varies from round to amoeba-like with a large, round to kidney-shaped basophilic nucleus. The cytoplasm is usually blue and may present with vacuoles (see **Figs. 8A** and **9A**). Fish monocytes also migrate into the tissue, where they are referred to as macrophages. The term macrophage is occasionally used to describe monocytes in fish because the appearance of the cell is similar to its stages during the migration into the tissue.[22]

Thrombocytes

Thrombocytes in fish are similar to mammalian platelets, and are important in the coagulation process and clot formation. Thrombocytes vary in shape among the species, but generally are round to elliptical and have a centrally positioned nucleus. The cytoplasm is usually clear but may have occasional, sparse, slightly eosinophilic granules, in which case they may be referred to as reactive. The cell margins are usually smooth, but cell clumping can also be seen (see **Figs. 8C** and **9B**).

Complete Blood Count (Hemacytometer)

As previously mentioned, the preferred method for establishing the total WBC count is by a manual method. This relatively easy, inexpensive, and potentially valuable diagnostic process is underused in practice. The equipment needed is a microscope, hemacytometer, counter, and the Natt-Herricks kit (the Natt-Herricks solution is used in fish because of their abundance of lymphocytes). To determine the total WBC count, the steps for determining the RBC count through step 5 listed earlier are followed, except that advancement to the 40× objective may not be necessary. Next, all the leukocytes with or without the thrombocytes in all 9 large squares of the grid in both chambers are counted (see **Fig. 7**). If the difference between counts in both chambers is greater than 10%, the process should be repeated. It is challenging to discern the thrombocytes from leukocytes; therefore, including them can be adjusted for in the calculation after the differential is performed. If only the leukocytes are counted, a total WBC count can be immediately calculated using the equation: WBC count/mm^3 (or μL) = (total count in 9 squares + 10%) × 200.[16] If the thrombocytes are included in the count, the thrombocytes are counted independent of the leukocytes during the differential while still counting until reaching 200 leukocytes. The percentage that is made up by the thrombocytes is then subtracted from the hemacytometer count.[19] The reference intervals for fish leukocytes varies, and normal variations from those respective intervals may occur based on species, season (water temperature), age, sex, diet, or stress. Reference intervals for select teleosts and elasmobranchs are shown in **Tables 3** and **4**. Because the basophil counts are low for both types of fish, they are not included in the tables.

Blood Smear and Differential

A blood smear can provide a wealth of information; therefore, even if only a drop of blood is collected, it should not go to waste. The blood smear is evaluated after processing the slide through any Romanowsky stain, which helps to visualize and identify different cell types. Viewing the slide at low power initially can subjectively offer an idea of cell type distribution, which is especially useful information if insufficient blood has been collected for a complete blood count. At higher power, the cells can be evaluated more closely. Owing to the diversity of fish and, consequently, their cells, it is recommended to scan over the slide initially to see which cells are present and to check the quality of the smear. Once a comfort level is established among cell types, the differential can be more effectively performed. Each cell is counted individually until a total leukocyte count of 200 is reached. The percentage of each cell type is used to calculate the absolute number using the total leukocyte count obtained from the hemacytometer.

Morphologic evaluation of the cells and identifying any inclusions, toxicity, polychromasia (noted by the presence of immature cells), pathogens, or artifacts should also be performed when viewing the blood smear. Toxic changes to neutrophils or heterophils appear during systemic illness and may aid with prognosis (**Fig. 10**). The degree of toxicity should be noted, because the greater the number of toxic cells present, the poorer the prognosis.[22] Intracellular or extracellular parasites may be present. For example, apicomplexan hemoparasites may be seen in the cytoplasm of RBCs (**Fig. 11**).[46,49] Depending on the history of the animal's health and the environmental conditions, some parasites may be incidental findings or contribute to alterations in cell counts (anemia, eosinophilia). Viral diseases represent another disorder that may alter the cell morphology whereby a blood smear evaluation would contribute to the diagnosis. Several diseases have been reported in which intracellular inclusions have been observed, such as viral erythrocytic necrosis, erythrocytic inclusion body syndrome, and intraerythrocytic viral disease.[49] The quality of the blood smear preparation or anticoagulant may negatively affect the cells. Often in an aquatic environment, humidity or water contamination can affect the preparation or the cell architecture. Certain anticoagulants may also affect the cells. For example, Na_2EDTA has been reported as inducing RBC swelling, anisocytosis, anisonucleosis, and hemolysis.[20]

Interpretation of Results

Although there is a growing database of reference intervals and information regarding cellular ultrastructure and chemistry, interpreting the results can be difficult. Some strategies to overcome this challenge may be to extrapolate from a similar species with known information, collect a sample from a tank mate of the same species to use as a control, extrapolate from general knowledge, or plan on collecting sequential samples to analyze the trend in a particular fish. **Tables 3** and **4** provide a summary of publications with established reference intervals for particular species. There are also publications that provide extensive tables with reference values.[19,31] Regardless, the interpretation is difficult because the functionality of many cell types is still uncertain.

Table 5 summarizes reports of intrinsic and extrinsic factors that affect hematologic parameters, and the direction (increased or decreased) in which they were affected. Many of the disease conditions affecting PCV that cause anemia have been described,[25] and therefore are not repeated here. In cases of anemia, fish are treated similarly to other animals. Blood transfusion is an option that has been reported on occasion. Elasmobranchs of the same species had no reaction to transfusion,[66] and

Table 3
Reference intervals for erythrocyte parameters of select teleosts and elasmobranchs

	PCV (%)	RBC (×10⁶/μL)	Hb (g/dL)	MCV (fL)	MCH (pg)	MCHC (g/dL)
Teleosts						
Acipenser brevirostrum Shortnose sturgeon[37]	26–46	0.65–1.09	5.7–8.7	307–520	65.9–107.1	15–30
Acipenser fulvescens Wild Lake Sturgeon[38]	17–38	—	—	—	—	—
Carassius auratus Goldfish[18]	21.3–23.3	0.8–2.4	6.45–6.95	134.4–139.6	40.6–43.4	0.3
Cichlasoma dimerus South American cichlid[39]	22.5–39.12	1.68–4.27	5.23–8.33	70.14–198	14.51–40.59	17.43–30.31
Colossoma brachypomum Red pacu[40]	20–32	0.98–2.95	—	—	—	—
Cyprinus carpio Common koi carp[18,32]	31.9–34.9	1.59–1.75	7.84–8.56	196.5–207.5	49.1	0.24
Ictalurus punctatus Farmed channel catfish[41]	27–54	1.5–4.1	4.4–10.9	88.6–186.7	—	15.7–28.7
Lutjanus guttatus Spotted rose snapper[42]	33.53–71.14	0.75–3.71	7.29–17.03	135.66–369.80	20.1–91.47	11.16–31.09
Oreochromis hybrid Tilapia[43]	27–37	1.91–2.83	7.0–9.8	115–183	28.3–42.3	22–29
Pterois volitans Red lion fish[44]	27–44	—	—	—	—	—
Elasmobranchs						
Alopias vulpinus Common thresher[45]	28.5–46.4	—	11.2–16.1	—	—	34.3–39.3
Carcharhinus obscurus Dusky shark[45]	9.4–25	—	3.1–8.7	—	—	32.4–38

Carcharhinus plumbeus Sandbar shark[36,45]	9.4–24	—	3.2–8.4	—	25.7–41.2
Carcharodon carcharias Great white shark[45]	22–49	—	8.2–16.2	—	31.2–43.1
Dasyatis americana Captive southern stingrays[46]	21–36	—	—	—	—
Galeocerdo cuvieri Tiger shark[45]	9.4–33	—	3.2–10.1	—	27.9–40
Isurus oxyrinchus Atlantic shortfin mako[45]	22.5–60	—	9.6–21.1	—	33.1–41.1
Mustelus canis Smooth dogfish[47]	20.1–28.3 (F) 27.3–32.1 (M)	—	—	—	—
Prionace glauca Blue shark[45]	9.4–22.5	—	3.1–7.6	—	27.9–40.4
Rhinoptera bonasus Captive cownose stingray[47]	27–35	0.38–0.64	—	—	—
Rhizoprionodon terraenovae Atlantic sharpnose[48]	18.9–30.8	—	—	—	—
Squalus acanthias Spiny dogfish[48]	15–22.8	—	—	—	—
Sphyrna lewini Scalloped hammerhead shark[45]	26.5	—	10	—	37.7
Sphyrna tiburo Bonnethead shark[48]	22–35	—	—	—	—

Hrubec and Smith[19] provide a list of additional teleosts, and Filho et al[31] provide a comparative study of 80 different marine teleosts and elasmobranchs.
Abbreviations: F, female; M, male.

Table 4
Reference intervals for leukocyte parameters of select teleosts and elasmobranchs

	WBC ($\times10^3/\mu$L)	Heterophil ($\times10^3/\mu$L)	Neutrophil ($\times10^3/\mu$L)	Eosinophil ($\times10^3/\mu$L)	Lymphocyte ($\times10^3/\mu$L)	Monocytes ($\times10^3/\mu$L)
Teleosts						
Acipenser brevirostrum Shortnose sturgeon[37]	28.4–90.8	—	3.8–33.6	0–1.5	9.1–56.7 (sm) 2.1–10.4 (lg)	0–7.1
Acipenser fulvescens Wild lake sturgeon[38]	2.7–23.2	—	0.2–6.1	0–0.6	1.4–14.0	0.1–1.7
Carassius auratus Goldfish[18]	47.4–57.2	—	1.74–2.86	0.0–0.2	23.1–29.6	0.1–0.3
Cichlasoma dimerus South American cichlid[39]	6.64–18.59	1.87–5.24	—	1.02–2.85	2.55–7.14	1.19–3.34
Colossoma brachypomum Red pacu[40]	13.5–57.5	0.2–19.1	—	0.13–0.3	7.8–35.9	0.38–0.518
Cyprinus carpio Common koi carp[18,32]	34.9–40.7*	—	3%–10%	0.5%–1%	88%–93%	0.5%–2.0%
Lutjanus guttatus Spotted rose snapper[42]	25.19–111.22	—	0.19%–8.40%	0.64%–7.8%	82.58%–100%	0.55%–5.37%
Oreochromis hybrid Tilapia[43]	21.56–154.69	—	0.56–9.87	0.04–1.65	6.78–136.4 (sm) 2.85–30.8 (lg)	0.4–4.29
Pterois volitans Red lion fish[44]	2.0–8.2	13%–72%	—	—	7%–67%	16%–51%

Elasmobranchs						
Dasyatis americana Captive southern stingray[46]	3.8–27.9	1.0–8.9	0–0.9	0.1–3.1	1.1–30.1	0–1.0
Mustelus canis Smooth dogfish[47]	11.24–19.42 (F) 7.86–20.74 (M)	2.37–8.21 (F) 1.57–4.69 (M)	2.33–4.41 (F) 2.06–4.69 (M)	0.28–0.92 (F) 0.4–1.28 (M)	3.08–6.74 (F) 1.69–8.87 (M)	0.42–1.91 (F) 0.6–2.75 (M)
Rhincodon typus Captive whale shark[30]	5.09	2.01	0.05	0.33	2.37	0.32
Rhinoptera bonasus Captive cownose stingray[47]	0.17–1.98	0–72 (seg) 0–55 (non)	—	0–77 (seg) 0–83 (non)	0.14–1.88	0–26
Rhizoprionodon terraenovae Atlantic sharpnose[45]	34.6–119.6	5.7–26.8	0.0–2.6	2.2–22.7	10.4–47.4	0.0–6.5
Squalus acanthias Spiny dogfish[48]	21.4–55.9	2.0–11.2	1.3–18.2	1.1–11.4	7.6–23.4	0.41–3.3
Sphyrna tiburo Bonnethead shark[48]	35.3–83.1	4.7–19.1	6.7–8.5	0.34–12.1	10.4–37.5	0.47–4.6

Hrubec and Smith[19] provide a list of additional teleosts, and Filho et al[31] provide a comparative study of 80 different marine teleosts and elasmobranchs.
Abbreviations: F, female; lg, large; M, male; non, nonsegmented; seg, segmented; sm, small.

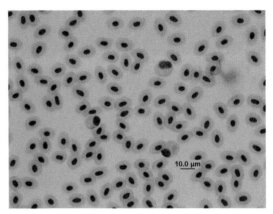

Fig. 10. An example of toxic neutrophils in a koi (*Cyprinus carpio*). Wright-Giemsa stain, 100×. (*Courtesy of* Terry Campbell, DVM, PhD, Fort Collins, CO.)

similar success has been documented in teleosts within the same taxonomic group[67]; however, cross-matching is recommended. Of course, similar conditions and diseases will also affect the other erythrocyte parameters. Hemoglobin is elevated in endothermic sharks in comparison with ectothermic sharks,[45] induced starvation,[53] and elasmobranchs in comparison with teleosts,[31] and is decreased in trout (*Oncorhynchus mykiss*) with viral hemorrhagic septicemia (VHS)[50] and in common carp (*C carpio*) with *Aeromonas* infection.[54] Similarly, the RBC indices also increased with induced starvation in traíra (*Hoplias malabaricus*)[53] and decreased with VHS in trout (*O mykiss*).[50]

The factors affecting leukocyte count are also represented in **Table 5**. In general, a stress leukogram is often defined as a relative leukocytosis with a lymphopenia. Elevated leukocytes as a result of a neutrophilia or heterophilia may also be associated with an inflammatory disease, although the actual function of such cells is unclear. Various disease processes have shown changes in total WBC count from low to high or high to low during different stages of the disease or severity of the insult. For example, channel catfish (*I punctatus*) showed a decrease in total WBC count when fed lower concentrations of *Fusarium moniliforme*, and increased counts

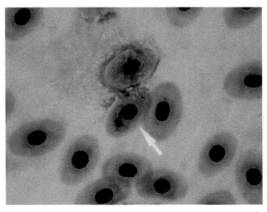

Fig. 11. *Light green arrow*: Hemogregarine parasite in the cytoplasm of a red blood cell in a southern stingray, *Dasyatis americana*. Diff Quik stain, 100×.

Table 5
Summary of some intrinsic and extrinsic factors that affect primary hematologic parameters

Parameter	Increased	Decreased
PCV	Stress: splenic contraction[16] Capture stress or inadequate anesthesia inducing RBC swelling[19] Male vs female smooth dogfish[51] Endothermic vs ectothermic sharks[45] Teleosts > sharks > rays[21,31] Increased activity level[21,31] Exposure to herbicide[56] Dactylogyrid monogenean infestation[42] Coccidiosis in carp[59]	Stress: increased water intake[16] VHS in trout[50] Younger fish[52] Starvation in traira[53] Dietary *Fusarium moniliforme*[54] Southern stingray in tourists sites (diet, parasites, crowding)[55] Sea louse infection in trout[57] *Aeromonas* infection in carp[58]
Hemoglobin	Endothermic vs ectothermic sharks[45] Induced starvation[53] Elasmobranchs vs teleosts[31]	VHS in trout[50] *Aeromonas* infection in carp[58]
RBC count	Coccidiosis in carp[59] Summer seasons in trout[60]	VHS in trout[50] Dietary *Fusarium moniliforme*[54] Sea louse infection in trout[57] *Aeromonas* infection in carp[58] Induced starvation[53]
MCV	Induced starvation[53]	VHS in trout[50]
MCHC	Induced starvation[53]	VHS in trout[50]
Total WBC count	Spring and summer seasons[61] Young fish[52] Stress[25] *Aeromonas hydrophila* injection[58] Higher concentrations of dietary *Fusarium moniliforme*[54] Dactylogyrid monogenean infestation[42] Exposure to herbicide[56] Zinc exposure[65] Traumatic clasper lesions[37]	Autumn and winter seasons[60] In low temperatures[62] Induced starvation[53] Stress (confinement, low water, chasing, netting)[63] Lower concentrations of dietary *Fusarium moniliforme*[54] Acute copper exposure[64]
Heterophils/ neutrophils	Day 8 coccidiosis infection[59] Female vs male[51] (FEG, CEG) Chronic copper exposure[64]	Initial (day 5) coccidiosis infection[59]
Eosinophils	Dactylogyrid monogenean infestation[60]	
Monocytes	Day 8 coccidiosis infection[59]	Initial (day 5) coccidiosis infection[59]
Lymphocytes	Initial (day 5) coccidiosis infection[59]	Day 8 coccidiosis infection[59] Stress[25] Sea louse infection in trout (stress or increased cortisol)[57] Chronic copper exposure[64]
Thrombocytes	Dactylogyrid monogenean infestation[42] Chronic copper exposure[64]	

Abbreviations: CEG, G$_3$ leukocytes (coarse eosinophilic granulocyte); FEG, G$_1$ leukocytes (fine eosinophilic granulocyte); VHS, viral hemorrhagic septicemia; WBC, white blood cells.

when fed high concentrations of the fungal toxins.[54] Another study showed an increase in leukocytes in common carp after 10 days of being infected with an *Aeromonas hydrophila* injection.[58] The leukocyte count continued to increase through the 30th day of the infected fish, whereas the leukocyte count of treated fish came down after the 10th day. Carp infected with a coccidian (*Goussia carpelli*) initially (by day 5) showed an increase in lymphocytes and a decrease in granulocytes and monocytes, but showed opposite results by day 8.[59] White-spotted bamboo sharks (*Chiloscyllium plagiosum*) with traumatic clasper lesions had increased total WBC counts as a result of heterophilia when compared with their tank mates without lesions (Carlson E. White-spotted bamboo sharks [*Chiloscyllium plagiosum*]: clasper removal and hematology findings. Unpublished data presented at the Regional Aquatics Workshop, 2012). As a potential treatment option, the claspers of the affected sharks were removed, and subsequently the WBC counts returned to their presumed normal range. There are many other documented disease processes that presumably affect WBC counts, some of which are presented in **Table 5**.

REFERENCES

1. Available at: https://www.flmnh.ufl.edu/fish/education/questions/questions.html. Accessed July 27, 2014.
2. Claver JA, Quaglia AI. Comparative morphology, development, and function of blood cells in nonmammalian vertebrates. Journal of Exotic Pet Medicine 2009; 18(2):87–97.
3. Available at: http://www.petplace.com/dogs/how-many-pets-are-in-the-us/page1.aspx. Accessed July 14, 2014.
4. Roberts HE. Physical examination of fish. In: Roberts HE, editor. Fundamentals of ornamental fish health. Ames (IA): John Wiley & Sons; 2010. p. 161–5.
5. Dyer SM, Cervasio EL. An overview of restraint and blood collection techniques in exotic pet practice. Vet Clin North Am Exot Anim Pract 2008;11(3):423–43.
6. Ross LG. Restraint, anaesthesia and euthanasia. In: Wildgoose WH, editor. BSAVA manual of ornamental fish. Gloucester (United Kingdom): British Small Animal Veterinary Association; 2001. p. 75–89.
7. Brooks EJ, Sloman KA, Liss S, et al. The stress physiology of extended duration tonic immobility in the juvenile lemon shark, *Negaprion brevirostris* (Poey 1868). J Exp Mar Bio Ecol 2011;409(1):351–60.
8. Henningsen AD. Tonic immobility in 12 elasmobranchs: use as an aid in captive husbandry. Zoo Biol 1994;13(4):325–32.
9. Watsky MA, Gruber SH. Induction and duration of tonic immobility in the lemon shark, *Negaprion brevirostris*. Fish Physiol Biochem 1990;8(3):207–10.
10. Stamper MA. Elasmobranchs (sharks, rays, and skates). In: West G, Heard D, Caulkett N, editors. Zoo animal and wildlife immobilization and anesthesia. Ames (IA): Blackwell Publishing; 2007. p. 197–203.
11. Carter KM, Woodley CM, Brown RS. A review of tricaine methanesulfonate for anesthesia of fish. Reviews in Fish Biology and Fisheries 2011;21(1):51–9.
12. Neiffer DL, Stamper MA. Fish sedation, anesthesia, analgesia, and euthanasia: considerations, methods, and types of drugs. ILAR J 2009;50(4):343–60.
13. Neiffer DL. Boney fish (lungfish, sturgeon, and teleosts). In: West G, Heard D, Caulkett N, editors. Zoo animal and wildlife immobilization and anesthesia. Ames (IA): Blackwell Publishing; 2007. p. 147–266.
14. Sneddon LU. Clinical anesthesia and analgesia in fish. Journal of Exotic Pet Medicine 2012;21(1):32–43.

15. Roberts HE. Anesthesia, analgesia, and euthanasia. In: Roberts HE, editor. Fundamentals of ornamental fish health. Ames (IA): John Wiley & Sons; 2010. p. 166–71.
16. Campbell TW, Ellis CK. Avian and exotic animal hematology and cytology. Ames (IA): John Wiley & Sons; 2007.
17. Roberts HE, Weber SE, Smith SA. Nonlethal diagnostic techniques. In: Roberts HE, editor. Fundamentals of ornamental fish health. Ames (IA): John Wiley & Sons; 2010. p. 172–84.
18. Groff JM, Zinkl JG. Hematology and clinical chemistry of cyprinid fish. Common carp and goldfish. Vet Clin North Am Exot Anim Pract 1999;2(3):741–76.
19. Hrubec TC, Smith SA. Hematology of fishes. In: Weiss DJ, Wardrop KJ, editors. Schalm's veterinary hematology. Ames (IA): John Wiley & Sons; 2010. p. 994–1003.
20. Walencik J, Witeska M. The effects of anticoagulants on hematological indices and blood cell morphology of common carp (*Cyprinus carpio* L.). Comp Biochem Physiol C Toxicol Pharmacol 2007;146(3):331–5.
21. Walsh CJ, Luer CA. Elasmobranch hematology. In: Warmolts D, Thoney D, Hueter R, editors. The elasmobranch husbandry manual: captive care of sharks, rays and their relatives. Columbus (OH): Ohio Biological Survey; 2004. p. 301–23.
22. Fánge R. Fish blood cells. Fish Physiol 1992;12:1–54.
23. Wingstrand KG. Nonnucleated erythrocytes in a teleostean fish *Maurolicus mülleri* (Gmelin). Z Zellforsch Mikrosk Anat 1956;45(2):195–200.
24. Campbell TW. Hematology of fish. In: Thrall MA, Weiser G, Allison R, et al, editors. Veterinary hematology and clinical chemistry. Ames (IA): John Wiley & Sons; 2012. p. 298–312.
25. Clauss TM, Dove AD, Arnold JE. Hematologic disorders of fish. Vet Clin North Am Exot Anim Pract 2008;11(3):445–62.
26. Available at: http://www.genomesize.com/cellsize/fish.htm. Accessed July 31, 2014.
27. Gregory TR. The bigger the C-value, the larger the cell: genome size and red blood cell size in vertebrates. Blood Cells Mol Dis 2001;27(5):830–43.
28. Maciak S, Janko K, Kotusz J, et al. Standard metabolic rate (SMR) is inversely related to erythrocyte and genome size in allopolyploid fish of the *Cobitis taenia* hybrid complex. Functional Ecology 2011;25(5):1072–8.
29. Mylniczenko ND, Curtis EW, Wilborn RE, et al. Differences in hematocrit of blood samples obtained from 2 venipuncture sites in sharks. Am J Vet Res 2006;67(11):1861–4.
30. Dove AD, Arnold J, Clauss TM. Blood cells and serum chemistry in the world's largest fish: the whale shark *Rhincodon typus*. Aquatic Biology 2010;9(2):177–83.
31. Filho DW, Eble GJ, Kassner G, et al. Comparative hematology in marine fish. Comp Biochem Physiol Comp Physiol 1992;102(2):311–21.
32. Tripathi NK, Latimer KS, Burnley VV. Hematologic reference intervals for koi (*Cyprinus carpio*), including blood cell morphology, cytochemistry, and ultrastructure. Vet Clin Pathol 2004;33(2):74–83.
33. Tavares-Dias M, Moraes FR. Leukocyte and thrombocyte reference values for channel catfish (*Ictalurus punctatus* Raf), with an assessment of morphologic, cytochemical, and ultrastructural features. Vet Clin Pathol 2007;36(1):49–54.
34. Cannon MS, Mollenhauer HH, Eurell TE, et al. An ultrastructural study of the leukocytes of the channel catfish, Ictalurus punctatus. J Morphol 1980;164(1):1–23.
35. Ainsworth AJ. Fish granulocytes: morphology, distribution, and function. Annual Review of Fish Diseases 1992;2:123–48.

36. Arnold JE. Hematology of the sandbar shark, *Carcharhinus plumbeus*: standardization of complete blood count techniques for elasmobranchs. Vet Clin Pathol 2005;34(2):115–23.

37. Knowles S, Hrubec TC, Smith SA, et al. Hematology and plasma chemistry reference intervals for cultured shortnose sturgeon (*Acipenser brevirostrum*). Vet Clin Pathol 2006;35(4):434–40.

38. DiVincenti L, Wyatt J, Priest H, et al. Reference intervals for select hematologic and plasma biochemical analytes of wild Lake Sturgeon (*Acipenser fulvescens*) from the St. Lawrence River in New York. Vet Clin Pathol 2013;42(1):19–26.

39. Rey Vázquez G, Guerrero GA. Characterization of blood cells and hematological parameters in *Cichlasoma dimerus* (Teleostei, Perciformes). Tissue Cell 2007; 39(3):151–60.

40. Tocidlowski ME, Lewbart GA, Stoskopf MK. Hematologic study of red pacu (*Colossoma brachypomum*). Vet Clin Pathol 1997;26(3):119–25.

41. Tavares-Dias M, Moraes FR. Haematological and biochemical reference intervals for farmed channel catfish. J Fish Biol 2007;71(2):383–8.

42. Del Rio-Zaragoza OB, Fajer-Ávila EJ, Almazán-Rueda P, et al. Hematological characteristics of the spotted rose snapper *Lutjanus guttatus* (Steindachner, 1869) healthy and naturally infected by dactylogyrid monogeneans. Tissue Cell 2011;43(3):137–42.

43. Hrubec TC, Cardinale JL, Smith SA. Hematology and plasma chemistry reference intervals for cultured tilapia (*Oreochromis hybrid*). Vet Clin Pathol 2000;29(1): 7–12.

44. Anderson ET, Stoskopf MK, Morris JA Jr, et al. Hematology, plasma biochemistry, and tissue enzyme activities of invasive red lionfish captured off North Carolina, USA. J Aquat Anim Health 2010;22(4):266–73.

45. Emery SH. Hematological comparisons of endothermic vs ectothermic elasmobranch fishes. Copeia 1986;1986(3):700–5.

46. Campbell TW, Grant KR. Clinical cases in avian & exotic animal hematology & cytology. Ames (IA): Wiley-Blackwell; 2010.

47. Ferreira CM, Field CL, Tuttle AD. Hematological and plasma biochemical parameters of aquarium-maintained cownose rays. J Aquat Anim Health 2010;22(2): 123–8.

48. Haman KH, Norton TM, Thomas AC, et al. Baseline health parameters and species comparisons among free-ranging Atlantic sharpnose (*Rhizoprionodon terraenovae*), bonnethead (*Sphyrna tiburo*), and spiny dogfish (*Squalus acanthias*) sharks in Georgia, Florida, and Washington, USA. J Wildl Dis 2012; 48(2):295–306.

49. Noga EJ. Fish disease: diagnosis and treatment. Ames (IA): John Wiley & Sons; 2010.

50. Rehulka J. Haematological analyses in rainbow trout *Oncorhynchus mykiss* affected by viral haemorrhagic septicaemia (VHS). Dis Aquat organ 2003; 56(3):185–93.

51. Persky ME, Williams JJ, Burks RE, et al. Hematologic, plasma biochemistry, and select nutrient values in captive smooth dogfish (*Mustelus canis*). J Zoo Wildl Med 2012;43(4):842–51.

52. Hrubec TC, Smith SA, Robertson JL. Age-related changes in hematology and plasma chemistry values of hybrid striped bass (*Morone chrysops* × *Morone saxatilis*). Vet Clin Pathol 2001;30(1):8–15.

53. Rios FS, Oba ET, Fernandes MN, et al. Erythrocyte senescence and haematological changes induced by starvation in the neotropical fish traíra, *Hoplias*

malabaricus (Characiformes, Erythrinidae). Comp Biochem Physiol A Mol Integr Physiol 2005;140(3):281–7.

54. Lumlertdacha S, Lovell RT, Shelby RA, et al. Growth, hematology, and histopathology of channel catfish, *Ictalurus punctatus*, fed toxins from *Fusarium moniliforme*. Aquaculture 1995;130(2):201–18.

55. Semeniuk CA, Bourgeon S, Smith SL, et al. Hematological differences between stingrays at tourist and nonvisited sites suggest physiologic costs of wildlife tourism. Biologic Conservation 2009;142(8):1818–29.

56. Modesto KA, Martinez CB. Effects of Roundup Transorb on fish: hematology, antioxidant defenses and acetylcholinesterase activity. Chemosphere 2010;81(6): 781–7.

57. Ruane NM, Nolan DT, Rotllant J, et al. Experimental exposure of rainbow trout *Oncorhynchus mykiss* (Walbaum) to the infective stages of the sea louse *Lepeophtheirus salmonis* (Krøyer) influences the physiologic response to an acute stressor. Fish Shellfish Immunol 2000;10(5):451–63.

58. Harikrishnan R, Nisha Rani M, Balasundaram C. Hematological and biochemical parameters in common carp, *Cyprinus carpio*, following herbal treatment of *Aeromonas hydrophila* infection. Aquaculture 2003;221(1):41–50.

59. Steinhagen D, Oesterreich B, Körting W. Carp coccidiosis: clinical and hematological observations of carp infected with *Goussia carpelli*. Dis Aquat organ 1997;30:137–43.

60. Morgan AL, Thompson KD, Auchinachie NA, et al. The effect of seasonality on normal haematological and innate immune parameters of rainbow trout *Oncorhynchus mykiss* L. Fish Shellfish Immunol 2008;25(6):791–9.

61. Houston AH, Dobric N, Kahurananga R. The nature of hematological response in fish. Fish Physiol Biochem 1996;15(4):339–47.

62. Sala-Rabanal M, Sánchez J, Ibarz A, et al. Effects of low temperatures and fasting on hematology and plasma composition of gilthead sea bream (*Sparus aurata*). Fish Physiol Biochem 2003;29(2):105–15.

63. Schreck CB, Contreras-Sanchez W, Fitzpatrick MS. Effects of stress on fish reproduction, gamete quality, and progeny. Aquaculture 2001;197(1):3–24.

64. Dick PT, Dixon DG. Changes in circulating blood cell levels of rainbow trout, *Salmo gairdneri* Richardson, following acute and chronic exposure to copper. J Fish Biol 1985;26(4):475–81.

65. Flos R, Tort L, Balasch J. Effects of zinc sulphate on haematological parameters in the dogfish, *Scyliorhinus canicula*, and influences of MS222. Mar Environ Res 1987;21(4):289–98.

66. Hadfield CA, Haines AN, Clayton LA, et al. Cross matching of blood in carcharhiniform, lamniform, and orectolobiform sharks. J Zoo Wildl Med 2010;41(3): 480–6.

67. Sakai DK, Okada H, Koide N, et al. Blood type compatibility of lower vertebrates: phylogenetic diversity in blood transfusion between fish species. Dev Comp Immunol 1988;11(1):105–15.

Evaluation of the Blood Film

Terry W. Campbell, MS, DVM, PhD

KEYWORDS

• Blood • Cells • Hematology • Mammal • Bird • Reptile • Amphibian • Fish

KEY POINTS

- A single drop of blood can provide valuable information in the assessment of the exotic animal patient by the examination of a properly prepared blood film.
- A blood film will reveal important erythrocyte abnormalities, such as changes in cell shape and color, presence of inclusions, and, in the case of lower vertebrates, changes in the position of the cell nucleus.
- A differential leukocyte count and detection of white blood cell abnormalities can be obtained from a stained blood film.
- Thrombocyte numbers and morphology are discerned from properly prepared blood films, in addition to mammalian platelets.
- A blood film can also reveal the presence of blood parasites and other infectious agents.

Evaluation of cell morphology in the stained blood film is an important part of hematology and the evaluation of the exotic animal patient. Often, the stained blood film is the only component of hematology available to the exotic animal veterinarian because of a small sample size. A single drop of blood can provide valuable information in the assessment of the patient.

A properly prepared blood film should not extend to the edges of the slide and will have a thick body that tapers into a feathered edge (**Fig. 1**). The best cell morphology lies just behind the feathered edge in the monolayer area. It is difficult to examine cells in the thick part of the blood film because they superimpose on each other, and the leukocytes appear rounded and not able to expand and flatten out (making them all resemble lymphocytes). Examination of cells in the feathered-edge area will reveal artifacts such as ruptured cells and, in the case of mammalian blood films, lack of erythrocyte central pallor.

A blood film made from a drop of non-anticoagulated blood placed on a slide immediately after collection is preferred over a blood sample exposed to an anticoagulant.

This article originally appeared in Veterinary Clinics of North America: Exotic Animal Practice, Volume 18, Issue 1, January 2015.

Department of Clinical Sciences, College of Veterinary Medicine and Biomedical Sciences, Colorado State University, 300 West Drake Road, Fort Collins, CO 80523, USA

E-mail address: Terry.Campbell@colostate.edu

Clin Lab Med 35 (2015) 703–721
http://dx.doi.org/10.1016/j.cll.2015.05.016
0272-2712/15/$ – see front matter © 2015 Elsevier Inc. All rights reserved.

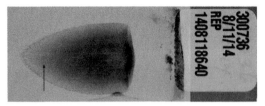

Fig. 1. Blood film with a thick body tapering to a feathered edge from a lizard (*Pogona vitticeps*) stained with Wright-Giemsa stain. The best cell morphology lies just behind the feathered edge in the monolayer area (*arrow*).

Anticoagulants, such as heparin and citrate, may affect the staining quality of the blood film. The anticoagulant EDTA (ethylenediaminetetraacetic acid) may cause hemolysis or cause the blood to clot in some species, such as birds in the crow family (corvids) or cartilaginous fish (elasmobranchs), rendering the sample useless. Once the film has been prepared, it should be dried immediately. In most settings, this is accomplished by waving the slide in the air; however, in high humidity the use of a commercially available slide warmer or a hair dryer set on a low (warm) setting held in front of the slide may be needed to properly dry the slide to prevent drying artifacts, such as excessive crenation of the red blood cells. Blood slides should be labeled with the animal identification information and the date. Romanowsky stains, such as Wright or Wright-Giemsa, are commonly used for the evaluation of hemic cytology.

At low magnification (using a 10× or 20× objective), an experienced cytologist can subjectively estimate the leukocyte concentration on a blood film as being low (leukopenia), normal, or high (leukocytosis) before examination of the cells using the 100× (oil-immersion) objective (**Fig. 2**). Several formulas for estimating the total leukocyte and thrombocyte concentrations from a blood film have been proposed; however, none are accurate or precise and should not be used in reporting leukocyte and thrombocyte numbers. The morphology of the 3 major cell types (erythrocytes, leukocytes, and platelets or thrombocytes) is best evaluated at higher magnifications.

A differential leukocyte count is obtained by counting a minimum of 100 consecutively encountered white blood cells in the monolayer area of the blood film. For most species, the cells are classified as neutrophils or heterophils (depending on species), eosinophils, basophils, lymphocytes, and monocytes, to obtain a relative percentage for each leukocyte type. Cells not readily identified can be placed into a sixth category of "other." Abnormalities in leukocyte morphologies are noted.

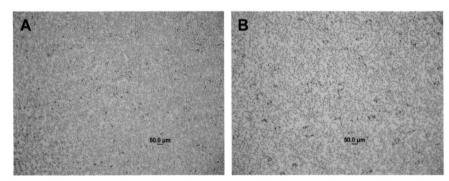

Fig. 2. (*A*) Leukocytosis in the blood film of a ferret (*Mustela putorius furo*) (Wright-Giemsa stain). (*B*) Leukocytosis in the blood film of a turtle (*Graptemys versa*) (Wright-Giemsa stain).

Evaluation of erythrocyte morphology is also made using high magnification. Important erythrocyte abnormalities include changes in cell shape, color changes, presence of inclusions, and, in the case of lower vertebrates, changes in the position of the cell nucleus.

Thrombocytes and mammalian platelets are evaluated under high magnification. Their numbers can be estimated as being adequate, low (thrombocytopenia), or high (thrombocytosis). In mammalian blood films, an average of 8 to 12 platelets per oil-immersion monolayer field is considered to be adequate. In lower vertebrates, such as birds and reptiles, an average of 1 to 2 thrombocytes per oil-immersion monolayer field is considered to be adequate, as these cells are larger than mammalian platelets. Lower numbers may indicate a true thrombocytopenia or excessive platelet clumping; the latter of which can be identified in the feathered-edge portion of the blood film. Evaluation of platelet morphology is made with special attention to size.

ERYTHROCYTES

Romanowsky-stained erythrocytes in mammalian blood films are anucleated, round (except those from camelids), biconcave discs that stain pink and often have a central area of pallor. As mammalian erythrocytes develop, there is an increase in hemoglobin synthesis, and during the final stages of maturation the nucleus undergoes degeneration and is extruded from the cells along with the organelles involved in metabolism. Reticulocytes are young erythrocytes in their final stage of maturation that have lost the nucleus, but have yet to lose ribosomes and mitochondria. When stained with new methylene blue or brilliant cresyl blue, these residual organelles aggregate into clumps of granular material referred to as reticulum, thus giving the cell the name reticulocyte. Reticulocytes in Wright-stained blood films appear blue and are called polychromatic cells.

Polychromatic cells in mammalian blood films are larger than mature erythrocytes and have a blue to reddish-blue cytoplasm. These cells may lack the classic discoid shape of mature red blood cell and have membranous folds.

The mean erythrocyte diameter of many small mammals ranges between 5 and 7 μm. The erythrocytes of small mammals, such as true rodents (ie, rats, *Rattus norvegicus*; mice, *Mus musculus*; gerbils, *Meriones unguiculatus*; and hamsters, *Mesocricetus auratus*) have a relatively short half-life (45–68 days) compared with larger mammals, such as dogs (100–115 days) and cats (73 days); as a result, their blood comparatively has a higher concentration of reticulocytes, so the presence of a greater degree of polychromasia and anisocytosis on the blood film is expected.[1–3] In general, 1% to 5% reticulocytes are expected in adult nonanemic rodents. On the opposite end of the spectrum, horses (with an erythrocyte life span of 140–145 days) do not release reticulocytes.

Diagnostically, the important morphologic characteristics of mammalian erythrocytes include polychromatic, hypochromatic, microcytic, and macrocytic erythrocytes; poikilocytosis; and red blood cell inclusions. Knowing the packed cell volume is important in the detection of anemia, and evaluation of the blood film will aid in the determination of a regenerative or nonregenerative anemia. Polychromatic erythrocytes (reticulocytes) are young erythrocytes that have been released into circulation early, and therefore are larger and more basophilic in color compared with mature erythrocytes (**Fig. 3**). The degree of polychromasia (total number of polychromatic erythrocytes) will aid in the determination of the cause of an anemia. For example, an increase in polychromatic erythrocytes occurs with blood loss and blood-destruction anemias, whereas a decrease or lack of polychromasia is observed in anemias caused by erythroid hypoplasia or in an aplastic anemia.

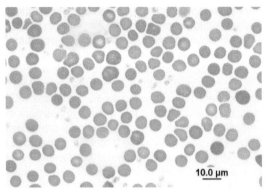

Fig. 3. Polychromatic erythrocytes (*blue-staining cells*) in the blood film of a domestic rat (*Rattus norvegicus*) (Wright-Giemsa stain).

Hypochromasia in the mammalian blood film is indicated by pale-staining erythrocytes with an increased area of central pallor. Hypochromatic erythrocytes indicate a state of iron deficiency. Iron deficiency in adult mammals is generally the result of chronic blood loss caused by bloodsucking parasites, gastrointestinal ulcers, inflammatory bowel disease, or neoplasms. Iron-deficiency anemia in very young mammals is due to inadequate dietary iron.

Electronic methods are better at determining the size of erythrocytes than are human eyes; however, when one has only a blood film to evaluate, the presence of large (macrocytic) and small (microcytic) red blood cells or anisocytosis may be apparent. Microcytic erythrocytes occur most commonly with iron-deficiency anemia or in iron-metabolism disorders. The most common cause of an increased number of macrocytic erythrocytes is an increase in polychromatic erythrocytes.

Poikilocytosis refers to an increased number of abnormally shaped erythrocytes. The important changes in the shape of mammalian erythrocytes include spiculated red blood cells and spherocytes. Fragmented red blood cells or schistocytes are spiculated cells caused by shearing forces during intravascular trauma, such as those caused by fibrin strands formed with disseminated intravascular coagulopathy or hemangiosarcoma, or from oxidative damage from iron-deficiency anemia. Keratocytes are iron-deficient red blood cells with 2 or more spicules that form during oxidative injury. Schistocytes form when the spicules fragment from the keratocytes.

Acanthocytes are spiculated mammalian erythrocytes that result from lipid metabolism changes in the cell membrane. Acanthocytes (also known as spur cells) possess unevenly distributed irregular spicules of variable lengths and diameters. Echinocytes or burr cells resemble acanthocytes, but have numerous short, evenly spaced spicules that are uniform in size and shape. Echinocytes are often artifacts and are a sign of crenation (a result of slow drying of blood films); however, they may also be seen with pathologic conditions such as renal disease, lymphoma, and rattlesnake envenomation.

Spherocytes appear as small, dark-staining erythrocytes that lack a central pallor. Spherocytes are more easily detected in species such as members of the family Canidae that have larger erythrocytes and prominent central pallor. Spherocytes are suggestive of immune-mediated hemolytic anemia.

Important structures in or on mammalian erythrocytes include Heinz bodies, basophilic stippling, nucleated erythrocytes, and Howell-Jolly bodies. Heinz bodies are small, eccentric, single to multiple pale structures that often protrude slightly from the red cell margins. Heinz bodies are caused by oxidative denaturation of hemoglobin, and can be associated with certain plant chemicals (onions and garlic), drugs (acetaminophen and propofol), and diseases such as lymphoma and hyperthyroidism. Basophilic stippling appears in the erythrocyte as small basophilic granules within the cytoplasm of the cell.

Basophilic stippling is commonly associated with erythrocyte regeneration, and is commonly found in blood films from healthy mammals such as gerbils. Basophilic stippling may also be associated with nonanemic animals with lead poisoning, but this is generally a rare finding.

Nucleated erythrocytes are immature red blood cells sometimes found in mammalian blood films (**Fig. 4**). These cells are released at an early stage of maturation from the bone marrow, usually as part of a regenerative response to anemia or hypoxia. An inappropriate release of nucleated erythrocytes may be seen with lead poisoning or a myelodysplastic condition.

Howell-Jolly bodies are small, variably sized, round, dark-blue inclusions present in the cytoplasm of the erythrocyte (**Fig. 5**). These inclusions represent nuclear remnants that occur as part of a regenerative response, or may indicate suppressed splenic function. Howell-Jolly bodies are found in low numbers of red cells in the blood films of normal mice and rats.

Other abnormalities such as Rouleaux formation and red blood cell agglutination should also be reported. Rouleaux formation appears as linear stacking of erythrocytes, and is often associated with increased plasma proteins, such as immunoglobulins, in domestic mammals. Rouleaux formation is uncommon in some mammals, such as rats and mice, with inflammatory disease. Erythrocyte agglutination may be identified by the irregular to circular clumping of erythrocytes, and is associated with immune-mediated hemolytic anemia.

Erythrocytes of lower vertebrates, such as birds, reptiles, amphibians, and fish, should be evaluated based on size, shape, color, nuclear morphology, and position, in addition to the presence of cellular inclusions. In general, the mature erythrocytes of these animals are elliptical and have an elliptical, centrally positioned nucleus. The immature erythrocytes begin as nucleated spheres that turn into flattened ellipsoids during the final stages of maturation. Unlike mammalian erythrocytes, erythrocytes of lower vertebrates retain their nuclei where the nuclear chromatin is uniformly clumped, and becomes increasingly condensed with age. In Wright-stained

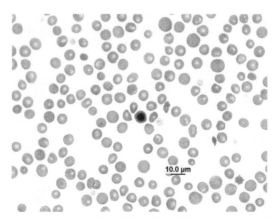

Fig. 4. Nucleated erythrocyte in the blood film of an African hedgehog (*Atelerix albiventris*) (Wright-Giemsa stain).

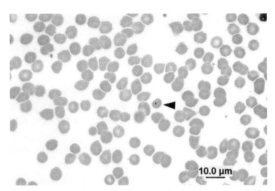

Fig. 5. A Howell-Jolly body (*arrowhead*) in the blood film of a ferret (*Mustela putorius furo*) (Wright-Giemsa stain).

blood films the nucleus stains purple, whereas the cytoplasm stains orange-pink with a uniform texture (**Fig. 6**).

Knowledge of avian hemic cytology in the blood film can serve as a model for evaluating the blood film from other lower vertebrate species. In most species of birds, erythrocyte shape is relatively uniform; however, the shape of the red blood cells from other lower vertebrates may be somewhat variable. Erythrocytes of reptiles are blunt-ended ellipsoidal cells with permanent, centrally positioned, oval to round nuclei containing dense purple chromatin. The erythrocytes of amphibians are large compared with those of other vertebrates, with sizes that vary from 10 to 70 μm in diameter. Most amphibian erythrocytes are nucleated and elliptical in shape, have a distinct nuclear bulge, and often have irregular nuclear margins. The erythrocytes of teleost fishes are similar in appearance to those of birds and reptiles (**Fig. 7**). The mature erythrocytes of elasmobranch fishes are also similar in appearance to avian and reptilian erythrocytes, but are much larger. Mature erythrocytes of some fish are biconvex with a central swelling that corresponds to the position of the nucleus, whereas other species have flattened biconcave erythrocytes.[4] The nuclei of fish erythrocytes can be large, and may occupy as much as one-fourth the cell volume or greater. The long axis of the nucleus is parallel to the long axis of the cell, except in a few species of fish that have round erythrocyte nuclei.

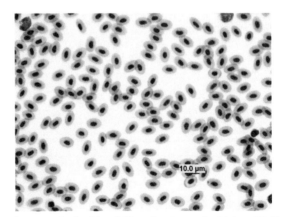

Fig. 6. Normal erythrocytes in the blood film of a domestic chicken (*Gallus gallus domesticus*) (Wright-Giemsa stain).

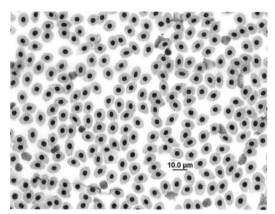

Fig. 7. Normal erythrocytes in the blood film of a fish (*Erimonax monachus*) (Wright-Giemsa stain).

Atypical erythrocytes may vary in both size and shape, and semiquantitative estimates of these changes can be made from evaluation of monolayer areas of the blood film (**Table 1**). The presence of macrocytes or microcytes should be noted during assessment of the blood film. The degree of variation in the size of erythrocytes (anisocytosis) can be scored from 1+ to 4+, based on the number of variably sized erythrocytes in a monolayer field (see **Table 1**).[5] Erythrocyte subpopulations have been reported in some species of birds (eg, ducks), in which larger erythrocytes most likely represent those most recently released from the hematopoietic tissue and smaller cells most likely represent the older, aging cells.[6] A slight variation in the size of erythrocytes (1+ anisocytosis) is considered normal for birds. A greater degree of anisocytosis, however, usually is observed in birds with a regenerative anemia, and is associated with polychromasia. Microcytic, hypochromic, nonregenerative anemia is often associated with chronic inflammatory diseases in birds, especially those with an infectious etiology.[7]

Minor deviations from the normal shape of avian erythrocytes (1+ poikilocytosis) are considered to be normal in the peripheral blood of birds, but marked poikilocytosis may indicate erythrocytic dysgenesis. For example, round erythrocytes with oval nuclei occasionally are found in the blood films of anemic birds and suggest a dysmaturation of the cell cytoplasm and nucleus, which may be a result of accelerated erythropoiesis.

Table 1
Semiquantitative microscopic evaluation of avian erythrocyte morphology[a]

	1+	2+	3+	4+
Anisocytosis	5–10	11–20	21–30	>30
Polychromasia	2–10	11–14	15–30	>30
Hypochromasia	1–2	3–5	6–10	>10
Poikilocytosis	5–10	11–20	21–50	>50
Erythroplastids	1–2	3–5	6–10	>10

[a] Based on the average number of abnormal cells per 1000× monolayer field.
Data from Campbell TW, Ellis CK. Avian and exotic animal hematology and cytology. 3rd edition. Ames (IA): Blackwell Publishing Ltd; 2007.

Variations in erythrocyte color include polychromasia and hypochromasia. Polychromatophilic erythrocytes are similar in size to mature erythrocytes and appear as reticulocytes when stained with vital stains, such as new methylene blue. The cytoplasm appears weakly basophilic, and the nucleus is less condensed than the nucleus of mature erythrocytes (**Fig. 8**). Polychromatophilic erythrocytes occur in low numbers (usually <5% of erythrocytes) in the peripheral blood of most normal birds. The degree of polychromasia can be graded according to the guideline presented in **Table 1**. Hypochromatic erythrocytes are abnormally pale in color compared with mature erythrocytes, and have an area of cytoplasmic pallor that is greater than half the cytoplasmic volume. These erythrocytes also may have cytoplasmic vacuoles and round, pyknotic nuclei. The degree of hypochromasia can be estimated using the scale presented in **Table 1**. The presence of many hypochromatic erythrocytes (ie, 2+ hypochromasia or greater) indicates an erythrocyte disorder such as iron deficiency.

The nucleus may vary in its location within the erythrocyte, and may contain indentions, protrusions, or constrictions. Micronuclei and nuclear budding are potential indices of environmental genotoxic exposure.[8,9] Chromophobic streaking suggestive of chromatolysis or achromic bands indicating nuclear fracture with displacement of the fragments may also be present.[10] Mitotic activity is occasionally noted in blood films, and is suggestive of a marked regenerative response or erythrocytic dyscrasia. Binucleate erythrocytes, when present in large numbers along with other features of red blood cell dyscrasia, are suggestive of neoplastic, viral, or genetic disease.[11] Anucleated erythrocytes (erythroplastids) or the presence of cytoplasmic fragments are occasionally noted in normal avian blood films.

LEUKOCYTES

The granulocytes of nondomestic mammals vary in appearance but can be classified as neutrophils or heterophils, eosinophils, and basophils.[12,13] Neutrophils contain cytoplasmic granules that stain neutral with Romanowsky stains, such as Wright or Wright-Giemsa stain. The 2 types of neutrophil commonly found in normal blood samples of most exotic mammal species are segmented neutrophils and small numbers of band neutrophils. Band neutrophils are immature neutrophils, and contain a smooth nucleus that has parallel sides and no constrictions in the nuclear membrane. Segmented neutrophils develop from band neutrophils. Neutrophils contain numerous

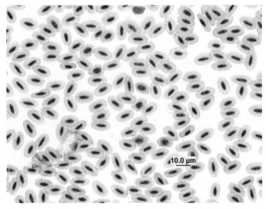

Fig. 8. Polychromasia (blue-staining erythrocytes) in the blood film of an eagle (*Aguila chrysaetos*) (Wright-Giemsa stain).

small granules that vary from colorless to pale-staining to dark-staining among different species of mammal. Neutrophils with a cytoplasm that typically stains diffusely pink with Romanowsky stains and contain variable numbers of larger eosinophilic granules are referred to as heterophils (**Fig. 9**). The granules of eosinophils become intensely eosinophilic with maturation as a result of the basic protein content with Wright or Wright-Giemsa staining. Mammalian basophils have characteristic cytoplasmic granules that are strongly basophilic in Romanowsky-stained blood films. In some species variation in the color of the granules occurs.

The avian heterophil is functionally equivalent to the mammalian neutrophil, and is the most abundant granulocyte of many species of birds. The nucleus (typically partially hidden by the cytoplasmic granules) of the mature heterophil is lobed (2–3 lobes), with coarse, clumped, purple-staining chromatin. The cytoplasm of normal mature heterophils appears colorless and contains granules that stain an eosinophilic color (dark orange to brown red) with Romanowsky stains (**Fig. 10**). Typically the cytoplasmic granules appear elongated (rod or spiculate shaped), but may also appear oval to round depending on the species.

Reptilian heterophils resemble those of birds, but are larger. These cells are typically round, with a colorless cytoplasm containing eosinophilic (bright orange), refractile, rod- to spindle-shaped cytoplasmic granules (**Fig. 11**). Occasionally degranulated heterophils can be found in the blood film of normal reptiles. The nucleus of the mature reptilian heterophil is typically eccentrically positioned in the cell, and is round to oval with densely clumped nuclear chromatin. However, some species of lizards have heterophils with lobed nuclei.

The nucleus of the avian eosinophil is lobed and usually stains darker than the nucleus of a heterophil, and the cytoplasm stains clear blue, in contrast to the colorless cytoplasm of normal mature heterophils (**Fig. 12**). The cytoplasmic granules are strongly eosinophilic in appearance and tend to stain more intensely in comparison with the granules of the heterophil on the same stained blood film. The granules are typically round in shape, although those of some avian species may be oval or elongated.

The eosinophils in most reptilian blood films are large round cells with light-blue cytoplasm, a round to oval (possibly lobed in some species of lizards), slightly eccentric nucleus, and large numbers of spherical eosinophilic cytoplasmic granules. The cytoplasmic granules of some reptilian species, such as *Iguana iguana*, stain blue with Romanowsky stains.

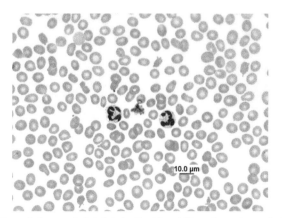

Fig. 9. Heterophils and clump of platelets in the blood film of a guinea pig (*Cavia porcellus*) (Wright-Giemsa stain).

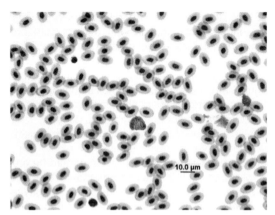

Fig. 10. Normal heterophil in the blood film of a domestic chicken (*Gallus gallus domesticus*) (Wright-Giemsa stain).

The basophils of birds and reptiles contain deeply metachromic granules that often obscure the nucleus. The nucleus is usually nonlobed, causing avian basophils to resemble mammalian mast cells (**Fig. 13**).

In general, amphibian granulocytes resemble those of mammals but are comparatively larger. Amphibian granulocytes are classified based on their appearance in blood smears stained with Wright-Giemsa and their resemblance to mammalian granulocytes; therefore, they have been classified as neutrophils, eosinophils, and basophils. Other classifications in the literature use heterophils instead of neutrophils.[12,14,15]

The term neutrophil has been frequently used to describe the predominant granulocyte of teleost fish, even if the granules in the cells do not stain neutral, because overall the cells resemble mammalian neutrophils when stained with Romanowsky stains. The cytoplasm of the mature piscine neutrophil is typically abundant and colorless, grayish, or slightly acidophilic in color, whereas the cytoplasm of immature neutrophils stains gray or blue-gray. Small granules may be present within the cytoplasm. Staining of the cytoplasmic granules is variable and depends on the species of fish or maturity

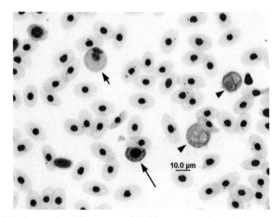

Fig. 11. Heterophils (*arrowheads*), eosinophil (*short arrow*), and basophil (*long arrow*) in the blood film of a turtle (*Trachemys scripta elegans*) (Wright-Giemsa stain).

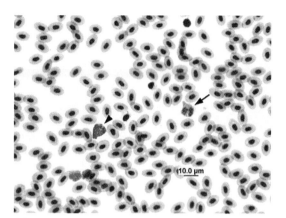

Fig. 12. An eosinophil (*arrow*) and normal heterophil (*arrowhead*) in the blood film of a domestic chicken (*Gallus gallus domesticus*) (Wright-Giemsa stain).

of the cell. The granules do not stain at all in most fish species, but may stain pale red, blue, or violet in others.[16] When present, eosinophils occur in low numbers that can be differentiated from neutrophils (or heterophils) by the presence of numerous round- to rod-shaped eosinophilic staining granules in a light-blue cytoplasm in films stained with Romanowsky stains. Basophils are rare in peripheral blood films of bony fish, and have been reported in only a few fish species.[17,18]

There is a considerable amount of confusion in the literature with regard to the naming of the various granulocytes found in the different species of elasmobranchs, partially because the granulocytes exhibit a marked variation in numbers and types between the species.[18–22] An attempt to standardize and simplify the nomenclature involving elasmobranch granulocytes has been offered using avian rather than mammalian terminology.[23] This system allows the granulocytes of elasmobranch fishes to be classified as heterophils, eosinophils, and basophils using the descriptive criteria for those cells in avian hematology. This scheme works well for some species; however, other elasmobranchs exhibit granulocytes that possess neutral-staining granules. These neutrophil-like granulocytes typically have an eccentric nonlobed

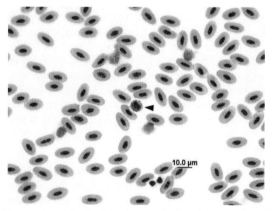

Fig. 13. A basophil (*arrowhead*) in the blood film of a hawk (*Buteo jamaicensis*) (Wright-Giemsa stain).

nucleus. It is not known whether these cells represent a fourth type of granulocyte or result from an artifact of the staining process.[23]

Monocytes are generally the largest leukocytes in peripheral blood films of animals, and do not vary grossly in appearance between species. The monocyte nucleus varies in shape (round or oval to lobed), and the moderately abundant cytoplasm is typically light blue-gray and may be vacuolated. The granules, when present, are very fine and appear azurophilic in Romanowsky-stained preparations.

The appearances of lymphocytes in the blood films of lower vertebrates resemble those of mammals. Their appearance may vary depending on the species, lymphocyte type, and degree of activation. Lymphocytes vary in size, color of cytoplasm (light to dark blue), and degree of nuclear chromatin condensation. Variability depends on the degree of antigenic stimulation and type of lymphocyte. The size of lymphocytes ranges from the size of an erythrocyte to the size a neutrophil or heterophil. The small lymphocytes are considered to be the inactive forms. Reactive lymphocytes have a slightly more abundant cytoplasm that stains basophilic, and nuclei that have clefts or are irregular in shape. These cells are considered to be B cells involved in immunoglobulin production.[24] Large lymphocytes that have an increased amount of light-blue cytoplasm and azurophilic granules that vary in size are considered to be T cells or natural killer cells.[25]

ACQUIRED CHANGES IN LEUKOCYTE MORPHOLOGY

In general, the leukocyte morphology is a reliable indication of disease. In mammalian blood films the presence of immature cells, toxic neutrophils or heterophils, and Döhle bodies are more reliable criteria for infectious diseases than are total leukocyte and differential counts. The same holds true for blood films of lower vertebrates. Immature heterophils of lower vertebrates have increased cytoplasmic basophilia, nonsegmented nuclei (in species that lobe the nucleus), and immature cytoplasmic granules in comparison with normal mature heterophils. Toxic changes are subjectively quantified according to the number of toxic cells and severity of toxicity present, as in mammalian hematology.[5] Toxic change in neutrophils/heterophils is a term referring to morphologic changes associated with inflammatory diseases that alter production of bone marrow in these types of cells. In response to the inflammatory disease, an acceleration of neutrophil/heterophil production occurs, resulting in the production and release of early-stage neutrophils/heterophils with retained organelles such as ribosomes. Retention of these organelles results in cytoplasmic basophilia and the presence of cytoplasmic vacuolation (**Fig. 14**). Döhle bodies may also be present. Döhle bodies are composed of aggregates of endoplasmic reticulum, and appear as gray-blue cytoplasmic inclusions.

In mammals and, presumably, lower vertebrates, eosinophils are particularly numerous in the peripheral blood when antigens are continually being released, as occurs in parasitic disease (especially those involving larvae of helminths) and allergic reactions (especially those associated with mast cell and basophil degranulation). In general, the presence of an eosinophilia is suggestive of one of these processes.

THROMBOCYTES AND PLATELETS

Mammalian platelets are cytoplasmic fragments (megakaryocytes) within the bone marrow, and participate in hemostasis. Platelets are flat discs of cytoplasm that contain cytoplasmic organelles; they tend to be round, but can vary slightly in shape and size. The anucleated cytoplasm contains variable amounts of small purple granules on Romanowsky-stained blood films. Because platelets are involved in

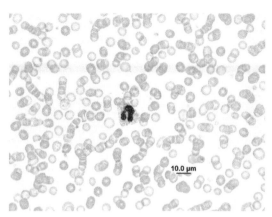

Fig. 14. A toxic heterophil in the blood film of a chinchilla (*Chinchilla lanigera*) (Wright-Giemsa stain).

the clotting process, they are often found in clumps on blood films. Mammalian platelets are much smaller than erythrocytes in the same blood film; therefore, the presence of platelets that are larger in size than erythrocytes (known as Shift platelets) indicate an accelerated thrombocytopoiesis, with early release of immature forms into the circulating blood and an indication of platelet regeneration in some species.

The thrombocyte is a nucleated cell that represents the second most numerous cell type (after erythrocytes) in blood films from lower vertebrates. Thrombocytes are typically small, round to oval cells (smaller than erythrocytes), with a round to oval nucleus that contains densely clumped chromatin. These cells tend to have a high nucleus-to-cytoplasm ratio. The appearance of the cytoplasm is an important feature used to differentiate thrombocytes from small, mature lymphocytes (**Fig. 15**). The cytoplasm of normal mature thrombocytes is colorless to pale gray, and may be reticulated in appearance compared with the homogeneously blue cytoplasm of the lymphocyte in the same Romanowsky-stained blood film. Thrombocytes frequently contain 1 or more distinct eosinophilic (specific) granules located in one area of the cytoplasm. Like mammalian platelets, thrombocytes are frequently found in clumps on the blood film.

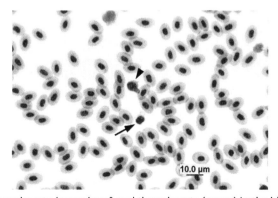

Fig. 15. A small lymphocyte (*arrowhead*) and thrombocyte (*arrow*) in the blood film of a domestic chicken (*Gallus gallus domesticus*) (Wright-Giemsa stain).

BLOOD PARASITES OF BIRDS

Parasites in the genera *Haemoproteus*, *Plasmodium*, and *Leukocytozoon*, and microfilaria of filarial nematodes are commonly found in avian blood films. Microfilarial nematodes are typically found between the cells. *Haemoproteus*, *Plasmodium*, and *Leukocytozoon* produce merozoites that invade erythrocytes, and their gametocytes are found within the erythrocyte. Most of the species of *Haemoproteus* and *Leukocytozoon* that infect birds are considered to be host specific. Many species of *Plasmodium* are capable of infecting a wide range of hosts.[26] Parasites of the genus *Plasmodium* can be pathogenic and are responsible for malaria. Certain species of birds, such as canaries, penguins, ducks, pigeons, raptors, and domestic poultry, are highly susceptible to avian malaria, whereas other species of birds seem to be asymptomatic carriers of the parasite and do not develop the clinical disease.[27]

In general, the presence of most blood parasites in wild birds has no effect on the health of the bird, although combined infections with *Haemoproteus* and *Leukocytozoon* can produce a fatal anemia.[28,29] Birds may be infected with a single blood parasite, or may have mixed infections based on examination of stained blood films.

Haemoproteus only appears in the peripheral blood of birds in the gametocyte stage. The appearance of the gametocyte is variable, and may range from small developing ring forms to the elongate crescent-shaped mature gametocytes that partially encircle the erythrocyte nucleus to form the characteristic halter shape (**Fig. 16**).[30] Mature gametocytes typically occupy greater than one-half of the cytoplasmic volume of the host erythrocyte and cause minimal displacement of the host cell nucleus: the nucleus is never pushed to the cell margin. *Haemoproteus* gametocytes contain refractile, yellow to brown to black pigment granules representing iron pigment deposited as a result of hemoglobin utilization. Erythrocytes parasitized by *Haemoproteus* are larger than normal erythrocytes, which likely causes the cells to become fragile.

Key features used to differentiate *Plasmodium* from *Haemoproteus* are the presence of schizogony in the peripheral blood, parasite stages within thrombocytes and leukocytes, and gametocytes (which also contain refractile pigment granules) that cause marked displacement of the erythrocyte nucleus. Identification of the *Plasmodium* species depends on the location and appearance of the schizonts, the number of merozoites present within the schizonts, and gametocytes.[30]

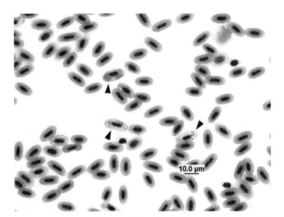

Fig. 16. *Haemoproteus* gametocytes (*arrowheads*) in the red blood cells of a bird (*Colaptes auratus*) (Wright-Giemsa stain).

Leukocytozoon only appears in the peripheral blood of birds in the gametocyte stage that grossly distorts the host cell (presumed to be an immature erythrocyte). The macrogametocyte appears as a parasite inclusion that occupies 77% of the area of the host cell–parasite complex (**Fig. 17**).[31] Microgametocytes are similar in morphology, but are usually 5% to 10% smaller.[31] The remainder of the life cycle occurs in the insect vector following ingestion of blood containing the gametes.[32]

Aegyptianella is a piroplasm that can affect several species of birds, usually those originating in tropical or subtropical climates. *Aegyptianella* appears as a minute parasite lacking pigment granules located within erythrocytes in blood films. Three forms can occur within the erythrocyte[30]: a small (<1 μm), round, basophilic intracytoplasmic, anaplasma-like inclusion; a *Babesia*-like round to piriform-shaped inclusion with pale blue cytoplasm and chromatin body at one pole; and a larger (2–4 μm) round to elliptical inclusion.

Atoxoplasma is a coccidian parasite often found in passerine birds. Atoxoplasmosis is identified by the presence of the characteristic sporozoites within lymphocytes in peripheral blood films. Affected lymphocytes contain small (3–5 μm), pale, round to oval eosinophilic intracytoplasmic inclusions or sporozoites that indent the host cell nucleus, resulting in a characteristic crescent shape in Romanowsky-stained preparations.

BLOOD PARASITES AND RED CELL INCLUSIONS OF HERPTILES (REPTILES AND AMPHIBIANS)

Commonly encountered blood parasites of reptiles include hemoprotozoa, piroplasmids, and microfilaria. Common hemoprotozoa include the hemogregarines, trypanosomes, and *Plasmodium* spp. Less commonly encountered hemoprotozoa include *Leishmania*, *Saurocytozoon*, *Haemoproteus*, and *Schellackia*. In general these parasites are considered to be incidental findings.

Parasites reported in amphibians include *Haemogregarina*, *Plasmodium*, *Aegyptianella*, *Haemoproteus*, and *Lankesterella*.[13] The common amphibian intraerythrocytic blood parasites include the hemogregarines and *Aegyptianella* spp.[33] These organisms are considered to be an incidental finding. Extracellular amphibian hemoparasites include trypanosomes and microfilaria, and are also considered nonpathogenic.

The hemogregarine parasites are the most common group of sporozoan hemoparasites affecting reptiles and amphibians. The 3 genera of hemogregarines commonly

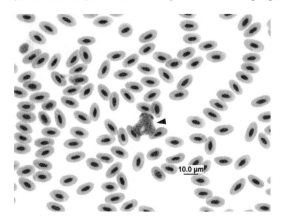

Fig. 17. *Leukocytozoon* (*arrowhead*) in the blood film of a hawk (*Buteo jamaicensis*) (Wright-Giemsa stain).

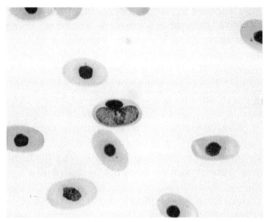

Fig. 18. Hemogregarine in the blood film of a reptile (Wright-Giemsa stain, original magnification of 1000x).

found in reptiles are *Haemogregarina, Hepatozoon*, and *Karyolysus*.[34,35] Hemogregarines are identified as sausage-shaped intracytoplasmic gametocytes in erythrocytes (**Fig. 18**). These gametocytes distort the host cell by creating a bulge in the cytoplasm, and are comparatively lacking in the refractile pigment granules found in the gametocytes of *Plasmodium* and *Haemoproteus*. Only one gametocyte is typically found per erythrocyte; however, when heavy infection occurs, 2 gametocytes may be found in 1 cell.

Round to irregular basophilic inclusions are frequently seen in the cytoplasm of erythrocytes in peripheral blood films from many species of reptiles and some amphibians (**Fig. 19**). These inclusions most likely represent an artifact of slide preparation or are considered to be normal findings.

Blood films from boid snakes affected with inclusion body disease (IBD) may reveal inclusions within the cytoplasm of erythrocytes, lymphocytes, or heterophils.[36,37] IBD inclusions stained with Wright-Giemsa appear as lightly basophilic homogeneous intracytoplasmic inclusions of varying size and shape (**Fig. 20**).

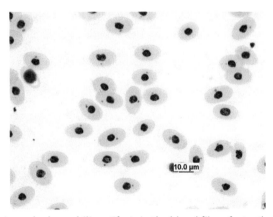

Fig. 19. Round to irregular basophilic artifacts in the blood film of a turtle (*Graptemys versa*) (Wright-Giemsa stain).

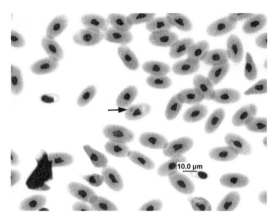

Fig. 20. Inclusion body (*arrow*) in an erythrocyte in the blood film of a snake (*Boa constrictor*) positive for inclusion body disease (Wright-Giemsa stain).

BLOOD PARASITES OF FISH

Little is known about the life cycle of fish hemogregarines. These hemoparasites are found most frequently in wild-caught fish, and probably require a blood-feeding intermediate host, such as leeches, copepods, and isopods.

Trypanosomes are found in all groups of animals worldwide, are usually considered to be an incidental finding, and are not typically pathogenic. Trypanosomes are large, extracellular, blade-shaped flagellate protozoa with an undulating membrane, a slender tapering posterior end, and a single short anteriorly directed flagellum.

REFERENCES

1. Moore DM. Hematology of the rat (*Rattus norvegicus*). In: Feldman BF, Zinkl JG, Jain NC, editors. Schalm's veterinary hematology. 5th edition. Philadelphia: Lippincott Williams & Wilkins; 2000. p. 1210–8.
2. Moore DM. Hematology of the mouse (*Mus musculus*). In: Feldman BF, Zinkl JG, Jain NC, editors. Schalm's veterinary hematology. 5th edition. Philadelphia: Lippincott Williams & Wilkins; 2000. p. 1219–24.
3. Everds NE. Hematology of the laboratory mouse. In: Foster HL, Small JD, Fox JC, editors. The mouse in biomedical research, vol. 3, 2nd edition. Amsterdam: Elsevier; 2006. p. 133–70.
4. Hibiya T. An atlas of fish histology, normal and pathological features. Tokyo: Kodansha Ltd; 1985.
5. Weiss DJ. Uniform evaluation and semiquantitative reporting of hematologic data in veterinary laboratories. Vet Clin Pathol 1984;13(2):27–31.
6. Herbert R, Nanney J, Spano JS, et al. Erythrocyte distribution in ducks. Am J Vet Res 1989;50:958–60.
7. Tell LA, Ferrell ST, Gibbons PM. Avian mycobacteriosis in free-living raptors in California: 6 cases (1997-2001). J Avian Med Surg 2004;18(1):30–40.
8. Wolf T, Niehaus-Rolf C, Luepke NP. Some new methodological aspects of the hen's egg test for micronucleus induction (HET-MN). Mutat Res 2002;514:59–76.
9. Gómez-Meda BC, Zamora-Perez AL, Luna-Aguirre J, et al. Nuclear abnormalities in erythrocytes of parrots (*Aratinga canicularis*) related to genotoxic damage. Avian Pathol 2006;35(3):206–10.

10. Lucas AJ, Jamroz C. Atlas of avian hematology, United States Department of Agriculture Monograph #25. Washington, DC: U.S. Government Printing Office; 1961.
11. Romagnano A. Binucleate erythrocytes and erythrocytic dysplasia in a cockatiel. In: Proceedings of the Association of Avian Veterinarians. Reno, September 28–30, 1994.
12. Hawkey CM, Dennett TB. A colour atlas of comparative veterinary haematology. London: Wolfe Medical Publications, Ltd; 1989.
13. Campbell TW, Ellis CK. Avian and exotic animal hematology and cytology. 3rd edition. Ames (IA): Blackwell Publishing Ltd; 2007.
14. Turner RJ. Amphibians. In: Rowley A, Ratcliffe N, editors. Vertebrate blood cells. Cambridge: Cambridge University Press; 1988. p. 129–209.
15. Pfeiffer CJ, Pyle H, Asashima M. Blood cell morphology and counts in the Japanese newt (*Cynops pyrrhogaster*). J Zoo Wildl Med 1990;21(1):56–64.
16. Zinkl JG, Cox WT, Kono CS. Morphology and cytochemistry in leucocytes and thrombocytes of six species of fish. Comp Haemat Inter 1991;1:187–95.
17. Saunders DC. Differential blood cell counts of 121 species of marine fishes of Puerto Rico. Trans Am Microsc Soc 1966;85:427–99.
18. Ellis AE. The leukocytes of fish: a review. J Fish Biol 1977;11:453–91.
19. Mainwaring G, Rowley AF. Studies on granulocyte heterogenicity in elasmobranchs. In: Mainwaring G, Rowley A, editors. Fish immunology. New York: Academic Press; 1985. p. 57–69.
20. Filho SW, Eble GJ, Kassner G, et al. Comparative hematology in marine fish. Comp Biochem Physiol 1992;102(2):311–21.
21. Hine PM. The granulocytes of fish. Fish Shellfish Immunol 1992;2:79–98.
22. Arnold J. Hematology of the sandbar shark, *Carcharhinus plumbeus*: standardization of complete blood count techniques for elasmobranchs. Vet Clin Pathol 2005;34(2):115–23.
23. Walsh CJ, Luer CA. Elasmobranch hematology: identification of cell types and practical applications. In: Smith M, Warmolts D, Thoney D, et al, editors. The elasmobranch husbandry manual: captive care of sharks, rays, and their relatives. Columbus (OH): Biological Survey, Inc; 2004. p. 301–23.
24. Weiser G. Introduction to leukocytes and the leukogram. In: Thrall MA, Weiser G, Allison RW, et al, editors. Veterinary hematology and clinical chemistry. 2nd edition. Ames (IA): Wiley-Blackwell; 2012. p. 118–22.
25. Weiser G, Thrall MA. Introduction to leukocytes and the leukogram. In: Thrall MA, Baker DC, Campbell TW, et al, editors. Veterinary hematology and clinical chemistry. Philadelphia: Lippincott Williams & Wilkins; 2004. p. 125–30.
26. Peirce MA, Lederer R, Adlard RD, et al. Pathology associated with endogenous development of haemoatozoa in birds from southeast Queensland. Avian Pathol 2004;33:445–50.
27. Castro I, Howe L, Tompkins DM, et al. Presence and seasonal prevalence of *Plasmodium* spp in a rare endemic New Zealand passerine (Tieke or Saddleback, *Philesturnus carunculatus*). J Wildl Dis 2011;47(4):860–7.
28. Evans M, Otter A. Fatal combined infection with *Haemoproteus noctuae* and *Leucocytozoon ziemanni* in juvenile snowy owls (*Nyctea scandiaca*). Vet Rec 1998; 143(3):72–6.
29. Michot TC, Garvin MC, Weidner EH. Survey for blood parasites in redheads (*Aythya americana*) wintering at the Chandeleur Islands, Louisiana. J Wildl Dis 1995; 31(1):90–2.
30. Soulsby EJ. Helminths, arthropods, and protozoa of domesticated animals. In: Soulsby EJ, editor. Helminths, arthropods, and protozoa of domesticated animals. 7th edition. Philadelphia: Lea and Febiger; 1982. p. 689–728.

31. Bennet GF, Pierce MA. Leucocytozoids of seven Old World passeriform families. J Nat Hist 1992;26:693–707.
32. Gardiner CH, Fayer R, Dubey JP. An atlas of protozoan parasites in animal tissues. U.S. Department of Agriculture, Agriculture Handbook. Washington, DC: U.S. Government Printing Office; 1988.
33. Desser SS, Barta JR. The morphological features of *Aegyptianella bacterifera*: an intraerythrocytic rickettsia of frogs from Corsica. J Wildl Dis 1989;25:313–8.
34. Telford SR. Haemoparasites of reptiles. In: Hoff G, Frye G, Jacobson E, editors. Diseases of amphibians and reptiles. New York: Plenum Book Co; 1984. p. 385–517.
35. Telford SR. The hemogregarines. In: Telford SR, editor. Hemoparasites of the Reptilia, Color Atlas and Text. Boca Raton (FL): CRC Press; 2009. p. 199–260.
36. Chang L, Jacobson ER. Inclusion body disease, a worldwide infectious disease of boid snakes: a review. J Exotic Pet Med 2010;19:216–25.
37. Banajee KH, Chang LW, Jacobson ER, et al. What is your diagnosis? Blood film from a boa constrictor. Vet Clin Pathol 2012;41(1):158–9.

Moving?

Make sure your subscription moves with you!

To notify us of your new address, find your **Clinics Account Number** (located on your mailing label above your name), and contact customer service at:

Email: journalscustomerservice-usa@elsevier.com

800-654-2452 (subscribers in the U.S. & Canada)
314-447-8871 (subscribers outside of the U.S. & Canada)

Fax number: 314-447-8029

Elsevier Health Sciences Division
Subscription Customer Service
3251 Riverport Lane
Maryland Heights, MO 63043

*To ensure uninterrupted delivery of your subscription, please notify us at least 4 weeks in advance of move.

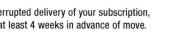

Printed and bound by CPI Group (UK) Ltd, Croydon, CR0 4YY

03/10/2024

01040391-0003